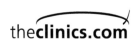

theclinics.com

CHILD AND ADOLESCENT PSYCHIATRIC CLINICS OF NORTH AMERICA

Pediatric Palliative Medicine

GUEST EDITORS
John P. Glazer, MD
Joanne M. Hilden, MD
Dunya Yaldoo Poltorak, PhD

CONSULTING EDITOR
Andrés Martin, MD, MPH

July 2006 • Volume 15 • Number 3

SAUNDERS

An Imprint of Elsevier, Inc.
PHILADELPHIA   LONDON   TORONTO   MONTREAL   SYDNEY   TOKYO

W.B. SAUNDERS COMPANY
A Division of Elsevier Inc.

Elsevier Inc. • 1600 John F. Kennedy Boulevard • Suite 1800 • Philadelphia, Pennsylvania 19103-2899

http://www.childpsych.theclinics.com

CHILD AND ADOLESCENT PSYCHIATRIC CLINICS	Volume 15, Number 3
OF NORTH AMERICA	ISSN 1056–4993
July 2006	ISBN 1-4160-3792-6

Editor: Sarah E. Barth

Reprints: For copies of 100 or more, of articles in this publication, please contact the Commercial Reprints Department, Elsevier Inc., 360 Park Avenue South, New York, New York 10010-1710. Tel. (212) 633-3813; Fax: (212) 462-1935; email: reprints@elsevier.com.

The ideas and opinions expressed in *Child and Adolescent Psychiatric Clinics of North America* do not necessarily reflect those of the Publisher. The Publisher does not assume any responsibility for any injury and/or damage to persons or property arising out of or related to any use of the material contained in this periodical. The reader is advised to check the appropriate medical literature and the product information currently provided by the manufacturer of each drug to be administered to verify the dosage, the method and duration of administration, or contraindications. It is the responsibility of the treating physician or other health care professional, relying on independent experience and knowledge of the patient, to determine drug dosages and the best treatment for the patient. Mention of any product in this issue should not be construed as endorsement by the contributors, editors, or the Publisher of the product or manufacturers' claims.

Child and Adolescent Psychiatric Clinics of North America (ISSN 1056-4993) is published quarterly by W.B. Saunders, 360 Park Avenue South, New York, NY 10010-1710. Months of publication are January, April, July, and October. Business and Editorial Offices: 1600 John F. Kennedy Boulevard, Suite 1800, Philadelphia, PA 19103-2899. Accounting and Circulation Offices: 6277 Sea Harbor Drive, Orlando, FL 32887-4800. Periodicals postage paid at New York, NY and additional mailing offices. Subscription prices are $185.00 per year (US individuals), $280.00 per year (US institutions), $95.00 per year (US students), $210.00 per year (Canadian individuals), $330.00 per year (Canadian institutions), $115.00 per year (Canadian students), $235.00 per year (international individuals), $330.00 per year (international institutions), and $115.00 per year (international students). International air speed delivery is included in all *Clinics* subscription prices. All prices are subject to change without notice. **POSTMASTER:** Send address changes to *Child and Adolescent Psychiatric Clinics of North America*, Elsevier Periodicals Customer Service, 6277 Sea Harbor Drive, Orlando, FL 32887-4800. **Customer Service: 1-800-654-2452 (US). From outside of the US, call 1-407-345-4000.**

Child and Adolescent Psychiatric Clinics of North America is covered in Index Medicus, ISI, SSCI, Research Alert, Social Search, Current Contents, and *EMBASE/Excerpta Medica.*

Printed in the United States of America.

CONSULTING EDITOR

ANDRÉS MARTIN, MD, MPH, Associate Professor of Child Psychiatry and Psychiatry, Yale Child Study Center, Yale University School of Medicine; and Medical Director, Children's Psychiatric Inpatient Service, Yale-New Haven Children's Hospital, New Haven, Connecticut

CONSULTING EDITOR EMERITUS

MELVIN LEWIS, MBBS, FRCPsych, DHC, Professor Emeritus, Senior Research Scientist, Yale Child Study Center, Yale University School of Medicine, New Haven, Connecticut

GUEST EDITORS

JOHN P. GLAZER, MD, Director, Pediatric Psychiatry Consultation-Liaison Service, Department of Psychiatry and Psychology, Cleveland Clinic, Cleveland, Ohio

JOANNE M. HILDEN, MD, Chair, Department of Pediatric Hematology/Oncology; Medical Director, Pediatric Palliative Medicine, The Children's Hospital at The Cleveland Clinic, Cleveland; and Associate Professor of Pediatrics, The Cleveland Clinic Lerner College of Medicine, Cleveland, Ohio

DUNYA YALDOO POLTORAK, PhD, Director, Pediatric Behavioral Medicine Hospital Consultation Service, Section of Behavioral Medicine, Children's Hospital, Cleveland Clinic, Cleveland, Ohio

CONTRIBUTORS

ANNAH N. ABRAMS, MD, Instructor in Psychiatry, Harvard Medical School; Staff, Child Psychiatry Consultation Liaison Service, Massachusetts General Hospital, Boston, Massachusetts

ETHAN BENORE, PhD, Staff Pediatric Psychologist, NeuroDevelopmental Center, Akron Children's Hospital, Akron, Ohio

MICHELLE R. BROWN, PhD, Clinical Assistant Professor of Psychiatry, Stanford University School of Medicine, Stanford; Pediatric Psychologist, Psychiatry Consultation-Liaison Service, Lucile Packard Children's Hospital at Stanford, Stanford, California

DAVID M. BROWNING, MSW, BCD, FT, Senior Research Associate, Education Development Center, Inc., Newton; Director, Initiative for Pediatric Palliative Care, Education Development Center, Inc., Newton, Massachusetts

BRIAN S. CARTER, MD, FAAP, Co-Director, Pediatric Advance Comfort Team, and Associate Professor, Department of Pediatrics, Vanderbilt Children's Hospital (Neonatology), Nashville, Tennessee

JOHN J. COLLINS, MBBS, PhD, FFPMANZCA, FRACP, Head, Pain, and Palliative Care Service, The Children's Hospital at Westmead, Westmead, New South Wales, Australia

JANET DUNCAN, MSN, CPNP, Nursing Director, Pediatric Advanced Care Team, Children's Hospital Boston and Dana-Farber Cancer Institute, Boston, Massachusetts

DAVID R. FREYER, DO, Director, After-Care and Transition (ACT) Program, Division of Hematology/Oncology/Bone Marrow Transplantation, DeVos Children's Hospital, Grand Rapids, Michigan; Associate Professor of Pediatrics, Michigan State University College of Human Medicine, East Lansing, Michigan

JOHN P. GLAZER, MD, Director, Pediatric Psychiatry Consultation-Liaison Service, Department of Psychiatry and Psychology, Cleveland Clinic, Cleveland, Ohio

JOANNE M. HILDEN, MD, Chair, Department of Pediatric Hematology/Oncology; Medical Director, Pediatric Palliative Medicine, The Children's Hospital at The Cleveland Clinic, Cleveland; and Associate Professor of Pediatrics, The Cleveland Clinic Lerner College of Medicine, Cleveland, Ohio

CHRIS HUBBLE, MD, Medical Director, Pediatric Advanced Comfort Care Team (PACCT), Children's Mercy Hospital and Clinics, Kansas City, Missouri

DAN HUDSON, MDiv, BCC, Chaplain, Spiritual Care Department, Childrens Hospital Los Angeles, Los Angeles, California

NANCY HUTTON, MD, Associate Professor of Pediatrics, Division of General Pediatrics and Adolescent Medicine, The Johns Hopkins University School of Medicine; and Medical Director, Harriet Lane Compassionate Care, Johns Hopkins Children's Center, Baltimore, Maryland

BARBARA JONES, PhD, MSW, Assistant Professor of Social Work and Co-Director, The Institute for Grief, Loss and Family Survival, University of Texas at Austin School of Social Work, Austin, Texas

MARSHA JOSELOW, LICSW, Clinical Social Worker, Pediatric Advanced Care Team, Children's Hospital Boston and Dana-Farber Cancer Institute, Boston, Massachusetts

AURA KUPERBERG, PhD, LCSW, Teen Impact Program, Childrens Center for Cancer and Blood Diseases, Childrens Hospital Los Angeles, Los Angeles, California

RENÉE McCULLOCH, BMBS, MRCPaeds (UK), Dip Pall Med (Paeds), Palliative Care Fellow, The Children's Hospital at Westmead, Westmead, New South Wales, Australia

STEVEN L. PASTYRNAK, PhD, Psychologist, Division of Psychology/Psychiatry, DeVos Children's Hospital, Grand Rapids, Michigan

DUNYA YALDOO POLTORAK, PhD, Director, Pediatric Behavioral Medicine Hospital Consultation Service, Section of Behavioral Medicine, Children's Hospital, Cleveland Clinic, Cleveland, Ohio

KRISTEN M. POWASKI, RN, BSN, CPON, Registered Nurse, Pediatric Hematology and Oncology, The Children's Hospital at The Cleveland Clinic, Cleveland; Registered Nurse, Pediatric Palliative Medicine Team, The Children's Hospital at The Cleveland Clinic, Cleveland, Ohio

PAULA K. RAUCH, MD, Director, Child Psychiatry Consultation Service and MGH Cancer Center Parenting Program, Massachusetts General Hospital, Boston, Massachusetts

TOM RICHARDS, BA, CCLS, Child Life Specialist, Child Life Program, Department of Pediatric Hematology/Oncology, The Children's Hospital at The Cleveland Clinic, Cleveland, Ohio

EYAL SHEMESH, MD, Assistant Professor, Departments of Pediatrics and Psychiatry, Mount Sinai Medical Center, New York, New York

MILDRED Z. SOLOMON, EdD, Associate Clinical Professor of Social Medicine, Medical Ethics and Anaesthesia, Harvard Medical School, Boston; Vice-President, Education Development Center, Inc., Newton, Massachusetts

BARBARA SOURKES, PhD, Associate Professor of Pediatrics and Psychiatry, Stanford University School of Medicine; Kriewall-Haehl Director of Pediatric Palliative Care Program, Lucile Packard Children's Hospital at Stanford, Stanford, California

DAVID J. STERKEN, MN, CPNP, Pediatric Nurse Practitioner, Division of Hematology/Oncology/Bone Marrow Transplantation, DeVos Children's Hospital, Grand Rapids, Michigan

FREDERICK J. STODDARD, MD, Associate Clinical Professor, Harvard Medical School, Boston; Psychiatrist, Massachusetts General Hospital, Boston; Chief, Department of Psychiatry, Shriners Burns Hospital, Boston, Massachusetts

MARGARET L. STUBER, MD, Jane and Marc Nathanson Professor, Department of Psychiatry & Biobehavioral Sciences, University of California Los Angeles, Los Angeles, California

SUSAN D. SWICK, MD, MPH, Instructor and Clinical Assistant, Department of Psychiatry, Harvard Medical School, Massachusetts General Hospital, Boston, Massachusetts

CRAIGAN T. USHER, MD, Clinical Teaching Fellow in Psychiatry, Harvard Medical School, Boston; Child and Adolescent Psychiatry Fellow, Massachusetts General Hospital/McLean Hospital, Boston, Massachusetts

KATHRYN L. WEISE, MD, Pediatric Critical Care Medicine and Bioethics Co-Director, Pediatric Palliative Medicine, The Cleveland Clinic Foundation, Cleveland, Ohio

Cover art courtesy of Socorro Rivera, Mexico City, Mexico.

CONTENTS

Barriers to effective pain management include poor assessment and measurement of pain and a lack of specialist knowledge. Fears regarding the use of opioids and their association with the end of life must be addressed openly and with clarity. Day-to-day management should include continual appraisal of pain issues if quality of life is to be maximized. The clinician must be vigilant and take responsibility for all aspects of pain management in these patients.

The alleviation of symptoms, with the ultimate intention of improvement of quality of life, is a fundamental component of pediatric palliative medicine. Several psychological factors can exacerbate physical symptoms or influence perceptions of symptoms. This article reviews cognitive-behavioral principles and interventions that show good promise for the amelioration of symptoms in children with advanced diseases. These interventions promote healthy cognitions and behaviors that facilitate coping with physical and psychological discomfort and improve quality of life.

Optimum palliative care for dying adolescents exceeds what may be provided by any single clinician, owing to the diversity of developmental tasks and correlative needs that arise. In adolescents, life-limiting illness may result in severe alterations in appearance, stamina, self-image, psychosexual maturation, peer and family relationships, educational achievement, and gaining of independence. To assist in the care of this challenging population, this article describes the distinct but interrelated roles of a multidisciplinary palliative care team comprising the physician, nurse, clinical psychologist, medical social worker, chaplain, and child life specialist. The unifying theme is respect for the developmental tasks of adolescence. Emphasis is placed on applying these considerations to support adolescent decision making at the end of life.

Parents and healthcare professionals face numerous challenges as they care for critically and chronically ill children and children who have a diagnosis associated with poor prognosis. Nursing staff must be available to foster hope, recognize each family's unique challenges, and advocate for specialized palliative care services to support the patient and family. This article outlines opportunities for nurses to work with patients and families through treatment, decline, and death of a child. Ways that nurses can foster hope, provide quality of life, offer support, facilitate a good death, and develop their own coping skills are covered. The importance of working with a palliative care team is emphasized.

Program Interventions for Children at the End of Life and Their Siblings

Janet Duncan, Marsha Joselow, and Joanne M. Hilden

An analogy may be drawn between readying a family for the birth of a child and readying a family for the death of a child. Both experiences bring about an intense fusion of the emotional, physical, and spiritual realms for those bearing witness. Preparation, communication, and collaboration are essential to provide optimal support for the children at the end of life, the parents, and the brothers and sisters.

Palliative Medicine in Neonatal and Pediatric Intensive Care

Brian S. Carter, Chris Hubble, and Kathryn L. Weise

Although palliative care services for children are becoming an accepted element of comprehensive, family-centered care, the nature of the ICU presents special challenges to providers and families in need of these services. Potential barriers include implicit expectations of families and providers for curative medicine; the belief that these expectations exclude palliative medicine team consultation; commonplace use of highly technical equipment and often painful procedures; and providers self-selected and trained for provision of aggressive, often invasive, life-extending care. Despite these challenges, palliative care should be provided concurrently with aggressive, curative care for all patients, especially patients at highest risk of dying. This article addresses issues of providing palliative care in the ICU and offers examples of how several current programs have integrated these approaches.

Children Facing the Death of a Parent: The Experiences of a Parent Guidance Program at the Massachusetts General Hospital Cancer Center

Susan D. Swick and Paula K. Rauch

Children facing the death of a parent are facing a major upheaval, a loss that will bring them emotional pain and will resonate in different ways at important points throughout their lives. Given the proper supports, most children can expect to adjust well to this enormous change and live happy, productive, and meaningful lives. The goal is to help parents relocate their bearings and realize they can use the parenting skills they already have in helping their children make this adjustment. Guided by the goal of protecting their children, these parents can find purpose and strength. Reframing their circumstances as a painful and unavoidable challenge, but one that they can actively face, is organizing and fortifying for these families buffeted by loss.

The discrepancy between what is taught in formal educational settings and what is learned by practitioners in the informal flow of everyday practice has been called the hidden curriculum. In this article, the authors apply a well-documented range of concerns about the hidden curriculum and the erosion of professionalism to the arena of pediatric palliative care education. The authors propose that educational initiatives must always be grounded in the charged existential space of relationships among children, families, and practitioners, because the learning that matters most occurs within these relationships. The authors present an educational approach, which they call relational learning, and offer some preliminary strategies educators may wish to foster this kind of learning in their own health care organizations.

FORTHCOMING ISSUES

RECENT ISSUES

The CLINICS ARE NOW AVAILABLE ONLINE!

Access your subscription at:
http//www.theclinics.com

ELSEVIER
SAUNDERS

Child Adolesc Psychiatric Clin N Am
15 (2006) xiii–xv

CHILD AND
ADOLESCENT
PSYCHIATRIC CLINICS
OF NORTH AMERICA

Foreword

Off-Season Events

> and I think of each life as a flower, as common
> as a field daisy, and as singular,
>
> and each name a comfortable music in the mouth,
> tending, as all music does, toward silence,
>
> and each body a lion of courage, and something
> precious to the earth.
>
> —*Mary Oliver: When Death Comes*

Children are not meant to suffer. Children in pain, children in clinical settings away from family, peers, and school, and children who die all violate our notion of childhood–and theirs. The field of pediatric palliative medicine has risen in response to the unique needs of these children and their caregivers. The shift in pediatrics away from acute, mostly infectious diseases, to chronic, life-limiting illnesses is not new, but the advent of pediatric palliative medicine as an integrated clinical, academic, and educational enterprise is recent. Families and clinicians involved with children with life-limiting illness face complex and inevitable questions. These include whether and when to use life-prolonging interventions that may not necessarily result in an improved quality of life. Even prior, how to address the rights of children and adolescents to know about their prognoses and choose among available treatment options without overwhelming them with emotionally charged information. As noted in the preface that follows, a fundamental principle of pediatric palliative medicine, within which all other questions are embedded, is its focus not on dying children so much as on those with life-limiting illness who may or may not recover.

Communication and decision making options around pain and symptom management are at the forefront of the care of children facing life-limiting illness. Pediatric palliative care has taken an assertive position on the centrality of these issues, whether or not full recovery is in the cards. Indeed, the movement as a whole may be conceptualized as an active response to the inevitability of a child's death, a distinct counterpoint to an earlier stance of seeing the phases of grief, loss, and bereavement unfold, while offering little beyond words of comfort.

1056-4993/06/$ - see front matter © 2006 Elsevier Inc. All rights reserved.
doi:10.1016/j.chc.2006.04.001   *childpsych.theclinics.com*

Another distinctly recent change has been where end-of-life care actually takes place. Terminally ill children spend considerable amounts of time in technologically sophisticated and potentially alienating hospital settings. Pediatric palliative medicine has provided a concerted and organized effort to maximize continuity of care—and continuity of meaningful relationships in particular—at some of the more challenging and difficult times in a sick child's life.

Pediatric palliative medicine originally was developed in tertiary care settings delivering highly specialized care to children facing the very end of their lives. But it would be shortsighted to think of it in only those settings, as its lessons are applicable across a wide range of locations. Palliative care teams are often available for consultation in specialized referral centers, as welcome clinical service additions. Nevertheless, they can lead some to believe that the painful aspects of terminal illness and end-of-life care can be conveniently "consulted out" and so artificially extricated from primary, front-line management. In teaching environments where medical continuity can become a logistic and practical challenge, palliative care teams may come to serve as a major thread of human consistency, as a way of avoiding the fragmentation of therapeutic relationships into as many hospital admissions. In other settings, where such discretely organized services may not be available, the lessons of palliative medicine are just as relevant and applicable: attention to the physical, emotional, spiritual, and practical needs of terminally ill children and their families can be profoundly meaningful and helpful, and should never be seen as capitulation when it has been deemed that recovery is not possible.

Palliative medicine has also provided valuable lessons around the subtleties of timing. Specifically, a palliative approach should be implemented not near the end, once death looms large and unavoidable, but rather at the beginning of the journey into life-limiting illness, when a diagnosis has been made and the child and family first confront the burden of their newfound knowledge. The palliative care team can also provide indirect support by working with primary teams rather than patients and families, so as to provide perspective, organize clinical templates, and coordinate with other relevant services and colleagues.

It is here, around the interplay with others, that the lessons of pediatric palliative medicine are most relevant—and humbling. The care of terminally ill and dying children cannot be undertaken alone: it demands a team approach. Teams can be comprised of less-than-traditional liaisons: anesthesia and pharmacologic pain management alongside acupuncture, massage therapy, and reiki comes to mind as a recent example of ambassadorial goodwill and effective interdisciplinary work.

Paradigmatic of such effective cooperation is the Cleveland Clinic's guest editorial team for this issue: for just as pediatric palliative medicine cannot be a solo practice, it is fitting for this issue to be a joint editorial effort that seamlessly crosses specialty lines. May the combined efforts of the superb lineup of contributors assembled in this issue help us do better by those under our care—precious lions of courage too soon departed.

Andrés Martin, MD, MPH
Yale Child Study Center
Yale University School of Medicine
230 South Frontage Road
New Haven, CT 06520-7900, USA

E-mail address: andres.martin@yale.edu

**ELSEVIER
SAUNDERS**

Child Adolesc Psychiatric Clin N Am
15 (2006) xvii–xx

CHILD AND
ADOLESCENT
PSYCHIATRIC CLINICS
OF NORTH AMERICA

Preface

Pediatric Palliative Medicine

"Although the world is full of suffering, it is also full of the overcoming of it."

–Helen Keller

Introduction to pediatric palliative medicine: an interesting notion. How do we introduce this specialty to our trainees, to our colleagues, to our students, to our patients and their families? It depends on our definition, of course.

Pediatric palliative medicine clinicians usually begin with the World Health Organization (WHO) definition from 1990: "the active total care of patients *whose disease is not responsive to curative treatment.* Control of pain, of other symptoms, and of psychological, social, and spiritual problems is paramount. The goal of palliative care is achievement of the best quality of life for patients and their families [1]."

There are two shortcomings to this definition.

The first is "not responsive to curative treatment." If we limit palliative care to those children with a terminal prognosis, or those whose parents have come to believe that their child's prognosis is terminal, then no one will be served. This is *the* most important barrier to getting children referred to palliative medicine teams. When health care team members try to refer a child, they are frequently met with replies such as, "Not yet. We are still trying to cure Sally." Then, when the child is near death and the referral is made, the family meets strangers to help with the death, when instead they could have been re-introduced to familiar, trusted faces at this most crucial hour. Until we define the palliative medicine clientele as *all* children who have a life-limiting condition, even while they are receiving the most aggressive curative therapy possible, we will remain in the untenable position that we are in: palliative medicine teams are allowed in the door for children only when children are very close to death, far too late for the team to forge relationships.

The editors gratefully acknowledge the expert administrative and manuscript support of Ms. Theresa Neiden.

doi:10.1016/j.chc.2006.03.004
childpsych.theclinics.com

The second problem with the WHO definition is the goal of "achievement of the best quality of life," which is stated in the context of good symptom control. What health care team does not tend to the psychological, social, and spiritual well-being of patients, and what team does not strive for the best quality of life? Palliative care teams often find primary teams feeling that if a referral is suggested, the implication is that they are not doing their job well. The important message here is this: Palliative care teams work alongside of, not instead of, the primary team. Rather than taking over, they complement that team's efforts. They ease some of the burden of caring for and communicating with the family when complex medical and psychosocial decisions must be made.

To address the need to improve access to quality pediatric palliative care, the Institute of Medicine, the American Academy of Pediatrics, and The International Society of Pediatric Oncology, among others, have put forth position and policy statements and care standards. This process has generated an honorable flurry of studies and publications, out of our duty to educate and implement. This work leads to a new definition of Pediatric Palliative Medicine: "Viewed broadly, palliative care is a multidisciplinary approach that prevents or relieves the symptoms produced by a life-threatening medical condition or its treatment. The goal is to help patients and their families live as normally as possible, and *to provide them with timely and accurate information and support in decision-making.* Such care and assistance is not limited to people thought to be dying, and it can be provided concurrently with curative or life-prolonging treatments [2]."

For children with life-limiting conditions, it is imperative to attend to all of their symptoms, physical and psychological, in an integrated fashion, without resort to artificial boundaries. This volume is in the *Child and Adolescent Psychiatric Clinics* series; as editors, we recognize our duty to a primary psychiatric readership but, we hope, to a much broader one as well. As an editorial team, we comprise a pediatric psychiatrist (JPG), oncologist (JMH), and psychologist (DYP), and our contributors further include anesthesiologists, nurses, educators, social workers, ethicists, and child life specialists. We approach the task by bringing together expertise from the many disciplines our children, adolescents, and families require both in clinical practice and in the education of ourselves, our colleagues, and our community.

The provision of "*timely and accurate information and support in decision-making*" is the most crucial, the least discussed, and the most poorly understood aspect of pediatric palliative medicine. It is also the most rewarding one for caregivers. This is something that most physicians believe they do quite well, yet parents hear caregivers through the fog of fear, panic, bewilderment, or numbness. It is the privilege of the palliative medicine team, if allowed in the door early enough to build meaningful relationships, to come alongside the family and the primary health care team, to look at the exchange of information, and to make sure it is understood, despite inherent ambiguities. We liken it to being "medical interpreters." If we do it well, parents look back on having made difficult yet informed decisions (Ventilator? Another surgery? More chemotherapy?) with information that they understood and assimilated. They can say they were good parents, even though their child died! "I wouldn't change a thing about how my child died." To hear this means we provided information that parents could understand and that helped families make their decisions, decisions that they will look back upon for years, after the rest of us have moved on.

Yet an even greater privilege: to do as much for the child patient. Helping children to understand what is going on, encouraging them to express their fears and hopes while actively listening to them, and helping them to feel part of difficult decisions is especially rewarding. We must recognize that serious illness accelerates cognitive and psychological development, varying from child to child, and we must be sure that we include even younger children in decision making to the extent appropriate for that child and family (see the article by Yaldoo and Glazer in this issue). If the outcome is that a child dies, it is both empathic to child and family and rewarding for the clinician to allow the child or teen to be involved enough to say goodbye, but first, to have quality time on their own terms, free from pain, delirium, guilt, anxiety, and depression to the greatest extent possible. To be allowed to learn directly from the children themselves throughout this process is the true golden nugget of pediatric palliative medicine.

Can any one person or subspecialty do this? No. The pediatric palliative medicine team consists of nurses and nurse practitioners, pediatric and psychiatric physicians, pediatric psychologists, social workers, child life specialists, pharmacists, chaplains, and sometimes ethicists and attorneys. The challenge is to bring diverse expertise together in a manner at once collaborative and distinguishable. In *The Confluence of Psychiatry, the Law, and Ethics* [3], Lederberg speaks to the need for clarity in addressing clinical situations presenting vexing cross-discipline ambiguities. A case recently facing the Helping Hands Palliative Medicine Service at our institution is illustrative: The intensive care team conferred regarding medical indications for continuing or discontinuing ventilator support to a 9-month-old infant with a progressive neurodegenerative disorder. Simultaneously, biological and adoptive parents, with opposing views about medical management, engaged in a custody dispute in the courts. Until resolution of legal decision-making authority among biological and adoptive parents and the County child protective service agency was finalized, meaningful medical decision making and preparation could not occur.

About 55,000 children aged 0–19 die annually in the United States, and an estimated 384,000 live with "special health care needs" as defined by the Maternal and Child Health Bureau of the United States Department of Health and Human Services [1]. The palliative medicine team works with families over time, as they traverse an increasingly complex health care system. The child will have ups and downs as his condition waxes and wanes, relapses and responds, or slowly and inexorably worsens. The team may work with a child who is ultimately cured, and rejoice with the family, having made an excellent contribution during the worst of times. Even cured children have families who have been through a catastrophic experience and who may have experienced post-traumatic stress or other psychological symptoms over the years; we hope that those families of cured children who had access to a palliative medicine team along the way have more favorable psychological and biological outcomes—moreover an important topic for empirical research.

The palliative medicine team works hardest, of course, with the child who worsens to the point of dying. Some palliative medicine teams are able to become "the hospice team" and provide the true end-of-life care, and others make hospice referrals. The palliative medicine and hospice teams also have a crucial role in bereavement support.

For those who work in this field, we hope to have put together a collection of articles that teach and help in the work. We appreciate all those involved in pediatric palliative medicine and encourage their efforts. To them we say, "Well done." To the families of children with life-limiting conditions who might make their way to this volume, we hope to have provided some guidance and comfort. To them we say, "Well done. You honor your child."

John P. Glazer, MD
Joanne M. Hilden, MD
Dunya Yaldoo Poltorak, PhD
Department of Psychiatry and Psychology
The Children's Hospital Cleveland Clinic Lerner College of Medicine
Cleveland Clinic, 3500 Euclid Avenue
Cleveland, OH 44195, USA

E-mail addresses: glazerj@ccf.org; hildenj@ccf.org; yaldood@ccf.org

References

[1] Cancer pain relief and palliative care. WHO technical report series 804. Geneva: World Health Organization; 1990.
[2] Institute of Medicine of the National Academies. When children die: improving palliative and end of life care for children and their families. New York: The National Academies Press; 2003. p. 2.
[3] Lederberg M. The confluence of psychiatry, the law, and ethics. In: Holland JC, Rowland JH, editors. Handbook of psychooncology: psychological care of the patient with cancer. New York and Oxford: Oxford University Press; 1989. p. 694–702.

ELSEVIER
SAUNDERS

Child Adolesc Psychiatric Clin N Am
15 (2006) 567–573

CHILD AND
ADOLESCENT
PSYCHIATRIC CLINICS
OF NORTH AMERICA

The Development of Children's Understanding of Death: Cognitive and Psychodynamic Considerations

Dunya Yaldoo Poltorak, PhD[a],*, John P. Glazer, MD[b]

[a]Section of Behavioral Medicine, Children's Hospital, Cleveland Clinic,
9500 Euclid Avenue A120, Cleveland, OH 44195, USA
[b]Department of Psychiatry and Psychology, Cleveland Clinic, 9500 Euclid Avenue P57,
Cleveland, OH 44195, USA

Development is the cornerstone of childhood. A developmental approach informs everything we do as adult caregivers to children, from prescribing medication [1] to psychotherapy. Opioid analgesic doses for children are based on unique pediatric physiology and pharmacokinetics. Psychotherapy with a 5-year-old child is play-based rather than narrative-based. The pediatric house officer who meets a 5-year-old with pallor, bruises, and fatigue in the emergency room; the oncologist who performs the first bone marrow aspiration; the nurse who administers chemotherapy; and the psychiatrist who assesses delirium must all be equipped with a framework of developmental understanding to assure competent care is given. A pediatric patient's behavior, degree of physical and psychological function, and comfort are embedded in the childs cognitive and psychosocial development. When clinicians provide developmentally informed care, it facilitates patient histories, physical examinations, adherence to life sustaining treatment, and prevention of post-traumatic stress and other psychological sequelae associated with serious pediatric illness.

Developmental theory encompasses a rich tradition of schools of cognitive and developmental (eg, Jean Piaget, Jerome Kagan) and psychoanalytic (eg, Sigmund and Anna Freud, Erik Erikson, John Bowlby) thought. The 5-year-old "preoperational" (Piaget), "Oedipal" (Freud) boy who is hospitalized for inguinal hernia repair benefits both from a concrete description of what to expect after he awakens from anesthesia (eg, the personnel and

---

* Corresponding author.
E-mail address: yaldood@ccf.org (D.Y. Poltorak).

doi:10.1016/j.chc.2006.03.003   *childpsych.theclinics.com*

layout of the recovery room, what the wound will look like) and by reassurance that his genitals are outside of the surgical field. Consistent with prior reviews [2] regarding children's understanding of death, the authors draw on these mutually complementary traditions and briefly review relevant empiric and descriptive literature in an effort to establish a developmental lens through which the material in the following articles will be seen and integrated.

Development of a concept of death

It was long believed that children were incapable of comprehending death and that even if they were, discussing it with them would cause them great harm. As a result, it was common for both clinicians and parents to avoid discussions of death with children, including children who themselves were seriously ill. It has come to be understood, however, that children do indeed have important understandings of death, and their conceptualization of death changes as they progress developmentally.

The understanding of illness and death among children is intimately bound to cognitive and psychological development. Pioneering research in this regard occurred in the 1930s and 1940s [3,4] and has continued [2,5]. Much of the research through the years has focused on a child's understanding of the biological aspects of death of the physical body, including the concepts of universality, irreversibility, nonfunctionality, and causality [5]. Speece and Brent [6] proposed additional focus on the concept of noncorporeal continuation. These components of the death concept are defined in Table 1.

Jean Piaget's [7] theory of cognitive development has provided a language to describe the qualitative differences in children's understanding of illness and death at various developmental levels. In a review of the literature, Burbach and Peterson [8] concluded that understanding of illness is positively correlated with chronological age and cognitive maturity, consistent with Piagetian theory. Piaget [7] explained that as a result of biological maturation and the accumulation of experience, children progress through four sequential stages of cognitive development: (1) the sensorimotor stage (infancy, birth through about age 2), (2) the preoperational stage (early

Table 1
Components of the death concept

Universality	All living things must eventually die
Irreversibility	Once the physical body dies, it cannot be made alive again
Nonfunctionality	All functions of the living physical body cease at the time of death
Causality	The realistic, abstract understanding of the internal (eg, illness, old age) and external (eg, accident) factors that cause death
Noncorporeal continuation	Includes concepts such as resurrection, reincarnation, etc.

childhood, approximately ages 2 through 7), (3) the concrete operational stage (middle to late childhood, approximately ages 7 through 11), and (4) the formal operational stage (adolescence through adulthood). Extensive research has demonstrated that the nature and sequence of these stages is highly predictable. However, it is now generally understood that some children may progress through these stages more rapidly than others. In particular, children who have a life-threatening illness may be advanced in their understanding of death relative to their healthy peers of the same age [9]. This knowledge should help clinicians and parents to avoid making rigid assumptions based strictly on chronological age. It is important, rather, to understand a child's specific level of comprehension, cognitive and emotional, to appreciate what misconceptions and concerns may exist.

Birth through Age 2–3

The sensorimotor child experiences the world almost exclusively through the senses and motor activity. Children at this developmental stage seem to have no concept of death as such; that is, they cannot distinguish cognitively between death and separation [10,11]. In a specific reference to early infancy, Piaget [10] stated that the sensorimotor "infant lacks the symbolic function, that is, he does not have representations by which he can evoke persons or objects in their absence."

Ages 2–3 through 5–7

Nagy [12] used drawings, writings, and interviews to study the attitudes toward death of 378 children age 3 to 10-years-old in post-war Budapest. Nagy's work and application of Piagetian developmental theory suggest that the illogical thought characteristic of young, preoperational children results in many misconceptions about death.

Young children are likely to believe that death is not universal. They might believe that they themselves, family members, and friends may be spared. Preschoolers are just beginning to grasp the concept of cause and effect and are limited by their senses—what they see, hear, feel, and smell—and as such, they might wrongly infer causality. Preschoolers attribute life and consciousness to the dead and come to concrete and sometimes frightening conclusions. For example, the preschooler might fear that the deceased will not be able to breathe while underground and would miss loved ones. Children at this stage might also imagine the deceased mourning. As these examples illustrate, preschoolers generally consider death as continued life but under changed circumstances [4,11]. This can be attributed in part to the egocentric thought characteristic of preoperational children, who are unable to imagine anything other than what they themselves experience [7].

Furthermore, because remnants of separation anxiety often persist in preschoolers and even young school-aged children, they may describe death as "to go away" or "to go asleep." A further example of the preschooler or young school-aged child's concretization of death can be seen in Nagy's [4] description of a child who suggests that one cannot sing at a funeral because it would not allow the dead person to sleep peacefully. This illustrates why bereaved young children are often anxious to go to sleep or have a parent go on a trip. It is important that parents and caregivers do not equate death with sleep or travel, which would reinforce the child's cognitive distortion.

In psychodynamic terms, preschool children face the developmental task of mastering deeply felt aggressive and sexual feelings toward their parents, and by extension, caregivers. One can integrate Piagetian notions of concreteness and egocentricity with dynamic views of aggression and a sense of right and wrong to account for the common observation that young children who have a serious or chronic disease often wrongly infer that the illness was caused by misbehavior [13]. Preschoolers are unlikely to give verbal expression to such feelings (although they may through play) and the painful guilt with which they are associated. Yet, by their very concreteness and the omnipotence with which parents and caregivers are viewed, the important adults in a child's life can greatly reduce suffering by reassuring them that illness does not reflect retribution for wrongdoing. More biologic, simple, reality-based explanations can be substituted and may be reassuring.

Young children are unlikely to understand the permanence of death. They may even think that people can go back and forth between life and death [4]. The death of a parent or sibling can prove especially troubling, in part because the preoperational child thinks that dead people can return if they want to or if the child wishes it so. Hence, when a deceased parent does not return, the young child might feel abandoned. The parent and caregiver must provide the bereaved child with a reality-based explanation for a loss and yet simultaneously respect adaptive defenses. Adults are frequently troubled and confused that bereaved preschoolers often behave as if nothing had changed, don't seem sad, and go on with their usual activities. This is often true, though it says little about the long-term impact on psychological and personality development or the potential need for psychological intervention sooner or later [2].

Ages 5–7 through 10–11

As a child moves from the preoperational stage into concrete operational thought, the concept of death gradually continues to mature. Children who are early in the concrete operational stage distance themselves from and objectify death; they may think that only those people taken by the "death man" will die (animism) and that death might be avoided if one is clever or lucky [4]. In other words, death is personified and has a distinct personality. Death might be understood as a "boogie man" who takes bad people away [4]. Hence, some children will attempt to exhibit exemplary behavior after they have been exposed to the death of a loved one, to assure that they are spared [14]. Although the belief in illness and death as punishment may still be present, children at the upper end of this age range begin to understand the biological meanings of death (ie, the cessation of all bodily functions, both voluntary and involuntary). They are beginning to appreciate that death is caused by serious illness or injury and not by any behavior of their own. Concrete operational children may have some early capacity for logic in their thoughts about death. However, they are limited because they are able to reason only about present situations with which they have personal contact and are not yet able to think more abstractly or theoretically about the future.

Ages 10–11 through adolescence

As children advance from concrete operational thought into formal operational thought and thinking gradually becomes more abstract, concepts of death further evolve. However, the understanding of death even among older adolescents may still be more ambiguous and less mature than that of adults. Older children and adolescents understand the universality of death. Nevertheless, as is often illustrated by the risk-taking behavior of adolescents, they can at times be characterized by a sense of personal omnipotence which convinces them that they are invincible, as if "immune" to death [14]. The understanding of causality of death has become more realistic and abstract. Some formal operational thinkers have highly structured and complex images of death that arise from their capacity for hypothetical deductive reasoning and abstract thought. Adolescents' attitudes and beliefs about death gradually begin to take on the complex and varied meanings characteristic of adults' views about death, and they are further elaborated as a function of spiritual and ethical beliefs about notions such as an afterlife and heaven and hell. Showalter [15] captures an adolescent's struggle with his own terminal illness with particular poignancy in his discussion of the loss of physical functioning and the paradox of the need for greater care by and dependence on parents and other adult caregivers at just the point in development at which the emergence of autonomy is the age-expected norm [13], "a life snuffed out before it has unfolded" [16]. Consider the following vignette:

M was 11 years old when chest wall pain led to a diagnosis of Ewing's sarcoma of a rib. From the first hospitalization on, M fought mightily to maintain her autonomy during blood draws, bone marrow aspirates, placement of intravenous catheters, and other procedures. First viewed by staff and even her parents as stubborn and complaining, by the end of the second week of her initial hospitalization, M had educated her caregivers. She was not only stoic during painful procedures but was also a model of cooperation whenever a procedure was preceded by clear explanation of what was to happen and why it was needed. M showed a facility for using her emerging pre-adolescent capacity for formal operational, abstract reasoning to cope with pain, nausea, and discomfort, by applying a keen knowledge of the favorable odds of remission and return to family, friends, and school in the anticipated future. M underwent tumor resection, radiation, and chemotherapy, achieved remission, and was discharged 3 weeks after admission. M led a rich, cancer-free young adolescent life at home, with friends, and excelled in school for 3 years. She then relapsed and had pulmonary metastases which were unresponsive to aggressive treatment. Because of rapidly progressive dyspnea, intubation was considered before it was clear that the tumor was unresponsive. Fourteen-year-old M guessed that assisted ventilation had been discussed and asked to speak with her oncologist. "Don't put that tube in my throat. I'm dying. It would hurt me, and it wouldn't do any good. I just want to be comfortable and be with mom and dad." Opiates and methylphenidate were given to relieve air hunger and maintain alertness. M died peacefully the next day in her parents' arms; they thanked the pediatric caregivers.

Summary

The cognitive and emotional development of children and adolescents follows a biologically driven, environmentally mediated, and predictable but not entirely invariate sequence. Piagetian, psychoanalytic, and other schools of thought inform an understanding of child development; some of the theories are empirically validated, some not. This framework enables clinicians and parents to approach their children, ill or well, from a developmentally informed perspective. At the same time, as Spinetta's [17] case-controlled study of 6 to 10-year-old children hospitalized either with cancer or non-life limiting illness demonstrated, serious illness itself accelerates cognitive development in often unpredicted ways: "To equate awareness of death with the ability to conceptualize it and express the concept in an adult manner denies the possibility of an awareness of death at a less cognitive level. If it is true that the perception of death can be engraved at some level that precedes a child's ability to talk about it, then a child might well understand that he is going to die long before he can say so." In the following articles, the editors invite a critical reading of the empiric and descriptive literature of pediatric palliative medicine that allows an informed and individualized approach to these extraordinary children and their families.

References

[1] Glazer JP, Danish M, Plotkin SA, et al. Disposition of chloramphenicol in low birth weight infants. Pediatrics 1980;66(4):573–8.
[2] Lewis M, Schonfeld D. Dying and death in childhood and adolescence. In: Lewis M, editor. Child and adolescent psychiatry: a comprehensive textbook. Philadelphia: Lippincott Williams & Wilkins; 2002. p. 1239–45.
[3] Schilder P, Wechsler D. The attitude of children towards death. J Genet Psychol 1934;45: 406–51.
[4] Nagy M. The child's theories concerning death. J Genet Psychol 1948;73:3–27.

[5] Speece MW, Brent SB. Children's understanding of death: a review of three components of the death concept. Child Dev 1984;55:1671–86.

[6] Speece MW, Brent SB. The development of children's understanding of death. In: Corr CA, Corr DM, editors. Handbook of childhood death and bereavement. New York: Springer Publishing Company; 1996. p. 29–50.

[7] Piaget J. The child's conception of the world. New York: Harcourt Brace Jovanovich; 1929.

[8] Burbach D, Peterson L. Children's concepts of physical illness: a review and critique of the cognitive-developmental literature. Health Psychol 1986;5:307–25.

[9] Bluebond-Langer M. Meanings of death to children. In: Feifel H, editor. New meanings of death. New York: McGraw-Hill; 1977. p. 48–66.

[10] Yamamoto K. Death in the life of children. Kappa Delta Pi; 1978.

[11] Crenshaw D. Bereavement: counseling the grieving throughout the life cycle. New York: Continuum; 1990.

[12] Nagy M. The child's view of death. In: Feifel H, editor. The meaning of death. New York: McGraw Hill; 1959. p. 95–6.

[13] Glazer JP. Life threatening illness in a high technology age: the paradigm of childhood cancer. In: Michels R, editor. Psychiatry. Philadelphia: Lippincott; 1990. p. 1–10.

[14] Rosen H. Child and adolescent bereavement. Child Adolesc Social Work J 1991;8(1):5–16.

[15] Showalter J. The child's reaction to his own terminal illness. In: Schoenberg B, Carr A, Peretz D, et al, editors. Loss and grief: psychological management in medical practice. New York: Columbia University Press; 1970. p. 51–69.

[16] Solnit A. Changing perspectives: preparing for life or death. In: Showalter JE, editor. The child and death. New York: Columbia University Press; 1983. p. 3.

[17] Spinetta J, Rigler D, Karon M. Anxiety in the dying child. Pediatrics 1973;52:841–5.

ELSEVIER
SAUNDERS

Child Adolesc Psychiatric Clin N Am
15 (2006) 575–584

CHILD AND
ADOLESCENT
PSYCHIATRIC CLINICS
OF NORTH AMERICA

From Cure to Palliation: Managing the Transition

Nancy Hutton, MD[a,b,*], Barbara Jones, PhD, MSW[c], Joanne M. Hilden, MD[d,e]

[a]Associate Professor of Pediatrics, Division of General Pediatrics and Adolescent Medicine, The Johns Hopkins University School of Medicine, 200 North Wolfe Street, Baltimore, MD 21287, USA
[b]Medical Director, Harriet Lane Compassionate Care, Johns Hopkins Children's Center, Baltimore, Maryland
[c]Assistant Professor of Social Work and Co-Director, The Institute for Grief, Loss and Family Survival, University of Texas at Austin School of Social Work, 1 University St., D3500, Austin, TX 78712, USA
[d]Chair, Department of Pediatric Hematology/Oncology and Medical Director, Pediatric Palliative Medicine, The Children's Hospital at The Cleveland Clinic, 9500 Euclid Avenue, Desk S20, Cleveland, OH, USA
[e]Associate Professor of Pediatrics, The Cleveland Clinic Lerner College of Medicine, Cleveland, OH, USA

When a child is diagnosed with a life-threatening or life-limiting condition, their physical and affective world is immediately changed, regardless of the outcome of treatment. Upon diagnosis, physicians, nurses, and mental health providers focus on curing the child and reducing the amount of suffering. Advances in medical and surgical treatment and in the intensive care of critically ill children have successfully increased child survival in the United States.

Sometimes, despite the best medical efforts and significant treatment advances, children do not survive. Ideally, children who are facing this possibility will receive palliative and supportive care [1–4]. However, recent reports indicate that this care is often inadequate or unavailable [2,5–8]. Despite recent awareness of the importance of pediatric palliative care, there is little recognition that shifting the focus beyond cure to palliation is itself a significant transition warranting special attention and intervention.

* Corresponding author. Division of General Pediatrics and Adolescent Medicine, The Johns Hopkins University School of Medicine, 200 North Wolfe Street, Baltimore, MD 21287, USA.
E-mail address: nhutton@jhmi.edu (N. Hutton).

1056-4993/06/$ - see front matter © 2006 Elsevier Inc. All rights reserved.
doi:10.1016/j.chc.2006.05.014
childpsych.theclinics.com

Life-threatening, life-limiting, and incurable illnesses, injuries, and conditions occur during childhood and cause suffering among children and adolescents, their loved ones, and the health professionals providing their care. This suffering is multidimensional and includes physical pain and other distressing symptoms, emotional or psychologic distress, social isolation or separation, and spiritual questioning. The causes of this suffering go beyond the physical effects of the condition itself. Treatments cause side effects, toxicities, adverse events, and physical limitations. Even when all goes "well," there are burdens associated with hospitalization, frequent medical visits, numerous medications, and separation from family, friends, and usual routines (eg, attending school). Parents and professionals share the desire to heal children of childhood conditions. Yet for too many children, this is not possible. Sometimes this is clear at the time of diagnosis and sometimes it becomes apparent later in the course of treatment.

At this transition in the goals for care from cure to palliation, parents and professionals want the best for children. For each child and family, the definition of what is optimal quality of life may differ depending on the family and cultural value system and the medical realities of the diagnosis. However, children have the capacity for decision-making, connectedness, positive adaptation, hope, and joy even at the end of life. Mental health professionals serve an essential role in reducing psychologic and spiritual suffering in children and improving quality of life.

Transition as a stage of care is important to discuss because many children and families will face this moment with little preparation and few supports. "Transition" as a construct allows both medical and mental health providers to prepare children and families for the palliative approach to care which is quite different than curative approaches. Depending upon diagnosis, some children live with chronic complex conditions that put them in the "transition" phase for years or even decades. Examples of this extended transition phase can be found among children living with advanced cystic fibrosis, severe complications of premature birth, or advanced HIV/AIDS.

If medicine can recognize a transition phase of care as a critical stage of treatment, perhaps the shift to palliative care can be eased. Pediatric care providers are in a unique position to offer hope to children and families even when cure is not possible. This hope focuses not only on cure, but incorporates the understanding that quality of life is not commensurate with length of life and that compassionate care can be provided in all stages of treatment.

Acknowledge challenges to transition

Pediatric specialists and children's hospitals provide excellent care for a full array of complex conditions. Tertiary care settings are designed to provide state-of-the-art diagnosis and treatment with the goal of curing serious and life-threatening conditions. The expectation is one of success, restoring children to full function. These academic medical centers are fast-paced and cutting-edge in their research and practice.

The palliative medicine approach focuses on the child and his or her quality of life. Its pace and process may differ dramatically from the familiar tertiary care approach. This unfamiliarity poses a challenge for institutions to provide palliative care. Acknowledging this challenge is the first step in changing the institutional culture to one that embraces the opportunity for transition from cure to palliation for patients and families who will benefit from this shift in focus.

Health care professional practice may pose challenges to transition. For example, although pediatric oncologists report feeling competent to manage pain and coordinate the care of the child dying from cancer [5], research shows us that patient outcomes do not support this contention. Wolfe and colleagues [8] interviewed the parents of children who had died from cancer and determined that physical symptoms were common and caused suffering at the end of life. Studies of pediatric oncology social workers indicate that pain and symptom management is the most important psychosocial need of children with cancer at the end of life [7]. Although pediatric oncology social workers report a strong desire to provide palliative care to children and families at the end of life, they encounter barriers to providing that care, including the demands of the health care system and overly high case loads [9].

These findings indicate the need for further exploration of the barriers to transitioning a child from curative to palliative care. Providers themselves may be reluctant to "admit" that cure is not likely. Physicians often feel the burden of "failure" when there are few curative options. This internal sense may be a barrier to transitioning the child and family to palliative approaches. Lack of training has also been found to be a significant barrier to providing palliative care in pediatric settings [1,2,5,10].

Sometimes it is the patients and families who are not ready for transition toward palliation. Good palliative care clinicians will meet the patient and family "where they are" and support them along the disease course. This partnering can be the beginning of the transition, avoiding an abrupt shift in the style and content of care. A careful transition attends to the physical and emotional needs of the child and family.

Recognize opportunities for transition

It may be helpful to think of palliation as mitigation of symptoms and reduction of suffering. If this construct is used, then palliation can be introduced from the moment of diagnosis even while the initial focus is on cure. As disease progresses, the clinician may offer more palliation and less curative therapy, thus creating a natural transition in treatment goals. Throughout this treatment, honest, frank, culturally congruent conversations with children and families are critical. Pediatric medical and mental health providers can make explicit the concept that palliative and curative approaches are not mutually exclusive and will be offered in varying proportions throughout the illness. This duality of approach lessens the stigma of palliative care which families may still interpret as "giving up." In fact, parents want full information about their child's condition, treatment, and prognosis, and they desire a partnership with their physician to plan for the future [11].

Integrated transdisciplinary approach eases transition

Pediatric care demands a well-rounded and functioning transdisciplinary team to fully assess, respond, and care for the multiple needs of children facing life-limiting conditions, as well as their families. No one provider can carry the full responsibility for the care, because each discipline brings an approach that complements the other and provides a web of support to the family. Understanding the medical prognosis of the child will not alone provide the necessary information to the provider. It is important to understand both the medical facts and the meaning that the child and family ascribe to those facts. Mental health providers such as psychiatrists, psychologists, and social workers can provide the child and family with opportunities to identify and express the range of intense emotions they may be experiencing throughout the transition to palliative care. When a family faces the trauma of a child's serious illness, their coping strategies are severely challenged. Families must work together to build additional supports and develop adaptive ways of functioning within this new reality. Mental health providers can work individually with children to help them find ways to express their needs, desires, fears, and hopes. Children often protect their parents from their deepest concerns and may need an outlet for the expression of their inner world. Modalities such as play therapy, creative arts, music, and art therapy all can help a child find verbal and nonverbal means of expression in a developmentally appropriate way. It is not uncommon for children to have questions about their treatment, their symptoms, or their dying that they do not know how to express. Children often have spiritual concerns and beliefs that need unique focused attention.

Benefits of palliative medicine

Although palliative medicine is not limited to the care of the dying, the people who die before reaching adulthood have much to teach us about who might benefit from palliative medicine. We learn the conditions they have, their age, and where and from whom they receive their care. One approach uses publicly available vital statistics. In the State of Maryland, we see patterns that must be considered in planning appropriate care [12]. For instance, the age groups experiencing the most deaths are infants and older adolescents. These groups are distinctly different in how communication and decision-making is approached in the locations of care, in the training needs of health care staff, and in the equipment and supplies needed for care. We note that sudden unexpected injury is the most common cause of death in almost all age groups. This mandates that our trauma services provide expert pain and symptom management in emergency settings with concurrent expertise in communication, decision-making, and bereavement support for surviving family and friends. Conditions noted at birth, such as complications of prematurity and genetic or chromosomal conditions, continue to cause death in older age groups, reminding us that surviving infants and their families are living with these life-threatening conditions over many years. For them, the palliative medicine approach is mandatory because it emphasizes quality of life. The demographic data reveal evidence of health disparities, with an overrepresentation of minority children among those who die. Those who live outside major metropolitan centers will not have easy access to specialized pediatric palliative medicine services without explicit planning to meet that need.

In a scholarly analysis of public health data from the State of Washington, Feudtner and colleagues [13] derived a working definition of complex (severe single organ or multiorgan disease) chronic (at least 12 months duration) conditions in childhood and then determined the prevalence of these conditions in the population of children and adolescents who died. He noted that the majority of these deaths occurred in the hospital. To assure that dying children receive the benefits of pediatric palliative medicine, we must integrate its services with pediatric specialty and hospital care. If the principles of palliative medicine are applied to all patients, the quality of health care we provide will improve significantly.

To transition: assess the situation

Assessment and management of the full range of physical, psychologic, social, and spiritual concerns should be integrated into the care of every patient regardless of diagnosis. The medical approach to a new patient presenting with a new problem is to promptly and fully evaluate, to make a clear diagnosis and recommend a treatment plan. Yet many conditions are not amenable to this narrow approach. Sometimes the diagnosis is not clear or there is no specific disease-directed therapy. It is still important to identify and manage problems recognizing that the management plan is still a sequence of treatments or procedures that include risks, discomforts, and worry. The psychosocial approach to a new patient is to conduct a thorough assessment of the person, including their hopes, dreams, family structure, sources of support, cultural and spiritual context, history, and meaning of illness and beliefs about the current diagnosis. Combining the traditional medical assessment with a psychosocial–spiritual assessment facilitates the transition from cure to palliation. If palliation is concerned with reducing suffering and improving quality of life from the moment of diagnosis, then this holistic approach to care allows the interdisciplinary team to understand the meanings that dictate the difference between suffering and healing in each child and family and provide care accordingly.

Acknowledging that cure is not likely

Experienced clinicians know that there are diagnoses and disease milestones that mean no cure is possible. Certain cancers, chromosomal anomalies, severe head trauma, HIV, or genetic disorders cannot be cured. The only possible goals are to maximize the quality and quantity of life. Some of these conditions are progressive and will cause premature death. Before we can talk with families about what to expect and how to proceed, we must first acknowledge for ourselves the reality of the child's prognosis for minimal recovery or disease progression ending in death. This can be very difficult for pediatric professionals, because we subscribe to the same human premise that children should be healthy and grow into independent adults. Working with children for whom this never will be possible can be a source of distress. Those of us who work with critically ill children all the time may develop protective strategies that compartmentalize our personal feelings from the care we provide. Those of us unaccustomed to working with children with grave illness may feel unprepared for the emotional intensity of providing this type of care. Both extremes erect barriers to recognizing and engaging with the "whole picture." Until we fully understand, we cannot communicate honestly, clearly, and completely with children and families about what the future holds.

Similarly, parents (and older children and adolescents) fear incurability and premature death when hearing a new diagnosis known to be potentially life-shortening, such as cancer or HIV. The initial need to educate, support, and reassure should not replace or preclude the need to address these fears directly and to validate them. In fact, the fears themselves must be acknowledged and heard before an authentic discussion of goals of treatment can progress. This moment provides the opportunity to initiate a full discussion of values, hopes, and goals that builds a foundation for ongoing discussion throughout the course of treatment, whether of progress or of relapse, complication, or deterioration. It is easy to avoid the larger picture of deterioration when focusing on the day-to-day details of test results or new medications. However, families live with the concern that their medical providers may not be giving them the "whole picture." Establishing a context of honesty from the initial meeting lays the groundwork for the trust that is essential to make informed medical decisions that will be congruent with the child and family's hopes and values.

Even when cure is initially a possible goal, there are events along the way that signal a change in prognosis. Cancer relapse or lack of response to antiretroviral therapy are examples. These events provide opportunities to continue the transition to a possible palliative approach.

In transition: talking with children and families about health care decisions

We know how to obtain informed consent, though the quality of that process is unacceptably variable in content and style and outcome. This quality ranges from none in an emergency setting, to brief for an urgent procedure, to focused and detailed for a planned procedure or treatment, to overwhelmingly complex for an experimental trial. The requirements are to provide information describing the intervention and about the indications, benefits, risks, and alternatives to choosing this intervention. Conversations usually dwell on the physical or "medical" information and ignore the benefits and burdens in other domains. For instance, children and parents want to know if choosing a particular treatment will require hospitalization or isolation or if it will interfere with activities of daily living. Health professionals may become so accustomed to these accommodations/burdens that they forget to discuss them explicitly.

Any discussion of informed consent in childhood diseases must include the acknowledgment that consent is gained from the surrogate decision-maker, usually a parent or guardian. This presents an ethical dilemma for the care provider as we attempt to gain "assent" from children and adolescents in their treatment decisions. The true perplexity occurs when the child and his/her surrogate decision maker do not agree. Although the legal mandate is to honor the decisions of the adult, this is ethically challenging. These decisions often occur upon diagnosis and then later when there is a transition in care. It is at the moments of transition in which the palliative approach— including an assessment of quality of life for the child—becomes so important. Understanding the hopes and dreams of a child and family in their sociocultural context can facilitate the conversations between child and family when there is disagreement.

In assessing a child's ability to provide consent, the care provider must make an assessment of the child's mental and emotional status, developmental age, family structure, cultural values including the role of children, the length of treatment the child has been exposed to, and the child's desire to participate in decision-making. Chaitin offers a formula for competency assessment of children which suggests that children must meet the following criteria [14]:

- ability to relay and understand information
- ability to understand the risks and benefits of the treatment options
- ability to understand the severity of the current medical situation
- voluntariness of choice: free from any internal constraints that could impair judgment or external constraints that could restrict free choice
- ability to render a choice

Communicating prognosis

In Wolfe and colleagues' [15] survey of parents whose children ultimately died with cancer, almost half did not believe that cure was a likely outcome right from the time of diagnosis. Although the proportion of physicians was a bit higher, this clearly indicates the opportunity to discuss the possibility of death and the importance of maximizing quality of life through palliative medicine immediately. As they moved through the disease trajectory, physicians recognized that there was no realistic chance for cure an average of 7 months before the child's death. This provides the second opportunity to assure that palliative medicine is integrated into the child's care. Of note, half of parents reported having come to this realization in the absence of a medical discussion about prognosis.

In a study of pediatric oncology social workers providing palliative care, the most difficult ethical dilemmas occurred when the medical team knew more than the child and family, when there was disagreement between child and family or team and family, and when the child was not told of their prognosis [9].

Talking about death (including children in the discussion)

When discussing illness and death with a child, the provider must consider the child's developmental stage, the child's previous experiences with illness, loss and death, the family structure and roles, the cultural and spiritual background of the child, the child's individual personality and approach, the child's sense of safety and the provider's comfort level in discussing death with children. Children will talk about death before they fully understand what it means to die. So, language alone does not indicate an understanding of the finality of death. Children typically do not understand the temporal meaning of death until nine or ten years of age. This range can be quite variable depending upon the individual child and their exposure to death. For example, children who have witnessed a number of friends die from cancer may understand the finality of death well before nine years of age.

Families must be consulted when talking with children about death, because ultimately the goal is to support the child and family and ensure that they are supportive of each other. However, many parents have concerns about talking honestly with their children that may be founded in fear rather than fact. For example, some parents are concerned about introducing the concept of dying to a child who has not yet considered this possibility. Anecdotal and empirical reports suggest that children can sense their impending death, sometimes even before their parents do [16]. Parents need support and information about childhood understanding of death to help them in these difficult conversations. Kreicbergs and colleagues [16] reported that parents who talk with their children about death do not regret it. Parents may also need to have their medical provider explain the prognosis to the child either alone or in tandem with the parent. Part of the transition to palliative care begins in the first meeting, when discussions about speaking honestly with children can be initiated. Some providers state in the diagnostic meeting that they will be honest with children about their own bodies throughout care, regardless of the prognosis. As always, cultural factors must be considered, understanding that in some cultures, any honest discussion of death is taboo and can cause greater distress.

Through transition: maintaining presence and continuity

Children and families value the relationships they have with their health care team. Knowing they can depend on their team regardless of what the future holds provides much comfort through the transition from cure to palliation. Health care professionals who provide honest, compassionate care improve the quality of life of the children and families they serve, regardless of the course and outcome of life-threatening conditions.

Acknowledgment

The authors wish to thank Miriam Stewart for her kind assistance with the literature review.

References

[1] National Consensus Project for Quality Palliative Care. Clinical practice guidelines for quality palliative care. 2004. Available at: http://www.nationalconsensusproject.org. Accessed June 11, 2006.
[2] Field M, Behrman R, editors. When children die: improving palliative and end-of-life care for children and their families. Washington, DC: National Academies Press; 2003.
[3] American Academy of Pediatrics. Palliative care for children. Pediatrics 2000;106:351–7.
[4] Carter B, Howenstein M, Gilmer M, Throop P, France D, Whitlock J. Circumstances surrounding the deaths of hospitalized children: opportunities for pediatric palliative care. Pediatrics 2004;114:e361–6.
[5] Hilden J, Emanuel E, Fairclough D, Link M, Foley K, Clarridge B, et al. Attitudes and practices among pediatric oncologists regarding end-of-life care: results of the 1998 American Society of Clinical Oncology Survey. J Clin Oncol 2001;19:205–12.
[6] Himelstein B, Hilden J, Boldt A, Weissman D. Pediatric palliative care. N Engl J Med 2004; 350:1752–62.
[7] Jones B. Companionship, control and compassion: a social work perspective on the needs of children with cancer and their families at the end of life. J Palliat Med 2006;9:774–88.
[8] Wolfe J, Grier H, Klar N, Levin S, Ellenbogen J, Salem-Schatz S, et al. Symptoms and suffering at the end of life in children with cancer. N Engl J Med 2000;342:326–33.
[9] Jones B. Pediatric palliative and end-of-life care: the role of social work in pediatric oncology. Journal of Social Work in End-of-Life & Palliative Care 2006;1(4):35–62.
[10] Sahler O, Frager G, Levetown M, Cohn F, Lipson M. Medical education about end-of-life care in the pediatic setting: principles, challenges, and opportunities. Pediatrics 2000;105: 575–84.
[11] Wharton R, Levine K, Buka S, Emanuel L. Advance care planning for children with special health care needs: a survey of parental attitudes. Pediatrics 1996;97:682–7.
[12] State of Maryland Department of Health and Mental Hygiene. Child death report 2004. Available at: www.fha.state.md.us/mch/pdf/ChildDeathReport2004FINAL.pdf. Accessed June 2006.

[13] Feudtner C, DiGiuseppe D, Neff J. Hospital care for children and young adults in the last year of life: a population-based study. BMC Medicine 2003;1:3.
[14] Chaitin E. Ethical decision making, morality and the law. Presented at the Annual Meeting of the Association of Pediatric Oncology Social Workers. St. Louis (MO), May 22, 2004.
[15] Wolfe J, Klar N, Grier H, Duncan J, Salem-Schatz S, Emanuel E, et al. Understanding of prognosis among parents of children who died of cancer. JAMA 2000;284:2469–75.
[16] Kreicbergs U, Valdimarsdottir U, Onelov E, Henter J-I, Steineck G. Talking about death with children who have severe malignant disease. N Engl J Med 2004;351:1175–86.

ELSEVIER
SAUNDERS

Child Adolesc Psychiatric Clin N Am
15 (2006) 585–596

CHILD AND
ADOLESCENT
PSYCHIATRIC CLINICS
OF NORTH AMERICA

Psychotherapy in Pediatric Palliative Care

Michelle R. Brown, PhD[a],*, Barbara Sourkes, PhD[b,c]

[a]Division of Child Psychiatry, Stanford University School of Medicine, Stanford, CA, USA
[b]Stanford University School of Medicine, Stanford, CA, USA
[c]Pediatric Palliative Care Program, Lucile Packard Children's Hospital at Stanford,
Stanford, CA, USA

I felt much better because I knew that I had somebody to talk to all the time. Every boy needs a psychologist! To see his feelings! —(6-year-old child) [1]

The role of psychotherapy

Most children who have a life-threatening illness enter psychotherapy because of the stress engendered by the illness rather than more general intrapsychic or interpersonal concerns. On one hand, children are forced to confront life issues prematurely and conceptualize things that ordinarily lie beyond their grasp. On the other hand, by being sequestered by the illness, they miss out on normal developmental milestones (eg, moving into the world of peer relationships). As a result, adaptation must be judged by balancing the illness parameters with normal development.

Although it is true that psychologic treatment is not necessary universally, the ability to identify high-risk children and intervene in a timely fashion is crucial. Ideally, the psychologic status of each child admitted to palliative care should be evaluated to plan for optimal care in the same way as medical and nursing assessments are performed [2]. Healthy siblings also should be included in the psychologic evaluation (along with the parents) and integrated into the psychotherapy if indicated.

Children's adjustment to illness also is influenced by their understanding of their illness and how they make sense out of their world at that point in time. Most of the children described or quoted in this article are (or were)

* Corresponding author. Division of Child Psychiatry, Stanford University School of Medicine, 401 Quarry Road, Stanford, CA 94305-5719.
E-mail address: mbrown@stanfordmed.org (M.R. Brown).

1056-4993/06/$ - see front matter © 2006 Elsevier Inc. All rights reserved.
doi:10.1016/j.chc.2006.02.004   *childpsych.theclinics.com*

living with a life-threatening illness, wherein cure is a possible outcome. Nonetheless, these children and families live in great uncertainty, experiencing anxiety and anticipatory grief reactions to the potential loss of the child, if not ultimately the actuality. Responding to children's questions about death (such as, "What's happening to me?" and "Am I dying?") requires careful exploration of what already is known by the children, what is really being asked (the question behind the question), and why questions are being asked at a particular time and in this setting [3]. Psychotherapy may facilitate psychologic adjustment by providing explanation in developmentally appropriate ways and identifying interventions that match their developmental understanding. During infancy and toddlerhood, children possess little if any understanding of death. Rather, death is equated with separation from caregivers. Preschoolers demonstrate magical thinking; they believe that things can come back to life and that they may have caused the illness by thinking bad thoughts. Within the context of psychotherapy, such beliefs can be explored and misconceptions clarified. From ages 6 to 12, children develop logical reasoning skills, and most acquire a mature concept of death. They are able to understand more objective causes of death and understand that death is universal and inevitable among all living things. Yet, children's fears of death remain centered primarily on the concrete fear of being separated from parents and other loved ones. By adolescence, abstract reasoning enables them to anticipate the future in a way that younger children cannot [4]. In that way, their experience of death becomes more focused on existential issues related to an afterlife, considerations more common to adults. It also should be emphasized that although concepts of death generally correspond with these developmental stages across all children, those who have a life-threatening illness often possess a precocious understanding relative to their well peers.

Psychotherapy for children or adolescents who are dying can provide the opportunity for expression of profound grief and for integration of all that they have lived, albeit in an abbreviated lifespan. Through words, drawings, and play, children convey the experience of living with the threat of loss and transform the essence of their reality into expression. Furthermore, even for young children, considerations about remaining quality of life may be discussed. There is a shared knowledge between children and therapists of the fine line that separates living from dying, communicated either implicitly or explicitly. Psychotherapy allows for the containment of anxiety resulting from the balance between the two. Children also can derive profound comfort from the safety and ongoingness afforded within the framework of therapy [4].

Through play, children can approach and retreat from the intensity of their illness at will, thereby allowing some containment and mastery over the emotional experience. Fantasy should not be construed as avoidance but, rather, a reflection of core feelings, conscious and unconscious [4]. Play enables seriously ill children to re-enter childhood. In child psychotherapy, play is the essential conduit of communication. Trauma of any kind, including illness, can extinguish—at least temporarily—some children's capacity for play or reduce its range of expression into rigid patterns [5]. Within the context of psychotherapy, emotional restoration is evident when children's play reflects earlier patterns of activity and liveliness.

For older children and adolescents, psychotherapy is a time apart—to reflect, question, grieve, plan, and hope. During a time when children are beginning to separate and develop a sense of their own personal identity, ill adolescents are forced back to depending on others, at times requiring assistance with basic tasks, such as personal hygiene or eating. They lack privacy over their bodies and must endure frequent intrusion, physical and emotional, by others. Psychotherapy can provide adolescents with a space of their own where thoughts and feelings are protected and confidential. The therapeutic relationship between therapists and children in itself may be a profound intervention, even when issues of death and loss are not addressed explicitly. Through the relationship, children are able to experience a sense of stability and continuity in an otherwise chaotic life.

> Elle, a 17-year-old who had acute myelogenous leukemia, received a visit from her therapist after admission to a hospice facility. During their time together, which was spent on craft activities and television, an unassuming nurse interrupted to inquire if the therapist was a friend or family member. Elle replied nonchalantly, "Oh, don't mind her. She's just my shrink!" and then returned to her TV program.

As children may not understand a therapist's role or the process of psychotherapy, it is important that simple, nonthreatening explanations be offered. Terms, such as "the talking doctor," provide a functional description that clearly distinguishes therapists from other professionals on the medical team [4]. Anxiety about seeing a therapist often is reduced when children are told that their feelings are common to all children and that therapy can help them feel less distressed. By introducing the concept of confidentiality, or privacy, early on, children may feel relieved to disclose thoughts or feelings that they have been reluctant to share with others. Over time, even if not articulated, children come to understand therapists' role in their care. For older children and adolescents, the concept of the "psych doctor" as a team member—albeit with special bounds of confidentiality—helps to diminish the sense of stigma associated with psychotherapy.

> On one of her clinic visits, Karen's physician asked her how she was feeling. She answered: "Medically I'm fine, but psychologically I'm not so fine, but I'll discuss that with my psychologist" [1].

A focus on well siblings also must be an aspect of the work, including, at times, meetings between a therapist and these children. Too often, siblings stand outside the spotlight of attention, even though they have lived through the illness experience with the same intensity as the child and parents [6,7].

Healthy siblings share common questions and concerns. They raise some questions and concerns with parents, professionals, or other trusted adults; others, they harbor silently. In an attempt to make sense of an overwhelming event, children may confuse coincidence with causality. Salient themes include fear of becoming ill, guilt for escaping the disease, lack of information, and anxiety that their own actions played a causal role in the onset of the illness. Rarely mentioned but often present is the unacceptable feeling of shame at having a different family, marked by a child who is ill, disfigured, or dying. Siblings also may harbor anger around diminished attention and nurturance from their parents, especially when a child is in the hospital. Older siblings who themselves are feeling deprived may resent stepping in as surrogate parents for younger brothers and sisters. Once ill children are home, siblings may resent the extra attention and privileges accorded to them, shifting their complaint from that of "too little attention" to "preferential treatment." Parents, meanwhile, are struggling to maintain equality and normalcy when, in fact, a distinctly abnormal factor in the family constellation exists [2].

Mariesa, a 16-year-old well sibling, comments on her experience of differential attention throughout the course of her younger sister's illness [8]:

> Everyone in my family was always calling [and asking], "How's Mikaela doing? How is the little angel?" And then with me, I was like, "What about me?" No one ever asked about me. No one cared anymore. From that moment on, it was not about me anymore. It was, "Oh, you have another daughter? We didn't notice." From that point on, everyone always cared about Mikaela and it made me feel like no one cares about me just because I'm not the one who is physically sick.

With the intrusion of the illness, the relationship between child and parent revolves around the threat of loss. Thus, it is critical that therapist intervention not disrupt the bond between them inadvertently. Therapists can diminish this threat by creating an ongoing alliance with the parents from the outset. In fact, such collaboration is the essential piece of the process. Because parents must assist children in extending the therapeutic work to everyday life, their role cannot be underestimated. Terr, in her work with traumatized children, comes to similar conclusions [5].

> It is almost impossible for a [therapist] to treat a child without providing some access to parents...who participate in the child's life. Parents need the reassurance of visiting the [therapist]. They need to know what the [therapist] is doing, to know how the child is faring in treatment, and to know what specific plans for the child they must put into operation themselves. Once the [therapist] is out of the picture, the family has to take over. Much of the therapeutic process consists of preparing for that time.

Family therapy can play a pivotal role in sustaining, strengthening, and repairing family resources [3]. The profound and enduring impact of a child's illness on the family is addressed within this context. In no way does family therapy preclude or contradict individual psychotherapy with a child.

Rather, it affirms the family unit as a whole and provides a framework for healing.

Themes in psychotherapy

Themes of loss are central to psychotherapeutic work with ill children, siblings, and family. Critical losses can be conceptualized around control, identity, and, overwhelmingly, relationships. Loss of control is a pivotal fear of any individual confronting life-threatening illness. In the moment of diagnosis, the entire sense of control dissolves in coming face-to-face with the limits of finite time. Children experience a loss of control in many areas—over their bodies, over disease and pain, over emotional boundaries, and, ultimately, over life itself [1].

When facing the death of their child, many parents attempt to keep the reality of impending death hidden from the child, with the hope that the child can be protected from the harsh reality. In essence, their efforts to limit information are aimed at gaining control over the pain and suffering that their child must endure. Parents also may be reluctant to discuss impending death with their child because they personally feel overwhelmed by the reality of the prognosis and feel unable to provide requisite emotional support to the child, as they are struggling to cope with their own distress.

While respecting parental wishes, team members can help parents talk through their own terror. They can share their professional knowledge from work with other families caught in this same excruciating situation. In doing so, parents may begin to understand that many young children already know what is happening to them, even when it purposely has been left unspoken by the adults. Specific examples of a child's own awareness may even be provided to a parent through a drawing or a comment made by the child in therapy. Thus, parents come to appreciate how shielding children from the truth inadvertently may heighten their anxiety and cause them to feel isolated, lonely, and unsure of whom to trust. Because the most basic tenet of parenthood is absolute trust, most parents can realize the need for responding honestly to a child's questions or fears. Perpetuating the myth that "everything is going to be alright" takes away the chance to explore fears and provide reassurance. For example, children may blame themselves for their illness and the hardships that it causes for their loved ones. Their guilt can be addressed and resolved only by open, honest communication, requiring a sensitive response that takes into account a child's developmental stage and unique lived experience. As a caveat, overriding all of these factors must be sensitivity to cultural beliefs and traditions.

In general, an individual child's competence and vulnerability serve as the context for decisions regarding disclosure at any point in the illness trajectory. Considerations about what, how much, and how to tell children should be based on their age, cognitive and emotional maturity, family structure and functioning, cultural background, and history of loss. These same factors apply at end of life, with extreme sensitivity to how parents choose to inform the child throughout the illness experience, how the child has understood and processed information up to this time, and what the child is not asking—implicitly and explicitly—about his or her situation [4,9].

Despite their absolute centrality in the treatment course, children usually have little control over the decisions that are made regarding their treatment plan. Decisions during the terminal phase are difficult, because there no longer is any promise of prolonged time. Parents do not want their children to suffer more, yet often they cannot tolerate the thought of ending life-prolonging treatment or curative attempts, of leaving any stone unturned. The physician and the team role shifts from leadership in decision-making regarding a treatment plan to clarification of remaining options and consequences. The balance between experimental treatment and cessation of aggressive interventions usually revolves around a child's quality of life and the family's comfort with the idea of terminating life-prolonging treatment. In most instances, parents make the decision; however, to varying degrees, children may be involved in such discussions. As children often express their understanding, awareness, and thoughts about treatment options and about living and dying to individuals other than their parents or primary physician, psychotherapists can be an important liaison during various junctures in treatment. A 10-year-old child who had medulloblastoma deliberated the pros and cons of continuing chemotherapy after a second relapse and noted [2]:

> I had two choices and I didn't want to take either of them. One of the choices was to get needles and pokes and all that stuff to make the tumor go away. My other choice was letting my tumor get bigger and bigger and I would just go away up to heaven...My mom wanted me to get needles and pokes. But I felt like I just had had too much—too much for my body—too much for me...So I kind of wanted to go up to heaven that time...But then I thought about how much my whole entire family would miss me and so just then I was kind of like stuck....

Parents or treatment providers may hold differing opinions regarding treatment goals. Physicians may encourage a family to continue an aggressive course of treatment, whereas parents are concerned about the pain and suffering associated with such a treatment approach. Alternatively, physicians may hold little hope for cure and encourage a transition to comfort care, whereas a family wishes to exhaust every possible treatment option. Differing priorities also may lead to misunderstandings between the child/family and provider. This is true especially when curative and comfort care are perceived as mutually exclusive. For example, a child's behavior might be perceived as nonadherent when medications or procedures that are time consuming or painful are missed. A child, however, simply may value quality of life or comfort above curative efforts. Physicians committed to providing the highest standard of care often are reluctant to negotiate terms of a prescribed treatment regimen knowing that such changes may reduce the treatment effectiveness or jeopardize a child's long-term prognosis. In this vein, a psychologist plays a vital role as liaison between child, family, or treatment team to facilitate communication and reduce the risk of misunderstandings around the treatment plan.

> A seventeen-year-old boy with end-stage pulmonary disease was encouraged by the medical team to agree to a DNR (do not resuscitate) order given his advanced, terminal condition. However, the child and the mother refused, wanting the treatment team to pursue every available life-sustaining measure. Every day on rounds, the medical team tried to persuade them to change their minds, pointing out how much additional pain and suffering could be involved. Although their intention was caring, the team's persistence cause the boy and him mother to feel judged and unsupported throughout the remaining days of his life [2].
>
> A sixteen-year-old girl with cystic fibrosis intermittently refused ventilatory support during sleep due to the chest pain caused by the air pressure from the bi-pap machine. She also frequently declined at least one of the four scheduled respiratory therapy treatments each day and decided to postpone the recommended gastronomy tube to facilitate nutritional intake. The medical team perceived her "nonadherent behavior" as indifference toward a possible lung transplant. She, however, clearly lamented her quandary in stating, "Why should I try so hard and endure so much pain if, in the end, a lung is not available for transplant, or even worse, if I get a lung and the transplant fails?"

Too often, children are labeled as "difficult" or "noncompliant" by caregivers when their behavior is notable for anger or resistance to their treatment regimen. Yet, in most instances, these children merely are acting out their inordinate difficulty in coping with a sense of total powerlessness. Once the meaning of this anger is acknowledged and the caregiving environment is structured to allow for as much control as feasible, children's behavior changes dramatically.

> A six-year-old boy refused his oral medications, required physical restraint for daily blood draws, and prohibited the medical team from examining him. The psychologist determined that several factors contributed to his difficulties: Multiple, unexpected visits by staff he did not know; procedures done without any explanation of their purpose or forewarning before touching him; and no opportunity for him to make any decisions in his care. A plan was created such that the number of visits by treatment team members was limited and scheduled; his physicians and the child life specialist provided him with age-appropriate explanations of his illness and related treatment; and the boy was also given the choice of which arm to use for taking his blood pressure, as well as which stickers he wanted after taking his medications. Within a few days, the child was entirely

cooperative with his treatment regimen and demonstrated a remarkable decrease in anger, frustration, and anxiety [2].

Self-help techniques, including relaxation, guided imagery, and hypnosis, also are integral psychotherapeutic interventions in providing a sense of control over symptoms, such as anxiety, nausea, and pain. Children and caregivers report dramatic reductions in physical and emotional distress as a result of these strategies. Furthermore, regardless of the actual impact of such techniques on symptoms, most children report an increased sense of well being resulting simply from their perception of exerting control.

An 8-year-old girl complained of phantom limb pain after leg amputation. During hypnosis, she was instructed to identify the switch in her head that could turn off incoming pain messages from various parts of her body. After one session, she reported a greater sense of control over her pain, and her discomfort appeared significantly reduced.

Psychotherapeutic techniques also can assist children in restoring a sense of control over emotions that often are experienced as overwhelming. Specific techniques, such as play with a therapeutic stuffed animal, letter writing, and the creation of a book, allow unstructured associative communication to be combined with a highly focused intervention. Art therapy also can be a powerful tool to facilitate children's expression and integration of complex experiences. Structured art techniques allow therapists to pose questions earlier in the process and with more specificity than might be done through verbal means alone. Further, children who are unable or unwilling to articulate their feelings verbally often communicate their experiences through drawings.

Loss of control over time often is prominent from the point of diagnosis, as children and families live with a sense of borrowed time. Particularly in late childhood and adolescence, children use the time to identify and accomplish certain goals, such as a family vacation or graduation from high school. For this reason, it is important that children have the right to know their diagnosis and prognosis. The information can provide a time context within which to organize and reorganize priorities. Therapists can play a critical role by helping children formulate a hierarchy of goals, thereby immediately instilling an increased sense of control over time.

What are the implications of life-threatening illness for a sense of identity? Initially, a diagnosis is viewed as an external intruder. Children refer to "the illness, the cancer," as if to assert, "This illness is separate from me." Over time, children begin to speak naturally of "my illness, my cancer." The subtle shifts in language are testimony to a significant process—what began as an external entity is transformed into an internalized part of physical and emotional being. Thus, another task within psychotherapy is to create a balance whereby a child's identity as a patient is incorporated into the broader spectrum.

When asked about cancer's impact on her life, a 19-year-old responded, "I wasn't like this before. I had interests. I went out with my friends. I used to take acting and dance classes. I had goals. Now I can hardly get out of bed."

Physical manifestations of the illness often have a significant impact on children's sense of self. Compounding children's own difficulty in adjusting to an altered body image is the fear of others' shock and revulsion at their appearance. At a more hidden level, an illness that affects sexuality directly through symptoms and effects of treatment, or indirectly through general debilitation, can be particularly devastating. Most profoundly, physical changes, obvious or subtle, attest to the presence of disease, and so to the threat of loss.

After a long course of steroids, a 16-year-old expressed reluctance to participate in social activities with peers, stating that no one would recognize her since she had become so "fat."

A myth persists that in the battle for survival, sexuality is of little psychologic importance. In fact, concerns about sexuality are pronounced in children who have life-threatening illnesses. The body is the focus of illness, and sexuality is an integral part of that same body. Sexual identity and functioning and fertility—and the potential or actual losses thereof—are major issues. Although adolescents are more likely than younger children to address them, the effect on all age groups should not be overlooked [10].

Denial of sexual issues by therapists serves only to close off a crucial avenue of disclosure. Acknowledgment of sexual activity and the impact of the illness on it are necessary if adolescents are to communicate with candor.

> An 18-year-old who had had a leg amputated expressed fears about his sexual functioning and about how his girlfriend would react. On a clinic visit shortly after his surgery, he greeted the therapist: "You'll be glad to know I still work!" Before the therapist had time to respond, the boy added, laughing, "I was glad, too!" [10].

There are concerns more subtle than those about actual sexual performance. For example, most children undergoing chemotherapy temporarily lose body hair, a common side effect of many drugs. There is much over-focus on the visible loss of hair on the head, from both cosmetic and symbolic points of view. In contrast, adolescents rarely mention the impact of the loss of pubic hair. Yet, as a perceived threat to a newly emerging sexual identity, this actually may be a more devastating loss.

At another level is the pain therapists may feel at understanding implications that children are not yet capable of grasping or choose not to look at in the present. Future sexual dysfunction or infertility, as a direct result of the illness or as a side effect of treatment, is a sobering prospect. Therapists bear the knowledge that one cost of long-term survival is the negotiation of these losses.

A 3-year-old boy with a bladder tumor required radical surgery and extensive radiation therapy. Although the treatment would cause sexual dysfunction and sterility, the prognosis for cure was excellent. The parents consented immediately to the protocol. However, they questioned the therapist extensively on how their son would react when he reached adolescence [10].

A 17-year-old girl who had been treated for uterine cancer cried, "The biggest scar is not having babies." Her grief was palpable and profound [10].

Medical personnel often are unprepared to broach sexual issues with children. All the more pressure, therefore, falls on therapists to take on the subject. As evidenced in the examples offered in this article, children have to progress not only through the normal developmental milestones of sexuality but also through the inextricable overlay of the immediate and long-term effects of their illness or treatment. Therapists' discomfort in handling sexual concerns—or the denial of their importance—can handicap the therapeutic process.

Although issues of control and identity belong primarily to the children, the loss of relationships is shared with family. Anticipatory grief—defined as "grief expressed in advance when the loss is perceived as inevitable" [11]— often is profound. Although children grieve the loss of their future, it often is the fear of being alone and separated from loved ones that is most palpable.

Anticipatory grief may show itself as children's increased sensitivity to separation, without any specific reference to death. It also may present as comments or questions related to death that may be seen as a type of preparation or rehearsal. It certainly also may present as the undiluted and unmistakable grief of the terminal phase of the illness. Thus, although anticipatory grief is catapulted into being at the time of diagnosis, its manifestation throughout the illness trajectory differs depending on whether or not the child is living with a life-threatening diagnosis but doing well, is going to die but not imminently, or actually is dying.

Parents may struggle with feelings of grief, attempting to deny the reality rather than experience the pain associated with the inevitable loss. During these times, psychotherapy also is useful in providing children a place to share their thoughts and fears when the topic is too sensitive for the family to bear.

When discussing the challenges to long-term treatment planning, a 17-year-old poignantly stated, "My mom won't face the fact that I'm dying (M. Brown, personal communication, 2005)."

An upsurge of jealousy or resentment toward well siblings may manifest in sick children as the end of life approaches, often reflecting sick children's fear of replacement. This fear may find expression either directly or through play. Although children's fear of replacement cannot be eliminated entirely, it can be worked through in psychotherapy and assuaged by parents' reassurance. A preoccupation with being replaced usually signifies children's need to talk about their life-threatening situation, with particular focus on fear of death. In addition, children often are speaking for the family's diffi-culty in negotiating the possibility of loss (M. Brown, personal communica-tion, 2005).

> The mother of a seven-year-old boy who had recently relapsed noted that he had become unusually hostile to his younger brother. Although they pre-viously had been close playmates, the child had become bossy, argumenta-tive, and even physically assaultive toward his sibling. He also became extremely protective of his mother's time, limiting the individual attention she could provide her youngest son.

Anticipatory grief is not static but fluid, with periods of lesser and greater presence. Families may panic over separation when a condition is stable and death is not imminent. Or, in contrast, a denial of impending loss may occur when time is short. These seeming inconsistencies arise from the fact that children and families live with a dualistic realm of time—real time as mea-sured by the clock and calendar year, which adheres to finite limits, and magical time, the individual omnipotent belief in endless time. Although the context for psychotherapy is finite time, a shift into magical time does not necessarily imply denial or blocking.

In his final days before dying, a 20 year old who had end-stage pulmo-nary disease asserted that she was the most appropriate of the three siblings to attend to their ailing mother and described detailed plans for her long-term care. During the conversation, she noted spontaneously that her death likely would precede such plans and then returned to her hopes and wishes for the future.

Members of the treatment team who are unaware of children's ability to shift fluidly between real time and magical time often can mistake children's fantasy life for ignorance or denial. When a child facing death refers to fu-ture dreams, those individuals who struggle to balance the reality of progno-sis with hope rigidly may comment, "Doesn't that child know he is going to die? Someone needs to tell him." Adherence to magical time to the exclusion of impinging reality may signify fear and dysfunction. Most children and families, however, flow between the two sets of time, in a normal adaptive process of maintaining hope. Psychotherapy can play a vital role in support-ing this process.

A clinical nurse specialist reflects on her conversations with Rachel, a 17-year-old girl living with cystic fibrosis, during her stay at Canuck Place [8]. Canuck Place in Vancouver, Canada, is the first freestanding pediatric hos-pice in North America.

> Living with knowing that you are dying is a balancing act. And Rachel re-ally showed me this through one of her stories. We were having a very in-tense talk about what she wanted it to look like...her end of life. And she said very seriously that when she is to die, she wanted to be here in Canuck Place, in a hospice surrounded by friends and family, and surrounded by

people that knew how to take care of her...and she was talking about the nurses and the doctors that can help her not feel scared...and then she said, "but I have another way that I'd like to die...I would like to be sitting on my front porch, wrapped in an afghan in a rocking chair and my husband holding my hand." And all I did was reflect that that would be a nice way. And to me that just spoke about the hope that we always have—that we have a rich full life, we have relationships that matter, we are supported in our pain...with also hanging on to the fact that she knows that it might look very different for her.

Psychotherapy for children who have life-threatening illness is unique in its challenges and rich in its rewards. It requires therapists to walk in tandem with children on a journey where the future is unknown. As children are held precariously in the balance between life and death, therapists must negotiate a balance between intimacy and emotional reserve. Along with the efforts to ease children's suffering, therapists must tolerate the personal pain associated with the threat of eventual loss [12]. It is this accomplishment that enables children to maintain their hopes, explore their dreams, and live more freely throughout their final days.

References

[1] Sourkes B. The deepening shade: psychological aspects of life-threatening illness. Pittsburgh: University of Pittsburgh Press; 1982. p. 3, 11.
[2] Sourkes B, Frankel L, Brown M, et al. Food, toys, and love: pediatric palliative care. Curr Probl Pediatr Adolesc Health Care 2005;35:350–86.
[3] Liben S. Pediatric palliative care. In: Behrman R, Klegman R, Jenson H, editors. Nelson textbook of pediatrics. 17th ed. Philadelphia: Saunders; 2003.
[4] Sourkes B. Armfuls of time: the psychological experience of the child with a life-threatening illness. Pittsburgh: University of Pittsburgh Press; 1995.
[5] Terr L. Too scared to cry. New York: Basic Books; 1990. p. 307.
[6] Sourkes B. Siblings of the pediatric cancer child. In: Kellerman J, editor. Psychological aspects of childhood cancer. Springfield (IL): Charles C. Thomas Publishers; 1980. p. 47–69.
[7] Sourkes B. Siblings of the child with a life-threatening illness. J Child Contemp Soc 1987;19: 159–84.
[8] Kuttner L. Making every moment count: pediatric palliative care. Documentary film. Montreal: National Film Board of Canada; 2003.
[9] Abrahm J, Sourkes B. Palliative care. In: Hoffman R, Benz E, Shattil S, et al, editors. Hematology: basic principles and practice. Philadelphia: Elsevier Science; 2004.
[10] Sourkes B. The child with a life-threatening illness. In: Brandell J, editor. Countertransference in child and adolescent psychotherapy. New York: Jason Aronson; 1992. p. 267–84.
[11] Aldrich CK. Some dynamics of anticipatory grief. In: Schoenberg B, Carr A, Kutscher A, et al, editors. Anticipatory grief. New York: Columbia University Press; 1974. p. 3–9.
[12] Sourkes B. Witness through time. J Palliat Care 2000;6:55–6.

ELSEVIER
SAUNDERS

Child Adolesc Psychiatric Clin N Am
15 (2006) 597–609

CHILD AND
ADOLESCENT
PSYCHIATRIC CLINICS
OF NORTH AMERICA

Post-traumatic Stress Response to Life-Threatening Illnesses in Children and Their Parents

Margaret L. Stuber, MD[a],*, Eyal Shemesh, MD[b]

[a]Department of Psychiatry & Biobehavioral Sciences, University of California Los Angeles,
760 Westwood Plaza, Los Angeles, CA 90024-1759, USA
[b]Departments of Pediatrics and Psychiatry, Mount Sinai Medical Center,
New York, NY, USA

Post-traumatic stress disorder (PTSD) is a constellation of psychological and physiologic symptoms that are persistent in some individuals who have been exposed to a traumatic event. Similar to most psychiatric disorders defined in the *Diagnostic and Statistical Manual of Mental Disorders* (DSM) of the American Psychiatric Association [1], the diagnosis depends on a combination of specific symptoms, over a set period of time, severe enough to lead to clinical distress or functional impairment. In this case, to qualify for a formal diagnosis of PTSD, a child or adult must display one or more symptoms from each of three clusters: avoidance of reminders of the stressor (eg, a traumatized soldier who does not want to return to the battlefield), re-experiencing of the event (eg, "flashbacks"), and hyperarousal (eg, hypervigilance, persistent heightened level of anxiety). These symptoms need to persist at least 1 month after the event and to be associated with functional impairments or disability to qualify for a diagnosis of PTSD.

In contrast to most diagnoses in DSM, a diagnosis of PTSD also requires that the symptoms be in response to a specific precipitating event, or trauma. According to the definition in the fourth edition of DSM (DSM-IV), a traumatic event must involve "actual or threatened death or serious injury, or a threat to the physical integrity of self or others," and the

---

This article was supported by KO8-MH63755 award and R-34 MH071249 (E. Shemesh) and the Maternal and Child Health Bureau (Title V, Social Security Act), Health Resources and Services Administration, Department of Health and Human Services (R40 MC00120) (M.L. Stuber).

  * Corresponding author.
  E-mail address: Mstuber@mednet.ucla.edu (M.L. Stuber).

individual must have experienced "intense fear, helplessness, or horror" at the time it happened [1]. In the early 1990s, the diagnosis or treatment of a life-threatening illness first was considered as a possible precipitating event for PTSD. Field trials done in preparation for DSM-IV evaluated a group of 24 adolescent cancer survivors and their mothers for PTSD [2,3]. The results of this field trial and others provided data that prompted the inclusion of medical illness as a potential precipitating traumatic event for PTSD in the text of DSM-IV and thereafter DSM-IV-TR [4]. Since that time, studies of post-traumatic stress symptoms have been published about a variety of medically ill patient groups, mostly adult but some pediatric studies, including cancer, burns, heart disease, diabetes, human immunodeficiency virus, and organ transplantation. These studies have supported the hypothesis that post-traumatic stress reactions are seen in medically ill children and adults and their families during active treatment and long after in survivors.

There has been little examination of PTSD in the context of palliative care settings, where the aim is to alleviate suffering, rather than offer a cure (see the Preface of this issue for the complexities of this "distinction"). It could be argued that PTSD should be less common for the children and parents in situations at the end of life, in which there are fewer invasive or painful procedures, and the uncertainty about outcome has been resolved. The focus on excellent pain management would be predicted to reduce the likelihood of post-traumatic symptoms [5]. It is also possible, however, that post-traumatic symptoms could give way to hopelessness and grief in the less anxious, but more certain, setting of palliative care. This article provides an overview of the literature on post-traumatic stress responses in children and their parents who are dealing with life-threatening illness, with a special emphasis on issues that may be encountered in palliative care settings.

Epidemiology of post-traumatic stress symptoms in pediatric patients and their parents

Children with cancer are probably the best studied medically ill pediatric population with regard to post-traumatic stress. Studies of children who are undergoing active treatment for cancer indicate evidence of post-traumatic symptoms during and after treatment. In the earliest published research study, nine children undergoing bone marrow transplant for hematologic and malignant disorders were followed longitudinally for evidence of PTSD. Symptoms consistent with PTSD were observed in a clinical interview performed in the hospital immediately before the bone marrow transplant. The children experienced a 4- to 8-week hospitalization in an isolation room, with intensive chemotherapy and radiation. The number and severity of the symptoms were increased from the pretransplant level in interviews held in the children's homes at the 3-month postdischarge visit after the transplant. The symptoms decreased at the 6-month and 12-month home interviews. The number and severity of symptoms did not return to the pretransplant level by the 12-month interview, however, despite the fact that at this point the child's chance of survival was quite good. Parents were not assessed formally in this study, but interviews with them about their children suggested they were distressed, but did not discuss this with their children [6].

The presence of post-traumatic stress symptoms in childhood cancer survivors was studied in comparison with other traumatized groups. Pelcovitz and colleagues [2] compared symptoms of 23 adolescent cancer survivors with 27 adolescents who had been physically abused and 23 healthy, nonabused adolescents. The cancer survivors not only reported more symptoms than the healthy, nonabused teens, but also more than the physical abuse victims. Using a measure of lifetime symptoms, 35% of cancer patients versus only 7% of abused adolescents met PTSD criteria. Cancer survivors reported their families as being significantly more caring than did the victims of abuse. The low prevalence of PTSD in the physically abused controls is puzzling and beyond the scope of this article.

Later studies of PTSD prevalence showed mixed outcomes. A large survey of 309 disease-free childhood cancer survivors, 8 to 20 years old, 6 years (mean) after the end of cancer treatment represented the following diagnostic groups: 38% acute lymphoblastic leukemia, 10% Wilms' tumor, 9% sarcoma, 8% acute nonlymphoblastic leukemia, 8% lymphoma, and 6% Hodgkin's disease. These pediatric cancer survivors were compared with 219 age-matched healthy control children. Both groups completed the PTSD Reaction Index, a widely used self-report instrument designed for children and adolescents. Of the cancer survivors, 2.6% reported severe PTSD symptoms, and 12.1% reported symptoms in the moderate range. By contrast, in the comparison group, 3.4% reported severe PTSD symptoms, and 12.3% reported symptoms in moderate range [7,8], with no statistically significant difference between pediatric cancer survivors and controls.

This study was followed by investigations of young adult survivors of childhood cancer, with different results. Of 78 childhood cancer survivors age 18 to 40 years, 20.5% met DSM-IV criteria for PTSD at some point after the end of treatment. As a group, participants reported elevated state and trait anxiety. Subjects meeting criteria for PTSD reported higher perceived current life threat, more intense treatment histories, and higher levels of psychological distress than subjects who did not have PTSD [9,10]. A subset of 51 of this sample was assessed with a structured clinical interview to determine PTSD status and given self-report measures of quality of life (Rand Short-form 36) and psychological distress (Brief Symptom Inventory). On this more rigorous assessment, 20% of the sample met criteria for PTSD. On all domains, quality-of-life scores were significantly lower (indicating poorer quality of life) for the PTSD group compared with the non-PTSD group. The survivors with PTSD also reported clinically significant levels of psychological distress, whereas symptom levels for survivors without PTSD fell well within population norms [11]. Age-specific developmental challenges were hypothesized to account for this higher level of symptoms compared with younger cancer survivors. Young adult survivors faced completion of higher education, career success, search for life partners, and related tasks apt to be affected by cognitive impairment, organ toxicity, infertility, and other late effects of cancer treatment to a greater degree than younger survivors.

Given the findings with PTSD prevalence in these studies of childhood cancer survivors, it might be concluded that post-traumatic stress symptoms are experienced primarily during acute illness at the time of initiation of treatment and after treatment ends by older survivors. Studies of pediatric solid organ transplant recipients suggest, however, that the level of symptoms reported by older cancer survivors in earlier studies may be a better estimate of the overall impact of life-threatening illness on children at all ages. A study of 104 pediatric heart, liver, or kidney transplant recipients, age 12 to 20 years, at least 1 year post-transplant, found that more than 16% of the adolescents reported symptoms meeting criteria for PTSD. An additional 14.4% met two of the three symptom-cluster criteria. Regression analysis indicated no effect of gender, ethnicity, age at interview, organ type, time since transplant, or age at transplant [12].

Comparable prevalence is found in other pediatric studies. A group of 35 children, and their parents, who had been hospitalized in a pediatric ICU were compared with 33 child/parent pairs who had been hospitalized on general pediatric wards; 21% of pediatric ICU–discharged children developed PTSD compared with none of the ward admissions. Pediatric ICU children had significantly more PTSD features of irritability and persistent avoidance of reminders of the admission [13]. In another study, 22% of 143 children 7 to 15 years old who experienced motor vehicle injury met criteria for PTSD. There were no associations for presence or absence of PTSD with age, gender, race, injury, or cause of injury [14].

Parents of children with serious medical illness

The largest study of post-traumatic stress symptoms in parents of children with life-threatening illness compared 309 mothers and 213 fathers of childhood cancer survivors with 211 mothers and 114 fathers of a healthy control group. Of the survivors' mothers, 10.1% reported severe levels of current post-traumatic stress symptoms, and 27% reported moderate levels of symptoms. The mothers in the comparison group reported 3% severe and 18.2% moderate levels of symptoms ($P = .001$). Of the fathers, 7.1% reported severe and 28.3% reported moderate symptoms of PTSD compared with 0% severe and 17.3% moderate in the fathers in the comparison group ($P < .001$) [7].

Another large but uncontrolled study of parents included 170 caregivers (mostly mothers) of pediatric transplant recipients 10 to 38 months after their child's most recent transplant. Although the parents did not report elevated levels of depression or anxiety, they did report elevated levels of post-traumatic stress symptoms, with 27.1% of the parents meeting diagnostic criteria for PTSD. The rate of post-traumatic stress symptoms did not vary by type of transplant or by ethnic group [15].

A similar prevalence is found in populations of parents dealing with a more acute life threat to their children. A study of 272 parents of children in the pediatric ICU for more than 48 hours found that 32% met symptom criteria for acute stress disorder. At follow-up 2 months later with 161 of the parents, 21% met symptom criteria for PTSD [16]. A British study found that parents of children hospitalized in the ICU were more likely to screen positive for PTSD (27%) compared with parents of children admitted to the ward (7%) [13]. In another study of mothers of children experiencing acute life-threatening illness, 111 mothers of children who survived hematopoietic stem cell transplantation completed self-report measures of psychological functioning at the time of hematopoietic stem cell transplantation and self-report measures and a structured psychiatric interview 18 months later. Approximately 20% of mothers had clinically significant PTSD spectrum symptoms. This prevalence increased to nearly one third when subthreshold PTSD was included [17].

Predictors for the development of post-traumatic stress disorder in medically ill children and their parents

Children

Studies examining predictors of post-traumatic stress symptoms in children with life-threatening illness have found consistent factors similar to those found for other types of traumatic exposure. In a report from the largest study to date of childhood cancer survivors, 186 survivors age 8 through 20 years, off treatment for more than 1 year, significant, independent predictors of persistent post-traumatic stress symptoms included (1) the survivor's retrospective subjective appraisal of life threat at the time of treatment, and the degree to which the survivor experienced the treatment as "hard" or "scary"; (2) the child's level of trait anxiety; (3) history of other stressful experiences; (4) time since the termination of treatment (negative association); (5) female gender; and (6) family and social support (negative association). The survivor's anxiety and current appraisal of life threat, but not post-traumatic stress symptoms, were related to the mother's perception of stress of treatment and current life threat. The assessment of prognosis and treatment intensity made by the oncologist was not significantly related to the appraisals of life threat or treatment intensity by the survivor and did not predict post-traumatic stress symptoms in the survivor [18].

Even injuries that are not life-threatening seem to result in post-traumatic stress symptoms in some cases. In one study, 400 pediatric orthopedic trauma patients with an average age of 11 years were assessed an average of 36 days after injury. Of the children, 33% reported high levels of post-traumatic stress symptoms. Levels of symptoms were not related to the mean Injury Severity Score or summed Extremity Abbreviated Injury Score. The only identified predictor was that patients admitted to the hospital after injuries were significantly more likely to develop high levels of post-traumatic stress symptoms compared with patients not admitted [19].

The subjective appraisal of the traumatic event, rather than an objective measure of actual risk or exposure, is particularly significant for the palliative care setting. Although it could be argued that the prognosis is grim for all of the children in a palliative care setting, not all experience it as traumatic, and not all children receiving palliative care services die (see Preface). There are many stressful events in the course of a serious illness, however, which may have been experienced as traumatic by a child or parent. This appraisal is highly individual and is shaped significantly by developmental level and by the parent's, usually the mother's, appraisal of risk. Younger children are less likely to interpret the diagnosis or life threat as the most traumatic aspect of the illness because they are less likely to understand fully the potential implications. Younger children are more likely than older children and parents to find separation from friends and family to be a major traumatic event, however [20]. Exposure to traumatic events at different developmental stages is likely to result in different psychological outcomes and disorder profiles, but interpretation of studies published to date are limited by failure to stratify by age or stage of development. Studies are needed with the sample sizes necessary to examine this question by age and developmental level stratification.

Often the intrusive or painful medical procedures and treatments, such as transplantation and chemotherapy, are cited later as traumatic events by children of all ages who report medically related post-traumatic stress symptoms. Medical professionals may be perceived as "inflictors" of trauma, with parents as collaborators. Clinical experience suggests some children may experience medical treatment as akin to interpersonal violence, despite sensitive, well-intentioned caregivers Studies of children exposed to repeated, interpersonal traumatic events suggest these events are more likely to lead to blunting and dissociation, whereas an acute, noninterpersonal event, such as a natural disaster, are more likely to lead to hypervigilance and avoidance of reminders. Although this distinction has not been firmly established for medically related traumatic stress responses, it should be considered for seriously ill children in intensive medical settings whose withdrawal and "depression" may reflect traumatic dissociation, rather than a mood disorder.

Parents

Predictors for post-traumatic stress responses in parents resemble the predictors seen in childhood cancer survivors. Mothers and fathers of 331 survivors of childhood cancer age 8 to 20 years were surveyed using the Posttraumatic Stress Disorder Reaction Index, a validated instrument used for self-report of traumatic stress symptoms in adults and adolescents. Trait anxiety as reported at 5 years after the end of treatment was the strongest predictor of post-traumatic stress symptoms for mothers and for fathers. Other significant contributors were the parent's perception of the life threat to the child, the parent's perception of the intensity of the child's treatment, and the parent's social support. Similar to the children, the oncologist's rating of life threat and treatment intensity did not contribute to post-traumatic stress symptoms in the parent. In contrast to the child survivors, there was a small but statistically significant correlation between the parent's and oncologist's rating of life threat and treatment intensity [21].

Similar predictors were found in the pediatric ICU study previously cited. Symptoms of PTSD and acute stress disorder at 2-month follow-up were associated with the parents' *perception* of life threat rather than *actual* life threat as measured by the Pediatric Risk of Mortality Scale. Other predictors of PTSD at 2 months were the symptoms of acute stress disorder assessed in the pediatric ICU, an unexpected admission, and the occurrence of another hospital admission or other traumatic event after the index admission [16].

The relationship between post-traumatic stress symptoms in children and their parents was studied in 209 children, age 6.5 to 14.5 years, interviewed 5 to 6 weeks after an accident or a new diagnosis of cancer or diabetes mellitus type 1. Of the children, 11.5% reported post-traumatic stress symptom levels in the clinical range of PTSD; 16% of the 175 fathers and 23.9% of the 180 mothers met full DSM-IV diagnostic criteria for current PTSD. Predictors of the development of PTSD in the children included accident-related injury (rather than cancer or diabetes) and the functional status of the child. The development of PTSD in the parents was associated with the diagnosis of cancer in their child (more commonly than injury). PTSD symptom scores of mothers and fathers were significantly correlated with each other. The children's PTSD symptoms were not significantly related to the symptoms of the mothers and fathers, however [22].

Implications for care

Children

Given the focus on quality of life and comfort care in a palliative care setting, what are the implications of PTSD in this setting? The study of Meeske and colleagues [11] of 51 young adult survivors of childhood cancer, 20% of whom met symptom criteria for PTSD, lends support to PTSD as an indicator of distress, finding that the summative score for psychological distress was in the upper 97th percentile compared with a normative population.

Of importance to children in palliative care, in this study subjects with moderate and severe "late effects" of treatment (eg, cardiovascular or pulmonary complications) were more likely to have PTSD. This finding suggests that a more severe medical outcome might act to sustain chronic symptoms of PTSD and be an indicator of more traumatic exposure over time [11]. In the pediatric oncology setting and by implication with other life-limiting illnesses, a substantial proportion of children sick enough to reach the point of palliative care are likely to have experienced multiple risk factors for PTSD and associated distress. These patients also are likely to experience functional impairment and reduced quality of life, which may be improved if PTSD symptoms are addressed.

Post-traumatic stress symptoms also seem to be related to nonadherence to treatment. A study of 19 pediatric liver transplant recipients found that 6 reported symptoms consistent with a diagnosis of PTSD. Three of these, and none of the others, had been rated as significantly nonadherent by their medical care team. The children with PTSD had significant fluctuations in their blood levels of immunosuppressive drugs. In this study, no significant differences were found in perception of disease threat or demographic variables between the subjects reporting PTSD and the subjects who did not. Most importantly, the three children who had been nonadherent became adherent to their medications when they were treated successfully for PTSD, using a cognitive-behavioral therapy (CBT) approach with an imaginal exposure component. Nonadherence to medications seemed to be related to the avoidance dimension of PTSD (patients avoid taking the medication because it is a traumatic reminder of the illness), as the avoidance dimension of PTSD accounted for much of the association with nonadherence [23].

Parents

The impact of post-traumatic stress on the parents is at least as serious a problem, given the higher prevalence of post-traumatic stress symptoms in parents than in their ill children and the added impact of grief and loss if the child dies. A small study found potentially adverse physiologic correlates of chronic PTSD in mothers of childhood cancer patients, even when the child survived. Participants included 21 mothers of pediatric cancer survivors with ($n = 14$) and without ($n = 7$) PTSD and control mothers of healthy children ($n = 8$). The PTSD group showed higher total urinary cortisol and a trend for higher total urinary norepinephrine than the non-PTSD group, who were no different from controls. This finding is consistent with findings in other populations of PTSD patients and suggests these mothers have a chronic stress response [24]. These findings are of even greater concern with the speculation that the parent's PTSD symptoms may affect the child's perception of threat and influence his or her risk for PTSD and other psychological symptoms. Parental functioning is unquestionably important for medically ill children, who might be dependent on their parents to administer medical treatments, make and transport to medical appointments, and perform related essential practical and psychological support functions.

Interventions

In the palliative care setting, some of the known contributors to psychological trauma and PTSD already have been reduced or eliminated, including painful medical interventions and the side effects of curative chemotherapy. Life threat is, by definition, always present. As noted elsewhere in this issue, adequate pain management, psychopharmacotherapy, CBT, and psychodynamic psychotherapy, with varying and emerging evidence bases, are cornerstones in the treatment of children with life-limiting illness. PTSD and acute stress disorder can be conceptualized as major symptom clusters with which children with life-limiting illness may present. Although controlled clinical intervention trials of PTSD treatment options in the unique setting of life-limiting pediatric illness have not been performed, other pediatric (and adult) research offers guidance until more definitive studies are conducted. The only rigorously investigated approach for the treatment of PTSD in children to date [25] used a manual to deliver an imaginal exposure–based CBT treatment in nonmedical PTSD. This was a randomized, multicenter, controlled trial of 229 children, age 8 to 14 years, all of whom had a history of sexual abuse. The trauma-focused CBT was superior to a form of "child-centered therapy" on all outcome measures, including depression, PTSD, and behavior. No other forms of treatment have been evaluated in large randomized trials. In adults, the best studied approaches include trauma-focused CBT (see later) and selective serotonin reuptake inhibitors (SSRIs). Paroxetine and sertraline are approved by the US Food and Drug Administration (FDA) for the treatment of PTSD in adults. A cautionary note is that for children, the use of SSRIs, as described in the FDA's "black box" warning, may be associated with an increase in suicidal ideation. An open trial [26] suggested the safety and efficacy of the SSRI fluvoxamine when given to children with cancer; fluvoxamine is the only SSRI studied in depressed children with cancer. At present, trauma-specific CBT techniques and, in selected cases, SSRIs are the best justified interventions for medically ill children who experience significant distress or impairment related to PTSD based on a growing, if incomplete, evidence base and with appropriate FDA-mandated precautions.

A different set of interventions may hold promise for PTSD prevention in medically ill children by addressing presymptomatic risk factors. Interventions can be made to decrease the fear and helplessness associated with illness and treatment. Although there has been limited formal study of family interventions in such settings [27], principles of humane family-centered care mandate psychosocial child and family support in pediatric palliative care, as exemplified by novel multidisciplinary team approaches such as the Helping Hands Service at the Cleveland Clinic Children's Hospital (JM Hilden, JP Glazer, and DY Poltorak, personal communication, 2006).

The following guidelines are offered to help clinicians develop a sensible approach to intervention for children in palliative care and their parents as a broader base of empirical evidence is awaited:

1. Given that perceptions of life threat and treatment intensity are a major contributor to symptoms, and that these perceptions vary greatly among child, parent, and physician, open and careful communication among the child, parents, and medical team about the child's medical condition is essential. This is not primarily to ensure the child has "the truth" so much as for the parents and medical care team to understand the child's perspective. It is often difficult for the medical team to comprehend that treatments that are aimed at palliation of symptoms (eg, placement of an intravenous catheter for administration of opiate analgesics) could be perceived as traumatic by the pediatric patient and his or her family, as reminders of past traumatic events.

2. When it is clear which specific reminders or treatments are distressing to a given child, interventions can be designed to help minimize this distress. Such an intervention may be improved pain control, but more often it is a matter of decreasing a sense of helplessness. Interventions often can be set up that restore more control and choice for the child or parents even with seriously or terminally ill children. Not every medical intervention can be eliminated or postponed, but some can, and such small changes as moments of privacy for child and family unencumbered by medical intervention can make a great difference.

3. Pretreatment with medications that decrease pain without causing confusion or perceived loss of control may be helpful in decreasing trauma symptoms. Pain and anxiety seem to amplify the imprinting of traumatic reminders and the conditioning of specific reactions. Increasing the morphine given to a burn-injured child while in the hospital diminishes the risk of PTSD 6 months after discharge [5]. As discussed elsewhere in this issue, desensitizing interventions, based on established behavioral principles, also can be useful.

4. Identification of traumatic reminders can help minimize avoidance by directly addressing the symptoms associated with re-experiencing. The child, family, and medical team can be helped by the psychiatric consultant to recognize traumatic reminders and develop ways of dealing with and minimizing these.

The staff can be trained to recognize and help with symptoms of PTSD. A toolkit has been created by the National Child Traumatic Stress Network (NCTSN), with support from the Substance Abuse and Mental Health Services Administration of the National Institute of Mental Health. These materials were designed to be useful for hospital-based health care providers, including physicians, nurses, and emergency care providers, and for parents. The toolkit includes the following:

1. An introduction to traumatic stress as it relates to children facing illness, injury, and other medical events.
2. Practical tips and tools for health care providers.
3. Handouts that can be given to parents with evidence-based tips for helping their child cope.

These materials can be downloaded free of charge from the NCTSN website, www.nctsnet.org.

Summary

Symptoms of PTSD have been reported in response to a variety of life-threatening medical illnesses and injuries in adults and children. Emerging data suggest that children often experience medical treatment and hospitalization as traumatic, putting caregivers and medical personnel in the role of the unintended accomplice. Adequate pain control by pharmacologic and behavioral means; child and family psychological support using evidence-based CBT, dynamic psychotherapy, and other techniques; and meticulous attention to communication via a team-based approach are the cornerstones of pediatric palliative care in general and PTSD prevention and treatment in particular. Emerging evidence suggests that PTSD in life-limiting pediatric illness can be ameliorated, if not prevented, and treated when it occurs, contributing materially to the quality of life of a child and family. A landmark finding of PTSD research with medically ill children and their families is that parents are at least as symptomatic, or more, as their children, underlining the importance of a family-directed approach addressing every family member. Pediatric caregivers increasingly recognize their therapeutic role when curative therapy is no longer possible is as pivotal as in the setting of acute illness.

References

[1] American Psychiatric Association. Diagnostic and statistical manual of mental disorders. 4th edition. Washington, DC: American Psychiatric Association; 1994.
[2] Pelcovitz D, Goldenberg B, Kaplan S, et al. Posttraumatic stress disorder in mothers of pediatric cancer survivors. Psychosomatics 1996;37:116–26.
[3] Alter CL, Pelcovitz D, Axelrod A, et al. Identification of PTSD in cancer survivors. Psychosomatics 1996;37:137–43.
[4] American Psychiatric Association. Diagnostic and statistical manual of mental disorders. 4th edition, text revision. Washington, DC: American Psychiatric Association; 2000.
[5] Saxe G, Stoddard F, Courtney D, et al. Relationship between acute morphine and the course of PTSD in children with burns. J Am Acad Child Adolesc Psychiatry 2001;40: 915–21.

[6] Stuber ML, Nader K, Yasuda P, et al. Stress responses after pediatric bone marrow transplantation: preliminary results of a prospective longitudinal study. J Am Acad Child Adolesc Psychiatry 1991;30:952–7.

[7] Barakat LP, Kazak AE, Meadows AT, et al. Families surviving childhood cancer: a comparison of posttraumatic stress symptoms with families of healthy children. J Pediatr Psychol 1997;22:843–59.

[8] Kazak AE, Barakat LP, Meeske K, et al. Posttraumatic stress, family functioning, and social support in survivors of childhood leukemia and their mothers and fathers. J Consult Clin Psychol 1997;65:120–9.

[9] Hobbie WL, Stuber M, Meeske K, et al. Symptoms of posttraumatic stress in young adult survivors of childhood cancer. J Clin Oncol 2000;18:4060–6.

[10] Rourke MT, Stuber ML, Hobbie WL, Kazak AE. Posttraumatic stress disorder: understanding the psychosocial impact of surviving childhood cancer into young adulthood. J Pediatr Oncol Nurs 1999;16:126–35.

[11] Meeske KA, Ruccione K, Globe DR, Stuber ML. Posttraumatic stress, quality of life, and psychological distress in young adult survivors of childhood cancer. Oncol Nurs Forum 2001;28:481–9.

[12] Mintzer LL, Stuber ML, Seacord D, et al. Traumatic stress symptoms in adolescent organ transplant recipients. Pediatrics 2005;115:1640–4.

[13] Rees G, Gledhill J, Garralda ME, Nadel S. Psychiatric outcome following paediatric intensive care unit (PICU) admission: a cohort study. Intensive Care Med 2004;30: 1607–14.

[14] Zink KA, McCain GC. Post-traumatic stress disorder in children and adolescents with motor vehicle-related injuries. J Spec Pediatr Nurs 2003;8:99–106.

[15] Young GS, Mintzer LL, Seacord D, et al. Symptoms of posttraumatic stress disorder in parents of transplant recipients: incidence, severity, and related factors. Pediatrics 2003;111 (6 Pt 1):e725–31.

[16] Balluffi A, Kassam-Adams N, Kazak A, et al. Traumatic stress in parents of children admitted to the pediatric intensive care unit. Pediatr Crit Care Med 2004;5:547–53.

[17] Manne S, DuHamel K, Ostroff J, et al. Anxiety, depressive, and posttraumatic stress disorders among mothers of pediatric survivors of hematopoietic stem cell transplantation. Pediatrics 2004;113:1700–8.

[18] Stuber ML, Kazak AE, Meeske K, et al. Predictors of posttraumatic stress symptoms in childhood cancer survivors. Pediatrics 1997;100:958–64.

[19] Sanders MB, Starr AJ, Frawley WH, et al. Posttraumatic stress symptoms in children recovering from minor orthopaedic injury and treatment. J Orthop Trauma 2005;19:623–8.

[20] Stuber ML, Nader KO, Houskamp BM, Pynoos RS. Appraisal of life threat and acute trauma responses in pediatric bone marrow transplant patients. J Trauma Stress 1996;9: 673–86.

[21] Kazak AE, Stuber ML, Barakat LP, et al. Predicting posttraumatic stress symptoms in mothers and fathers of survivors of childhood cancers. J Am Acad Child Adolesc Psychiatry 1998;37:823–31.

[22] Landolt MA, Vollrath M, Ribi K, et al. Incidence and associations of parental and child posttraumatic stress symptoms in pediatric patients. J Child Psychol Psychiatry 2003;44: 1199–207.

[23] Shemesh E, Lurie S, Stuber ML, et al. A pilot study of posttraumatic stress and nonadherence in pediatric liver transplant recipients. Pediatrics 2000;105:E29.

[24] Glover DA, Poland RE. Urinary cortisol and catecholamines in mothers of child cancer survivors with and without PTSD. Psychoneuroendocrinology 2002;27:805–19.

[25] Cohen JA, Deblinger E, Mannarino AP, Steer RA. A multisite, randomized controlled trial for children with sexual abuse-related PTSD symptoms. J Am Acad Child Adolesc Psychiatry 2004;43:393–402.

[26] Gothelf D, Rubinstein M, Shemesh E, et al. Pilot study: fluvoxamine treatment for depression and anxiety disorders in children and adolescents with cancer. J Am Acad Child Adolesc Psychiatry 2005;44:1258–62.
[27] Kazak A. Evidence-based interventions for survivors of childhood cancer and their families. J Pediatr Psychol 2005;30:29–39.

ELSEVIER
SAUNDERS

Child Adolesc Psychiatric Clin N Am
15 (2006) 611–655

CHILD AND
ADOLESCENT
PSYCHIATRIC CLINICS
OF NORTH AMERICA

Psychopharmacology in Pediatric Critical Care

Frederick J. Stoddard, MD[a,b,*],
Craigan T. Usher, MD[a,c], Annah N. Abrams, MD[a,d]

[a]Harvard Medical School, 25 Shattuck Street, Boston, MA 02115, USA
[b]Massachusetts General Hospital, 51 Blossom Street, Boston, MA 02114, USA
[c]Massachusetts General Hospital/McLean Hospital, 55 Fruit Street,
Yawkey Suite 6A, Boston, MA 02114, USA
[d]Child Psychiatry Consultation Liaison Service, Massachusetts General Hospital,
Boston, MA 02114, USA

This overview of psychopharmacology in pediatric critical care is timely because of the rapidly expanding use of psychopharmacologic drugs in pediatric populations and in critical care [1,2]. Compassionate prescribing of medications for children who are critically ill and who have injuries or life-threatening disease has reduced the pain and suffering they may endure dramatically [3]. Because they are critically ill, the potential benefits of psychotropic medications must be weighed against risks for severe adverse effects, toxicity, or drug interactions. Most clinical trials evaluating the safety and efficacy of psychotropic medications have not included children under 12 or those who are critically ill. Pediatric intensivists, therefore, often must rely on clinical experience as opposed to evidence-based medicine when selecting agents for optimal effectiveness, tolerability, and safety.

Drug selection and monitoring should take into account the organ system that is damaged: neurologic, cardiovascular, hematologic, pulmonary, gastrointestinal, genitourinary, musculoskeletal, endocrine, or integumentary. Impairment of any system can affect psychiatric symptomatology, drug metabolism, and drug response. The relevance of psychopharmacology in critical care is increased by the preparations, plans, and protocols to treat survivors of hurricanes, earthquakes, terrorism, and wars who are acutely injured [4,5]. This article addresses five areas of pediatric critical care: (1) psychopharmacologic principles; (2) classes of psychotropic drugs in

* Corresponding author. Massachusetts General Hospital, 51 Blossom Street, Boston, MA 02114.
E-mail address: fstoddard@partners.org (F.J. Stoddard).

1056-4993/06/$ - see front matter © 2006 Elsevier Inc. All rights reserved.
doi:10.1016/j.chc.2006.02.005
childpsych.theclinics.com

pediatric critical care; (3) child psychiatry consultation—assessment and developmental principles; (4) psychopharmacologic treatment of delirium, pain, and psychiatric disorders; and (5) palliative care in a critical care setting.

Psychopharmacologic principles

Psychotropic drug use (stimulants, anxiolytics, antidepressants, and antipsychotics) is expanding rapidly in all pediatric practice despite the black box warning on antidepressants from the Food and Drug Administration (FDA) in 2004 [6,7]. The scientific basis for psychotropic use is limited, however, especially in young children [8]. Although the evidence is limited in child and adolescent psychopharmacology [9], it is limited even more in pediatric critical care [10]. Available evidence, however, is summarized in the practice guidelines of the American Academy of Child and Adolescent Psychiatry [11]. Psychopharmacologic research focuses on specific disorders (eg, posttraumatic stress disorder [PTSD], attention-deficit/hyperactivity disorder [ADHD], and psychotic, mood, or anxiety disorders), with little research in pediatric critical care settings. Nevertheless, these agents are in wide use in pediatric critical care and rational prescribing based on the best available evidence and clinical experience addressing benefits, alternatives, and risks is mandatory. Finally, unique age-dependent variables in pharmacokinetics and pharmacodynamics and genetic influences on protein binding, metabolism, and elimination are central to the prescription of psychopharmacologic agents to children in pediatric critical care [12].

Child and adolescent psychiatrists play an important role with other medical, surgical, and mental health colleagues [13]. They may assist pediatric, nursing, psychology, and social service and other staff who may be unfamiliar with children.

Information technology

Psychopharmacologic treatment is aided increasingly by information technology monitoring critical care. Most critical care units or ICUs either have or are implementing electronic medical records, physician order entry, automated devices for drug dispensation, bar coding, and point of care testing, allowing for constant detailed monitoring of treatment and response, even from a distance. New child and adolescent psychopharmacology studies, in part using such IT, aim to increase the practical empiric evidence base, including efficacy and safety [14].

Developmental neurobiology

Developmental neurobiology now is being delineated from infancy through adulthood with major implications for diagnosis and treatment in critical care [15–18]. The discoveries of how the glutaminergic, endorphin, γ-aminobutyric acid (GABA)-ergic, dopaminergic, serotonergic, and cholinergic neural networks develop and interrelate are transforming understanding children's responses to drugs [19]. Understanding the developmental mechanisms of neural growth, injury, and repair also is being transformed. This is leading to discoveries in a wide range of areas relevant to pediatric critical care, including pain pathways and pain responses in infants and children, the effects of psychologic trauma (including medical illness) on development, developmental psychopathology and critical care outcomes, and adult psychiatric disorders associated with childhood trauma. Although genetic understanding of the mechanisms of drug actions and interactions still is young [20], explanations for how genes and environment interact to orchestrate human development, particularly under stress [21], have implications for clinician selection and dosing of drugs. The empiric success and improved outcomes from aggressive pain management [22] has led one of the authors (FJS) to advocate similar empiric approaches to preventing stress disorders and depression in critical care [23].

Pharmacokinetics and drug-drug interactions

Pharmacokinetic data in children are limited but increasing rapidly. In critical care, children's metabolism of psychotropic drugs may be increased because of the stress response or decreased because of injury or illness. Metabolism also is affected by medical and surgical treatments, such as anesthesia, fluid and electrolyte replacement, pressors, and antibiotics. The pharmacokinetics of a given drug for a specific patient affect dosage selection, paradoxic responses, potential side effects, and ability to produce desired effect [24]. One main factor in dosing associated with growth and development is children's age. There is a greater need, especially near puberty, for higher weight–adjusted doses of medications than in adults because of increased rates of hepatic and renal metabolism and excretion.

Pharmacokinetics play a role in decisions of which drug to select and how much and how often to administer them. Unavailablity of the oral route in some children who are critically ill narrows the selection of analgesic, anxiolytic, antidepressant, and antipsychotic drugs and expands the use of others, such as the sedative, midazolam [25]. Drugs with short half-lives, such as midazolam or sertraline, rather than diazepam or fluoxetine, tend to be preferred to minimize the duration of any adverse effects and allow rapid switching to another drug (Table 1) [26–63].

Elimination half-life

The time required for the plasma concentration of a given drug to be reduced by one half is called the elimination half-life. The two main processes that affect elimination half-lives are renal excretion and hepatic metabolism. Drugs are described as following zero-order kinetics when a fixed amount of drug is eliminated per increment of time. Alcohol consumed in excessive quantities, such that the eliminating mechanisms become saturated, follows

Table 1
Half-lives of the major metabolites of selected psychopharmacologic agents encountered in pediatric critical care

Antidepressants	Antipsychotics	Benzodiazepines	Mood stabilizers	ADHD treatment/other
Amitriptyline Adult: 36.1 h [26]	Aripiprazole Adult: 47–68 h [27]	Alprazolam Adult: 9–16 h [28]	Carbamazepine Pediatric: 32 h on initiation, 3 h after long-term use [29]	Atomoxetine Pediatric: 3.28 h (at steady state), 3.12 h (after one-time dose) [30]
Bupropion SR Pediatric: bupropion—12.1 h, threohydrobupropion—26.3 h [31]	Chlorpromazine Pediatric: 7.74 ± 0.65 h [32]	Clonazepam Adult: 20–80 h [33]	Gabapentin Pediatric: 5.5 ± 0.8 h [34]	Clonidine Pediatric: 8–12 h [35]
Citalopram Adult: 33 h [36]	Clozapine Adult: 10.5 h for clozapine, 19.2 h for norclozapine, and 8.6 h for the N-oxide metabolite [37]	Diazepam Pediatric: 15–21 h [38]	Lamotrigine Pediatric: 32 h [39]	Dextroamphetamine Pediatric: 6.8 ± 0.5 h [40]
Fluoxetine [41][a] Adult: 3.9 days (fluoxetine) 15 days (norfluoxetine) [42]	Haloperidol Pediatric: 18.6 ± 12.2 [43]	Lorazepam Pediatric: 10.5 ± 2.9 h [44]	Lithium Pediatric: 18 h [45]	Diphenhydramine Pediatric: 5.4 ± 1.8 h [46]
Imipramine Adult: 22.8 ±6.4 h [47]	Olanzapine Pediatric: 37.2 ± 5.1 h [48]	Midazolam Pediatric: 0.8–1.8 h [49]	Oxcarbazepine (monohydroxy derivative) Adult: 8–10 h [50]	Methylphenidate Pediatric: 2.5–3.4 h [51]
Mirtazapine Adult: 20–40 h [52]	Quetiapine Adult: 7 h [53]	Oxazepam Adult: 5–15 h [54]	Topiramate Adult: 19–25 h [55]	Pemoline (off-market) Pediatric: 7.05 ± 1.99 h [56]

Nortriptyline
Pediatric: 20.8 ± 7.2 h [57]

Paroxetine
Child data: 11.1 h ± 5.2 h [59]

Sertraline
Pediatric: 50 mg po qd steady state 15.3 ± 3.5 h and 100–150 mg po qd steady state 20.4 ± 3.4 h [62]

Venlafaxine
Adult: 5 h and 11 h for O-desmethylvenlafaxine [63]

Risperidone
Pediatric: 3 h in quick metabolizers 17 h in poor metabolizers [58]

Ziprasidone
Adult: Oral administration, 6–7 h
IM administration 2–5 h [60,61]

Valproic acid
Pediatric: 5 h on initiation 14 h after long-term use [28]

Pediatric data refer to studies in subjects ages 0 to 18.
Although amitryptiline is included, this should not be regarded as endorsement of its use in children who are critically ill.
a Data suggest that the half-life is similar for children and adolescents.

zero-order kinetics. In contrast, most psychotropics follow first-order kinetics, in which the amount of drug cleared per unit of time is proportional to the amount of drug in the circulation. Meanwhile, plasma steady-state concentration refers to an equilibrium that is achieved when the amount of drug coming into the bloodstream is equal to the amount of drug eliminated from the bloodstream. It requires 4.5 half-lives to achieve steady-state concentration and, once a drug is stopped abruptly, 4.5 half-lives to allow for near complete elimination of a drug. The half-life of a drug (that follows the first-order kinetics) given in a one-time dose that never reaches plasma steady-state concentration is different from the elimination half-life for a drug at steady-state concentration. The elimination half-life of various medications plays an important role in the management of patients after toxic ingestions and in other aspects of pediatric critical care. Table 1 summarizes child, adolescent, and adult data on drug elimination half-lives. Elimination half-lives may differ from the timing of pharmacodynamic effects; that is, the arrival of a drug at a steady state does not necessarily reflect its pharmacodynamic effectiveness. For example, although selective serotonin reuptake inhibitors (SSRIs) may reach steady-state concentration in a matter of days, their clinical antidepressant effects may not take place for weeks.

Pharmacokinetic phases

Pharmacokinetics can be divided into four functional phases: absorption, distribution, metabolism, and excretion.

Absorption. Psychotropics are able to reach their targets only if they enter the systemic circulation. All drugs administered intravenously (IV) reach the systemic circulation. Meanwhile, oral medications must be absorbed in the stomach or the small intestine, where they enter the portal circulation and then the systemic circulation. Drugs that slow intestinal motility, such as tricyclic antidepressants (TCAs), can alter absorption of other drugs, as they may be in contact with intestinal mucosa for a longer time. Binding agents, such as charcoal and cholestyramine, decrease absorption of other medications. Other factors involved in absorption include gastric pH, the action of enzymes within the gastrointestinal tract, and the properties of the drug (tablet, capsule, or liquid). First-pass metabolism also plays a significant role in the absorption process. This term refers to the process by which drugs absorbed through the gastrointestinal tract are carried first to the liver via the portal circulation. There they undergo substantial metabolism, thereby reducing the amount of drug that reaches the systemic circulation. Thus, medications that are not metabolized hepatically, such as lorazepam, as opposed to diazepam, are preferable in patients who have hepatic failure and portosystemic shunting. First-pass metabolism can be avoided completely by giving medication through IV or intramuscular routes. Rectal administration, which involves mesenteric and hemorrhoidal absorption, results in decreased first-pass metabolism.

Distribution. Once absorbed, drugs distribute throughout the body into various IV and extravascular spaces. How much drug is available at its target is determined by total body water and lipid stores, regional blood flow, binding of drugs to plasma proteins, permeability of cell membranes, acid-base balance, and physiochemical properties of the drug. Once a drug is absorbed and undergoes first-pass metabolism, generally it is circulated in two forms, protein-bound and unbound. Unbound, or free, drug is available to cross cell membranes. The equilibrium of unbound and bound drugs can be disturbed by an increased amount of circulating protein (such as in febrile illness) or by introducing a drug that competes for protein-binding sites. As these physiologic variables change more rapidly and unpredictably in children who are critically ill, unexpected drug effects are common, and close monitoring for efficacy and toxicity is crucial.

Metabolism refers to the biotransformation of drugs to different forms. Most drugs are lipid soluble, a feature necessary for them to be absorbed, distributed, and available at receptor sites, particularly in the central nervous system (CNS). These drugs need to be made more hydrophilic to be excreted. Although some drugs are excreted mostly (eg, topiramate) or completely (eg, lithium) in an unmetabolized form, most undergo biotransformation in the liver.

Phase I reactions involve oxidation, reduction, or hydrolysis and are mediated by the cytochrome P450 (CYP450) enzymes located in hepatocyte endoplasmic reticula. A drug that has undergone phase I metabolism is called a metabolite and may be more or less efficacious or toxic than the parent compound. Clinically relevant examples include diazepam, which has several active metabolites with long elimination half-lives, limiting the appropriateness of this benzodiazepine in critical care practice, and imipramine, whose demethylated metabolite, desipramine, may account for the cardiotoxicity of this tricyclic agent.

Drugs that are metabolized by a given CYP450 enzyme are substrates. Drugs that increase the activity of a CYP450 enzyme are inducers and those that reduce CYP450 activity are inhibitors. Understanding the genetics of the CYP450 system and the CYP450 relationship between drugs can help clinicians avoid toxicities or even enhance treatment. For example, patients who are treated with haloperidol (which is metabolized by the CYP1A2 enzyme) and develop a urinary tract infection for which ciprofloxacin (an inhibitor of CYP1A2) is prescribed should be monitored for increased haloperidol side effects, because it is not metabolized as quickly. Table 2 outlines some of the genetic polymorphisms and interactions of the CYP450 system.

Phase II metabolism involves the conjugation of compounds with glucuronic acid, sulfate, or glycine, thus making them excreted more readily in the urine. Clinically relevant drug interactions at the level of phase II reactions also occur. For example, lamotrigine is metabolized solely by glucuronidation, a process inhibited by valproate. Hence, coadministration of lamotrigine and valproate can increase lamotrigine levels significantly and

Table 2
Selected psychotropic, analgesic, and antibiotic/antifungal cytochrome P450 interactions and genetic variabilities often encountered in pediatric critical care

1A2	2B6	2C9, 2C19	2D6	2E1	3A4,5,7
Substrates	*Substrates*	*Substrates*	*Substrates*	*Substrates*	*Substrates*
Acetaminophen	Bupoprion	Barbiturates	Aripiprazole	General anesthetics	Alfentanil
Caffeine	Methadone	Diazepam	Atomoxetine	Acetaminophen	Alprazolam
Clozapine		Modafinil	β-blockers	Ethanol	Aripiprazole
Haloperidol		NSAIDs	Codeine		Buspirone
Mirtazapine		Phenytoin	Dextromethorphan		Carbamazepine
Naproxen		Propanolol	Haloperidol		Clozapine
Olanzapine		Tertiary TCAs	Hydroxycodone		Cyclosporine
Tertiary TCAs		(including	Lidocaine		Diazepam
(including amitriptyline,		amitriptyline,	Odansetron		Fentanyl
clomipramine, imipramine)		clomipramine,	Phenothiazines		Methadone
theophylline		imipramine)	(including		Midazolam
		THC	thioridazine,		Pimozide
			perphenazine)		Prednisone
			Risperidone,		Progesterone
			SSRIs		Quetiapine
			TCAs		Tacrolimus
			Tramadol		Testosterone
			Trazadone		Tertiary tcas
			Venlafaxine		Triazolam
					Zaleplon
					Ziprasidone
					Zolpidem

Inducers Charbroiled meats Cigarettes	*Inducers*	*Inducers* Rifampin	*Inducers* Dexamethasone Rifampin	*Inducers* Ethanol Isoniazid	*Inducers* Carbamazepine Glucocorticoids Modafinil Oxcarbazepine Phenobarbitol Phenytoin Rifampin St. John's wort
Inhibitors Cimetidine Fluoroquinolones (ciprofloxacin levofloxacin) Fluvoxamine Grapefruit juice	*Inhibitors* Phenobarbitol Rifampin	*Inhibitors* Fluoxetine Fluvoxamine Ketoconazole Modafinil Oxcarbezepine Sertraline	*Inhibitors* Antimalarials Bupropion Cimetideine Duloxetine Fluoxetine Methadone Metoclopramide Paroxetine Phenothiazines Sertraline TCAs	*Inhibitors* Disulfiram	*Inhibitors* Antifungals Cimetidine Clarithromycin Erythromycin Fluvoxamine Fluoxetine (norfluoxetine) Grapefruit juice Nefazadone Troleandomycin
	Whites: 3%–4% are poor metabolizers	Whites: 1%–3% are poor metabolizers of 2C19 substrates 3%–5% are poor metabolizers of 2C19 substrates, Asians: 15%–20% are poor metabolizers of 2C19 substrates	Whites: 7%–10% are poor metabolizers of 2D6 substrates		

Adapted from Flockhart D. Drug-interactions.com 14 June 2005. Available at: http://medicine.iupui.edu/flockhart/clinlist.htm. Accessed October 29, 2005; Alpert JE, Fava M, Rosenbaum JF. Psychopharmacologic issues in the medical setting. In: Stern TA, Fricchione GL, Cassem NH, et al, editors. Massachusetts General Hospital handbook of general hospital psychiatry. 5th edition. St. Louis: Mosby; 2004. p. 641–70.

place patients at greater risk for developing lamotrigine-related Stevens-Johnson syndrome [64].

Excretion. Renal excretion is responsible for ridding the body of drugs or their metabolites. Factors that effect renal function, specifically glomerular filtration, tubular reabsorption, and tubular secretion, can alter excretion. Agents that are excreted as active metabolites or that are nonmetabolized, such as lithium [65] or gabapentin, need to be dose adjusted for patients who have impaired renal function.

Drug-drug interactions

The two types of clinically significant drug-drug interactions are pharmacokinetic and pharmacodynamic interactions [66]. Pharmacodynamic interactions are those that occur when two or more drugs act on a particular receptor or target, sometimes producing benefits but other times producing bothersome or even lethal side effects. Pharmacokinetic interactions refer to those situations in which a drug alters the metabolism of another drug. An example of a pharmacodynamic interaction is serotonin syndrome (SS), in which an excess of serotonin is available in the CNS, resulting in mental status changes, autonomic disturbance, and neuromuscular abnormalities (see discussion later of toxicity and side effects) [67]. This may occur when the antibiotic, linezolid, a weak monoamine oxidase inhibitor (MAOI), is combined with a SSRI, resulting in excess synaptic serotonin [68,69]. The combination of MAOIs (including linezolid and procarbazine and, rarely in pediatric critical care, other MAOIs) and SSRIs should be avoided. No MAOIs should be used with SSRIs. Moreover, SS can result from a pharmacokinetic interaction. For example, CYP450 2D6–inhibiting agent fluoxetine used in combination with the CYP450 2D6 substrate 3,4-methylenedioxymethamphetamine (MDMA or "ecstasy") may result in increased levels of MDMA, producing SS [70]. Some common pharmacokinetic and pharmacodynamic interactions with antipsychotics and antidepressants are listed in Tables 3 and 4, respectively. Prevention of adverse drug-drug interactions may include pharmacogenomic research, physician education, avoidance of multidrug regimens, and use of physician order entry and personal digital assistants to detect and avoid potential adverse drug interactions [67].

Classes of psychotropic drugs in pediatric critical care

Anxiolytics and sedatives

Anxiety and stress are common in critical care patients. Protocols have been developed during the past 20 years to reduce or eliminate pain and anxiety in children who are critically ill. These have reduced the adverse psychologic sequelae (traumatic stress and depression) and adverse physical sequelae from untreated pain and anxiety. Different stages in the care of

Table 3
Potential interactions with antipsychotic medications

Drug	Potential interaction
Antacids (aluminum-magnesium containing), fruit juice	Interference with absorption of antipsychotic agents
Carbamazepine	Decreased antipsychotic drug plasma levels; additive risk of myelosuppression with clozapine
Cigarettes	Decreased antipsychotic drug plasma levels; reduced extrapyramidal symptoms
Rifampin	Decreased antipsychotic drug plasma levels
TCAs	Increased TCA and antipsychotic drug plasma levels; hypotension, depression of cardiac condution (with low-potency antipsychotics)
SSRIs	Increased SSRI and antipsychotic plasma levels.
Bupropion, duloxetine	Increased antipsychotic drug plasma levels.
Fluvoxamine,	Increased antipsychotic drug plasma levels
β-blockers	Increased antipsychotic drug plasma levels; reduced akathisia
Anticholinergic drugs	Additive anticholinergic toxicity
Antihypertensives, vasodilators	Hypotension (with low-potency antipsychotics and risperidone)
Guanethidine, clonidine	Blockade of antihypertensive effect
Epinephrine	Hypotension (with low-potency antipsychotics)
Class I antiarrhythmics	Depression of cardiac conduction; ventricular arrhythmias (with low-potency antipsychotics, ziprasidone)
Calcium channel blockers	Depression of cardiac conduction; ventricular arrhythmias (with pimozide)
Lithium	Idiosyncratic neurotoxicity; possibly increased risk of NMS

From Alpert JE, Fava M, Rosenbaum JF. Psychopharmacologic issues in the medical setting. In: Stern TA, Fricchione GL, Cassem NH, et al, editors. Massachusetts General hospital handbook of general hospital psychiatry. 5th edition. St. Louis: Mosby; 2004. p. 641–70.

patients require different dosing. A protocol was designed to fit the four clinical states and best multidisciplinary pharmacologic practices in the critically ill pediatric burn patient [71]. The four clinical states are (1) mechanically ventilated acute, (2) nonmechanically ventilated acute, (3) chronic acute, and (4) reconstructive surgery. For each clinical state, five subguidelines were developed: (1) background pain, (2) background anxiety, (3) procedural pain, (4) procedural anxiety, and (5) methods of transition from one clinical state to the next [71]. The published protocol was subjected to clinical trials and ongoing monitoring and modified in response to updating of best practices parameters. The dosing of agents, such as midazolam and lorazepam, progresses from IV to oral administration, with the occasional addition of longer-acting benzodiazepines, such as diazepam and clonazepam, when appropriate. Midazolam and lorazepam are metabolized adequately and

Table 4
Potential interactions with selective serotonin reuptake inhibitors and newer antidepressants

Drug	Potential interaction
MAOIs	Serotonin syndrome
Linezolid	Serotonin syndrome
Procarbazine (weak MAOIs)	
Secondary amine TCAs	Increased TCA levels when coadministered with fluoxetine, paroxetine, sertraline,
Tertiary amine TCAs	Increased TCA levels when coadministered with fluvoxamine, paroxetine, sertraline, bupropion, duloxetine
Antipsychotics (typical) and risperidone, aripiprazole	Increased antipsychotic levels with fluoxetine, sertraline, paroxetine, bupropion, duloxetine
Thioridazine	Arrhythmia risk with CYP450 2D6 inhibitory antidepressants
Pimozide	Arrhythmia risk with CYP450 3A4 inhibitory antidepressants
Clozapine and olanzapine	Increased antipsychotic levels with fluvoxamine
Diazepam	Increased benzodiazepine levels with fluoxetine, fluvoxamine, sertraline
Triazalobenzodiazepines (midazolam, alprazolam, triazolam)	Increased fluoxamine, nefazadone, sertraline (diazepam)
Carbamazepine	Increased carbamazepine levels with fluoxetine, fluvoxamine, nefazadone
Theophylline	Increased theophylline levels with fluvoxamine
Type 1C antiarrhythmics	Increased antiarrhtymic levels with fluoxetine, paroxetine, sertraline, bupropion, duloxetine
β-Blockers	Increased β-blocker levels with fluoxetine, paroxetine, sertraline, bupropion, duloxetine
Calcium channel blockers	Increased levels with fluoxetine, fluvoxamine, nefazadone

Adapted from Alpert JE, Fava M, Rosenbaum JF. Psychopharmacologic issues in the medical setting. In: Stern TA, Fricchione GL, Cassem NH, et al, editors. Massachusetts General Hospital handbook of general hospital psychiatry. 5th edition. St. Louis: Mosby; 2004. p. 641–70; with permission.

safely for acute IV administration [72]. Midazolam infusions tend to be the mainstay of sedation therapy in pediatric patients who are critically ill because of its brief duration of action, ease of dosage adjustment, and ready reversibility. Although more expensive, midazolam is not associated with lactic acidosis believed to result from the accumulation of propylene glycol, a problem seen occasionally with lorazepam infusions. Precautions to prevent respiratory arrest and withdrawal are essential, and weight-based therapy with strict protocols should be used. Other sedatives that provide anxiolysis and may be used as second- and third-line agents include chloral hydrate and pentobarbital.

There are other critical care medications that can be used in the pediatric ICU (PICU) as second- and third-line agents, including ketamine, chloral hydrate, haloperidol, propofol, and pentobarbital (Table 5). These

Table 5
Anxiolytics and sedatives used in pediatric intensive care patients who are acutely ill

Drug	Drug class	Initial dose	Concerning side effects
Lorazepam	Benzodiazepine	0.01–0.05 mg/kg/h IV	Lactic acidosis
Midazolam	Benzodiazepine	0.02–0.04 mg/kg/h IV	Rapid tachyphylaxis
Ketamine	Anesthetic	0.5–3 mg/kg/h IV or 0.5–2 mg/kg/dose IV Bolus PRN	Hallucinations
Haloperidol	Antipsychotic	0.2–0.5 mg/kg/dose IV q6h	Ventricular arrhythmias, extrapyramidal side effects
Chloral hydrate	Sedative/hypnotic	25–50 mg/kg/dose PO/PNGT/PR q8h	Hallucinations, nightmares, ventricular arrhythmias
Dexmedetomidine	α2 adrenergic agonist	0.3–2.5 µg/kg/h IV	Bradycardia and hypotension
Propofol	Anesthetic	0.5–3 mg/kg/h IV for pre-extubation sedation (<12 h)	Prolonged continuous infusions not recommended in children <16 y due to metabolic acidosis, cardiovascular collapse, and death

medications tend to have larger side-effect profiles requiring more intense monitoring and continuous assessment for toxicity.

A large literature, mainly in perioperative and emergency care [73], supports the use of ketamine to reduce procedural pain and anxiety, with subsequent amnesia. Because ketamine is one of the most well known psychotomimetic drugs [74] whose long-term neurodevelopmental effects are unknown, however, caution is advised.

Later in an acute patient's clinical course when specific diagnoses can be made, such as PTSD, generalized anxiety disorder (GAD), panic disorder, or phobia, psychopharmacologic treatment proceeds similarly to the outpatient setting. Combination cognitive behavior therapy (CBT) and benzodiazepines, with or without SSRIs, are common treatments.

Antipsychotics

The uses of antipsychotics in critical care, including sedation, delirium, and palliative care, is described here (Table 6) [75]. The number of antipsychotics available has increased dramatically, as has the promotion of different agents by pharmaceutical companies. Haloperidol is the typical antipsychotic used most widely. It is the least expensive and may be administered IV. Its use carries the risk, however, of cardiovascular and other adverse effects. Chlorpromazine also has a place, particularly when its hypotensive side effect is desirable.

Atypical antipsychotics are in wide use, but none can be administered IV, although their effects may occur within 2 hours. These include olanzapine,

Table 6
Selected: neuroleptics used in pediatric critical care

Drug	Formulation	Initiating dose (not approved for children under 18 y)	Concerning side effects and toxic effects[a]
Aripiprazole	Tablet	2.5 mg–5 mg PO QD	• Occasional agitation, anxiety + Hypotension 0 Hyperprolactinemia 0 Glucose intolerance 0 Weight gain + Risk of EPS + Risk of NMS
Haloperidol	Tablet, IM injection, IV	0.2–0.5 mg IV TID for 1–2 days	• QTc prolongation + Hypotension ++ Hyperprolactinemia + Glucose intolerance 0 Weight gain +++ Risk for EPS +++ Risk for NMS
Olanzapine	Tablet, oral disintegrating tablet, IM injection	2.5 mg PO BID	• Anticholingergic effects ++ Hypotension + Hyperprolactinemia ++ Glucose intolerance +++ Weight gain + Risk of EPS + Risk of NMS
Quetiapine	Tablet	25 mg PO BID	• Sedation ++ Hypotension 0 Hyperprolactinemia + Glucose intolerance ++ Weight gain 0 Risk of EPS + Risk of NMS
Risperidone	Tablet, solution, IM injection	0.25 mg PO QD	• Hepatotoxicity +++ Hypotension ++ Hyperprolactinemia + Glucose intolerance ++ Weight gain ++ Risk of EPS + Risk of NMS
Ziprasidone	Tablet, IM injection	20 mg PO/IM QD	• QTc prolongation + Hypotension + Hyperprolactinemia + Glucose intolerance 0 Weight gain + Risk of EPS + Risk of NMS

The dose guidelines provided are for general guidance and not intended to be definitive. Medication selection and dosing should be individualized and accompanied by appropriate clinical and laboratory monitoring.

Abbreviations: EPS, extrapyramidal side effects; NMS, neuroceptic malignant syndrome.

[a] •, Indicates slightly more unique side effect; +++, high risk; ++, moderate; +, low; 0, little or neglible [75].

risperidone, ziprasidone, quetiapine, and aripiperazole, among others. All of these medications are available as oral preparations. Olanzapine, risperidone, and ziprasidone also are formulated for intramuscular administration. They require close EKG monitoring [76]. Evidence-based medicine is lacking to guide the use of atypical antipsychotics in children who are critically ill. Many pediatric critical care settings use atypical antipsychotics because of the improved side-effect profiles compared with typical or conventional antipsychotics, particularly as they carry less risk for neuroleptic-related movement disorders.

Antidepressants

SSRIs have replaced TCAs as preferred agents for the treatment of depression, PTSD, obsessive-compulsive disorder (OCD), and GAD in children because of their benign side-effect profile and their comparative safety in the event of overdose compared with TCAs (Table 7) [77]. For depression, fluoxetine has to date seemed preferable to the other agents [78], based on the FDA approval of only fluoxetine for pediatric depression. Citalopram, sertraline, and other SSRIs, however, are in wide use in child psychiatry. Sertraline is found safe and effective in some studies for GAD [79], OCD, and depression [80,81]. Paroxetine, in December 2005, was given an FDA alert because of preliminary results of two studies indicating human fetal risk for congenital malformations, in particular cardiovascular malformations, and initiation of its use was discouraged for women in their first trimester of pregnancy or those who plan to become pregnant [82]. It was advised that discontinuing paroxetine therapy or switching to another antidepressant be considered for these patients. This drug has the advantage of sedative properties but because of its short half-life has a discontinuation syndrome, often with increased anxiety. Other antidepressants that sometimes are used but for which there is no evidence base include venlafaxine, buproprion, and mirtazepine.

Table 7
Selected antidepressants used in pediatric critical care

Drug	Formulation	Initiating dose	Side effects
Fluoxetine	Tablet, oral disintegrating tablet	5–20 mg PO daily	Irritability Akathisia Insomnia
Sertraline	Tablet, solution, IM injection	12.5–25 mg PO daily	Appetite decrease (acute use) or increase (chronic) Gastrointestinal symptoms
Citalopram	Tablet, oral solution	10–20 mg PO daily	Platelet dysfunction Sexual side effects
Escitalopram	Tablet, oral solution	2.5–5 mg PO daily	Suicidality*

The doses and side-effect profiles provided in this paper are general guidelines and are not intended to be definitive. Medication selection and dosing should be individualized and accompanied by appropriate clinical and laboratory monitoring.
* FDA box warning applies to all antidepressants in children and adolescents.

Cardiovascular risks, such as hypotension and cardiac arrythmias, associated with TCAs have limited their use in children who are medically ill, despite the safety and efficacy suggested in a pilot study of PTSD in burn patients [83]. TCAs also have value in potentiating analgesia and treating neuropathic pain. Unlike the SSRI's, TCAs are not shown effective in treating pediatric depression.

In the fall of 2004, the FDA directed pharmaceutical manufacturers to add a black box warning to the patient package inserts of all antidepressant medications to describe the risk for suicidality and emphasize the need for close monitoring of patients started on these medications [7]. This concern stems from data suggesting an increased risk for worsening depression and suicidal ideation in a small subset of children who have major depressive disorder [84]. The FDA also determined that a Patient Medication Guide (MedGuide) must be given to patients receiving any new antidepressant medication [7]. As noted, FDA approval for the treatment of pediatric major depressive disorder is limited to fluoxetine; however, clinical trials also support the safety and efficacy of sertaline in pediatric patients, which may be preferable to fluoxetine in pediatric critical care because of its shorter half-life and fewer CYP450 drug-drug interactions.

Stimulants

Psychostimulants are the psychoactive drugs prescribed most frequently and may be the safest class prescribed to children. Clinical trials data are nonexistent in pediatric critical care. Preliminary pediatric data and controlled adult studies confirm the usefulness of psychostimulants as opiate adjuvants in treating mood disorders in children who are critically ill and to reduce somnolence in the palliative care setting. When used to treat mood disorders, stimulants have the advantage of rapid onset of action, unlike SSRIs. Although appropriate caution about the cardiovascular effects of stimulants is required, most children who are not ventilated can receive stimulants safely when indicated. Stimulants also can be used to treat children who have ADHD if their symptoms are compromising their medical care. Stimulants also play a role in the care of children who are terminally ill (see discussion later of palliative care). Typically, methylphenidate is used because of its rapid onset and short half-life. Usually, other stimulant medications, such as the longer-acting forms, are used only if children have been taking them before their hospital admission.

Mood stabilizers and anticonvulsants

The range of mood stabilizers now in use with children is far greater than when carbamazepine first was introduced for bipolar disorder. As a result, children who have mood disorders or aggression [85] may be admitted already receiving a range of medications, known originally for their anticonvulsant properties but now used widely for mood stabilization. Occasionally, one of these agents is initiated to treat newly diagnosed patients who have bipolar disorder in critical care. These drugs include carbamazepine, valproic acid, lithium carbonate and gabapentin, although the latter is only a weak mood stabilizer. Carbamazepine and gabapentin also are helpful in treating neuropathic pain and, thus, may address two target symptoms at once.

α_2-Adrenergic agonists

The two α_2-adrenergic agonists available readily to treat children who are critically ill are clonidine and a new agent more potent than clonidine, dexmedetomidine [86,87]. Their uses are limited primarily to enhancing sedation and facilitating tapering of analgesics or to lessen withdrawal symptoms, including anxiety.

Toxicity and side effects

The most serious toxicities associated with psychotropic drugs in children are increased suicidality, cardiovascular arrythmias, extreme weight gain, seizures, neuroleptic malignant syndrome (NMS) [88], toxic epidermal necrolysis or Stevens-Johnson Syndrome, delirium (eg, lithium-induced), hepatotoxicity [89,90], pancreatitis [91], tardive dyskinesia, and psychosis. A potential cause of death is torsades de pointes, the ventricular tachyarrthythmia with syncope, cardiac arrest, or sudden death [92,93]. In addressing cardiovascular risk, Lebellarte and coworkers [94] recommend a cautious threshold of corrected QT prolongation (QTc) during treatment: increased QTc duration greater than or equal to 450 msec or greater than or equal to 10% increase in QTc duration, together with more detailed recommendations for specific QTc findings. The American Heart Association recommends EKG monitoring of the QTc duration for children treated with desipramine, imipramine, haloperidol, pimozide, thioridazine, and many other phenothiazines. Atypical antipsychotics, including olanzapine, risperidone, and ziprasidone, also require monitoring of the QTc duration.

Seratonin syndrome (SS) is a serious, iatrogenic, potentially life-threatening adverse drug reaction resulting from a serotonergic drug. Many different drugs, including SSRIs and meperidine, with serotonergic effects may cause SS. The symptoms include mental status changes, agitation, restlessness, myoclonus, hyperreflexia, diaphoresis, tremor, shivering, incoordination, autonomic disturbance, hyperthermia, and musclear rigidity (see Boyer and Shannon's decision tree [67]). This may lead to shock. SS is not rare, and symptoms range from mild to severe. It has a rapid onset after initiation of drug, dose change, or overdose. One early, tragic, and dramatic case caused by coadministration of meperidine and phenelzine was the death in the 1980s of an 18-year-old patient, Libby Zion, in New York City [95]. A survey in 2002 reported 93 deaths from SS, and it was reported to occur in 14% to 16% of people who overdosed on SSRIs [96]. The differential diagnosis includes anticholinergic poisoning, malignant hyperthermia, and NMS. A single dose of fluvoxamine caused SS in an 11-year-old boy [97], and cases are reported in infants. Only clinical recommendations based on few patients are available to date, no prospective studies. Treatment should be instituted in consultation with a clinical pharmacology service, toxicologist, or poison control center. Treatment includes removal of the causative agents, provision of supportive care, control of agitation probably with benzodiazepines, therapy with $5HT_{2A}$ antagonists (such as cyproheptadine), control of autonomic instability, and control of hyperthermia. For severe cases, further treatments often are required [67].

The most common side effects of the psychotropic medications include nausea, gastrointestinal disturbance, insomnia, rash, dystonias, and agitation. These effects occasionally are a reason for discontinuation or switching medications. Monitoring methods for adverse events are improving steadily and are reviewed by Greenhill and colleagues [98].

In assessing risks and benefits when psychotropic drug administration is considered for children who are critically ill, clinicians must weigh the risks for treatment and the risks for nontreatment. Delirium in a critical care setting, for example, bears significant risk for morbidity and mortality, even when treatable medical causes, such as infection, structural CNS, or metabolic disturbance, are addressed. Clinicians face a best practices decision when using an increasingly common intervention, such as IV haloperidol for delirium, even when the evidence base is suboptimal. Such clinical challenges underscore the important role of consulting child psychiatrists in pediatric critical care.

Child psychiatry consultation in the pediatric critical care setting

Reason for requesting consultation

In a pediatric critical care unit, child psychiatrists are consulted to address and evaluate several different issues, including assessment of primary psychiatric disorders, mental status and behavioral changes, psychiatric factors affecting a medical illness, behavior issues compromising optimal medical care, child abuse assessments, and supportive interventions for children who have acute and life-threatening illnesses and their families and for assisting with palliative care at end of life.

Assessment

When child psychiatrists are called to evaluate children in a critical care setting, a physician needs to consider whether or not the injury, disease, or treatment has led to the symptoms in question and whether or not patients have an underlying psychiatric disorder contributing to the presentation [99,100]. It is essential to perform a thorough psychiatric assessment before making recommendations on the use of medications in children who are acutely medically ill. When indicated, this should include laboratory tests, radiographic studies, psychologic testing, or neurologic or other evaluation. It is useful to explain that generally a minimum of 1 hour is required to obtain history from caretakers and a second hour is required to interview a child and present the results of the evaluation to parents or legal guardians. The interviews must be in a language comprehensible to parents and children (when old enough), with an interpreter if needed. Thorough evaluations include clarifying what led to a consultation request and to whom consultants should report findings and recommendations; a review of medical records, assuring that parent or guardian permission for psychiatric consultation is granted; interviewing children and performing a mental status examination; and seeking collateral information as warranted. It is important to contact the consulting physician or team on the phone or in person to discuss the assessment. It then is essential to provide legible documentation of the assessment, organized charting of medication dosages, clarification of desired response over time, laboratory studies requested, and plan for follow-up.

A formulation of children's psychiatric disorders can be made based on a *Diagnostic and Statistical Manual of Mental Disorders, Fourth Edition Text Revision (DSM-IV-TR)* multiaxial differential diagnosis [101]. Standard symptom rating scales, the Mini–Mental State Examination (which was found useful in children ages 4 to 15 [102,103]), and research diagnostic instruments are helpful additions in quantifying target symptoms and monitoring symptom response to pharmacologic treatment. For children who are medically ill, the decision of whether or not to use psychotropic medications to treat psychiatric symptoms is based on severity, duration, type, and overall patient clinical status. Prescription of psychotropic drugs may be indicated based on patient critical status; developmental and psychodynamic factors; assessment of the psychiatric, medical, and social history, including prior psychiatric, pediatric, legal, and school records; mental status; and physical and laboratory examinations. The principles of evidenced-based psychopharmacologic practice guide the selection, administration, and monitoring of medications.

Developmental considerations

When approaching children in a critical care setting, it is important to consider the age of the children being evaluated. How children experience and cope with medical illness is different based on age and stage of development. Frequently, children regress developmentally when ill. Reassuring parents and staff about this can relieve concerns. Typically, children regain these milestones when they are well.

Infants and toddlers (0–2.5 years old)

Infants and toddlers experience the world largely in the moment. Although the gravity of their illness, length of stay, or the prospect of getting better may weigh heavily on the minds of parents and staff, these do not concern infants and toddlers. They see the world only in terms of the pain or pleasure of the moment and seek out attachment from caregivers on whom they are fully dependent. This attachment can be disrupted by the procedures, monitoring, and general noise of a critical care unit or pediatric ward. As much as possible, these interruptions should be minimized so that attachment can flourish. Most pediatric teams encourage parents to sleep near their infants or toddlers and to be present and offer soothing touches or sounds during procedures, and they allow for quiet times where parent-child closeness can take place without interruption. Parental traumatic stress and depression are prominent problems that arise when young children are hospitalized, and parental concerns or impairment may be a secondary focus for the consultant.

Preschoolers (2.5–6 years old)

Preschool-aged children are egocentric, have magical thinking, and are preoccupied with body integrity. Egocentricity refers to children's belief that the world revolves around them and that others see the world from their perspective alone. Magical thinking refers to the interweaving of reality and fantasy such that medical events have magical causes.

Egocentricity and magical thinking combine to produce notions of guilt and punishment in hospitalized preschoolers. They may see injuries and medical illnesses as punishment for bad deeds and see treatments, such as blood draws, lumbar punctures, and fluid restriction, as penalties for not thinking the right thoughts in the hospital. Consultants should provide appropriate reassurance to children that they did not do anything wrong to deserve injury, medical illness, or treatment. Preschoolers also focus on maintaining body integrity, believing that blood, stool, pus, or essential "parts" can leak out of holes. For example, most 5 year olds are preoccupied with boo-boos, love adhesive bandages, and are frightened by surgical procedures, needle sticks, and catheters. Being aware of these and offering alternative and consistent explanations for medical phenomena is helpful. Finally, children 6 and under often want to be interviewed in the presence of a parent. It is helpful to work together with parents when asking children why they were injured or became ill and why they are getting treatment and when outlining with parents the principles of egocentricity, magical thinking, and body integrity.

School-aged children (7–12 years old)

At this age, children are able to understand their medical illness better and are more curious about the world outside themselves. Latency-age children are rules based in their life approach. They want to gain mastery over their illness and the hospital. Promoting this mastery is key to alleviating anxiety and dysphoria in hospitalized children. Children at this age often allow themselves to be interviewed alone, but it is important to ask.

Adolescents

Adolescents have the capacity to understand illness, its causes and treatments, and the ramifications disease has on their lives. Although this cognitive development offers the advantage of making a hospital experience meaningful, it allows the gravity of illness to take greater hold, including its impact on peer relationships. Adolescence is a time of puberty, rapid growth, and physical maturation, when children are worried about fitting in with peers; are concerned with romantic relationships and competence in athletic, academic, and artistic pursuits; and are trying out independence. From the initial meeting, identifying and providing verbal recognition of their areas of competence and skill provide a solid basis for later interventions.

Premorbid functioning

Premorbid functioning is a helpful predictor for how children fare during an acute medical crisis. A biopsychosocial understanding of children's functioning before admission is essential: (1) psychologic: how children coped with past insults, such as divorce or other medical problems, offers perspective on how they will cope with the stress of their medical illness; (2) social: it is important to know which other factors may be contributing to the stress children and their families experience in the hospital—for example, a patient recently may have experienced the loss of a grandparent or pet, or a parent may be unemployed; and (3) biologic: it is important to understand how children's illness or medical treatments affect their mental health—Is the child receiving steroids and, therefore, more likely to experience mood lability and irritability? Is the child being weaned from pain or sedating medications and possibly experiencing withdrawal symptoms?

Specific injuries and diseases

Understanding the medical work-up and treatment of major pediatric injuries and illnesses allows more effective work with a critical care team and with children and their parents. Children who have injuries [3] and chronic illnesses [104] are more likely than their peers to suffer psychiatric illness. Developing resources within comprehensive care planning to designate a specific psychiatrist as an integral part of the treatment team for children who have a given chronic disease or injury or as part of treatment or research protocols is recommended strongly.

Treatment considerations

When possible, pharmacotherapy usually follows psychosocial treatment interventions. Psychopharmacologic treatment is directed toward specific target symptoms of agitation, anxiety, delirium, perceptual disturbances, depression, and insomnia. Despite a suboptimal evidence base to guide psychopharmacotherapy in pediatric critical care, intervention often is mandatory and, as discussed previously, a clinical best practices approach should be the objective. Indications for psychopharmacotherapy include acute symptoms interfering with functioning, recovery, and *DSM-IV-TR* disorder based on these symptoms [102]. Palliative care may include psychopharmacologic agents to address specific target symptoms and increase patient comfort.

In this context, the authors' colleague and mentor, Dr. Ned Cassem, has a maxim, "start low, go slow," that applies to children even more than to adults, given the developmental variations in children and their critical condition in a critical care unit. Medical precautions: psychotropic drugs may affect any organ system, and adverse effects (as described previously) that affect neurological, hematological, cardiovascular, hepatic, genitourinary, gastrointestinal, musculoskeletal or dermatological systems must be considered when prescribing in critical care settings.

Guardianship and informed consent

When providing emergency care, psychopharmacologic treatment is included in consent for emergency treatment. In other circumstances, psychopharmacologic treatment requires consent from custodial parents or legal guardians. Inadvertently obtaining consent from someone other than a legal guardian may result in failed recommendations and unlawful treatment. Delay in instituting treatment may be required to obtain consent from a legal guardian. Assent by children beginning at age 7 also is desirable.

Off-label prescribing

In medical settings, as in general child psychiatry, many medications are used that are not officially FDA approved for the purpose they are being prescribed or for use in children under 12. As in any informed consent situation, a consulting child psychiatrist in pediatric critical care discusses the risks from, benefits of, and alternatives to a proposed treatment. This discussion should be detailed sufficiently and as appropriate to the setting of pediatric critical care. It is appropriate to clarify for parents and guardians that many psychotropic drugs used are off label, similar to other pharmacologic treatments in pediatric critical care.

Psychopharmacologic treatment of delirium, pain, and psychiatric disorders

Common concurrent or pre-existing psychiatric disorders in patients who have trauma, burns, cancer, inflammatory bowel disease, renal failure, cystic fibrosis, trauma, and other conditions that hospitalized children suffer include (1) pain, (2) delirium, (3) affective disorders, (4) anxiety disorders, (5) disruptive behavior disorders (ADHD, oppositional defiant disorder [ODD], and conduct disorder [CD]), (6) eating disorders, and (7) substance abuse disorders.

Acute pain

Undertreatment of pain may cause anxiety or depression in children and lead to requests to prescribe psychotropic medications or analgesics. For discussion of pain management, see article by Pottorak and Benore elsewhere in this issue. Rather than initiating psychotropic medications, it is critical that pain be assessed adequately and treated before psychopharmacologic intervention is considered. Pain often can be reduced or prevented, and child psychiatrists have a role as consultant in evaluating pain and anxiety, depression, and behavioral disturbances [21]. Historically, infants in surgical settings were not believed to feel pain and did not receive analgesics. This changed with the studies of Anand [105] and others, who found improved prognoses after major surgery for infants whose pain was treated with anesthesia and analgesia. Children from infancy through adolescence should be assessed and treated for pain and pain-associated stress and depression, including pharmacologic interventions as appropriate. Combined psychosocial and pharmacologic treatments are standard for procedurally related pain and anxiety.

Pain assessment

Assessment of pain in very young children requires evaluation and monitoring behavioral and physiologic parameters [106]. Prescribing is guided by use of pain rating scales appropriate to the age of the children. For children, like adults, the visual analog scales used most commonly rate pain intensity from 0 to a maximum of 10 (or 5) and are used for self-ratings or observer ratings of pain assessment. Other more detailed pain assessments also are possible and valuable for selected patients or patient populations.

Psychologic preparation and treatment

Preparation for painful procedures is demonstrated to reduce pain and anxiety, enhance compliance with procedures, and reduce the stress response. Children are able to manage their pain and cooperate with treatment better when they are participants in their care and have an appropriate sense of control. Psychologic interventions that can reduce pain and provide children with an added sense of control include relaxation, hypnosis, cognitive behavioral interventions, focused imagery, and patient-controlled analgesia (PCA).

Pharmacologic treatment

Pharmacologic treatment is the gold standard for treatment of severe pain in critical care. It is accomplished by administration of adequate doses of analgesics (especially opiates and nonsteroidal anti-inflammatory drugs [NSAIDs]) by various routes (oral, intramuscular, or IV) and methods (eg, spinal block or PCA). For refractory or neuropathic pain, although studied in children only on a limited basis, low doses of TCAs, stimulants, or anticonvulsants can be effective [107,108]. The dosages of morphine or other analgesics generally are proportional to the severity of (1) self-rated pain, (2) the injury (eg, leg amputation versus appendectomy wound), and (3) overall medical condition of the patient (eg, large acute burn versus elective skin graft).

What are major issues of psychotopic drugs and pain management?

There are issues of physiologic dependency on opiates or benzodiazepines. The discontinuation of these medications may lead to withdrawal symptoms. A gradual taper of these medications is recommended to avoid withdrawal symptoms. Serious withdrawal symptoms, such as seizures, require reinitiation of the inciting drug (eg, benzodiazepines). Milder withdrawal symptoms may be ameliorated by slowing the taper or adding other agents, such as clonidine. Another matter is that some pain medications cause psychiatric symptoms. These include sedation, delirium (opiates and benzodiazepines), depression (opiates), and disinhibition (benzodiazepines). The first treatment of psychiatric symptoms secondary to pain medications is not with psychotropic medication but, rather, the tapering, removal, or replacement of an analgesic or anxiolytic, which may be causing the psychiatric symptoms.

Delirium

Delirium is a common reason for psychiatric consultation. When delirium is suspected, an emergency evaluation should be performed. Usually it is a transient derangement of cerebral function with global impairment of cognition and attention, frequently accompanied by disturbances of the sleep-wake cycle and changes in psychomotor activity. Florid delirium often includes visual and auditory hallucinations, delusions, and paranoia. The Pediatric Anesthesia Emergence Delirium scale [109], a new 5-item scale that identifies "emergence delirium" in children after anesthesia, is the only scale specifically for children. The Mini–Mental State Examination [102] is used with adolescents and is valuable with children [103]. The Delirium Rating Scale is a 10-item scale used widely for children as young as 6 [110]. Delirium complicates acute medical-surgical treatment, often occurs postoperatively, and may be an early signal of a deteriorating medical condition; infectious, metabolic, or drug toxic insult; CNS injury; or acute delirious mania. Rapid psychiatric assessment, diagnosis, and treatment can be life saving [111].

Symptoms of delirium

The symptoms of delirium are (1) a disturbance of consciousness with reduced ability to focus, sustain, or shift attention; (2) a change in cognition (eg, memory deficit, disorientation, or language disturbance) or the development of a perceptual disturbance, such as visual or auditory hallucinations and delusions; (3) a disturbance developing over a short period of time and tending to fluctuate during the course of the day; and (4) evidence from history, physical examination, or laboratory findings that a disturbance is caused by the direct physiologic consequence of a general medical condition. One study of children under 62 months who were emerging from anesthesia suggests that symptoms differ depending on the age of the children. These children manifested higher rates of perceptual hallucination, perceptual disturbance, and agitation than older children [112].

Causes of delirium

Medical.

The causes of delirium include vascular, infectious, neoplastic, degenerative, toxic, congenital, central nervous system (CNS) pathologic, traumatic, vitamin deficiency, endocrinologic, metabolic, heavy metal, and anoxic phenomena [113].

Substance-induced or withdrawal.

Many therapeutic drugs and drugs of abuse are implicated in the etiology of delirium, including narcotics, benzodiazepines, ketamine, pressors, antibiotics, anticholinergics, anticonvulsants, antiarrhythmics, antihypertensives, antiviral agents, barbiturates, β- blockers, cimetidine, digitalis, diuretics, ergotamine, GABA agonists, immunosuppressives, MAOIs, NSAIDs, lithium, trazodone, sympathomimetics, corticosteroids, and corticotropin. Drugs of abuse are frequent causes, especially amphetamines and hallucinogens, as is withdrawal from alcohol or opiates. Sometimes there are multiple factors; in children, it is common for analgesics or analgesic withdrawal, antibiotics, and infection to contribute together to the onset of an acute delirium.

When a cause is being evaluated and determined, symptoms of confusion, agitation, and impulsive or aggressive behavior require emergency treatment. If behavioral and medical interventions fail to resolve a problem rapidly, antipsychotics are indicated. Antihistamines and benzodiazepines may worsen the symptoms of delirium.

Psychopharmacologic treatment of delirium

IV haloperidol has an established place in the treatment of delirium in adult critical care, but in children, brief use of haloperidol with substitution of an atypical antipsychotic increasingly is common [111,114]. Discussion follows of psychopharmacology of delirium in palliative care. In the authors' experience with older children, haloperidol is safe, inexpensive, and highly effective in the rapid remission of acute delirium and its associated risks, particularly in alleviating the effects of sleep deprivation associated with delirium [115,116]. In contrast, with children under 12, the occurrence of hypotension and cardiac irregularities discourages its use in this age group in one retrospective study of burned children. As a result, that group discontinued using haloperidol [117]. Another retrospective study of burned children, however, finds it useful even in young children. In the authors' experience, IV-administered haloperidol can be used safely for short periods in older children and adolescents who are selected carefully and monitored for cardiovascular and other adverse effects. This includes monitoring pulse, blood pressure, and EKG with QT interval corrected for heart rate (QTc) based on norms for the ages of the children. A cardiac consultation is indicated if cardiovascular symptoms or disease are present or if there is a strong family history of cardiac disease.

In the authors' center, haloperidol has been used to relieve the symptoms of various types of delirium, including that associated with burns in more than 80 older children, with excellent calming effects and no emergence of acute dystonia while the causes of the delirium were being sought and treated. Usually haloperidol is required for only 1 to 3 days until the delirium resolves. Low doses, between 0.5 and 3.0 mg given by slow IV push, usually are adequate and repeated every 6 to 8 hours once the appropriate dosage is identified; large adolescents may require larger doses, such as 3 to 10 mg every 6 to 8 hours. Monitoring for adverse effects is essential, particularly for dystonia. It is the authors' practice to keep an antiparkinsonian agent, either benadryl or cogentin, readily available should this occur. One center, in a retrospective study, while administering mainly haloperidol IV, also used oral and longer-term administration and reported adverse effects in 23% of 26 severely burned children studied (mainly dystonia and hypotension; hyperpyrexia, not believed to be NMS, was reported in two patients, one of whom died of respiratory and renal failure) and they no longer use it with children in that center [117]. To the authors' knowledge, after use for delirium in children, no case of tardive dyskinesia resulting from haloperidol has been reported or observed. Haloperidol, although approved for oral and intramuscular administration by the FDA, is not approved for IV administration for adults or children.

Other agents

Increasingly, if children are able to tolerate oral, nasogastric, or gastrostomy tube medications after brief treatment (24–48 hours) with IV haloperidol, there is substitution of an atypical antipsychotic, such as risperidone, olanzapine, or quetiapine. Many children now receive only an atypical antipsychotic instead of haloperidol, but these agents have risks (discussed previously). IV benzodiazepines, in particular midazolam and lorazepam, are safe and short-acting alternative agents, which in some cases relieve the symptoms of delirium but may be ineffective or complicate assessment by causing increased delirium, sedation, or paradoxic disinhibition. Diazepam is not favored because of its long half-life, making it more difficult to eliminate the sedation when desired.

Anxiety disorders

Children usually are anxious about being in the hospital. In 2002, the authors called attention to the potential of critical care settings as a source of fear-inducing stressors that trigger PTSD. Critical care settings are places where preventative measures can be taken to minimize later stress-related disorders and comorbid conditions [23]. Psychiatric consultation is indicated in two contexts. The first is assisting in designing and implementing preventive psychoeducational interventions within critical care protocols to prevent anxiety. There is extensive research evidence that preparation of children and parents for painful procedures reduces pain and anxiety associated with procedures and improves outcomes [118,119]. The second is that psychiatric consultation is indicated when anxiety persists, escalates, fails to respond to calming interventions, or interferes with children's medical care. Pediatric anxiety disorders seen in the medical setting include separation anxiety, acute stress disorder (ASD), PTSD, phobias, GAD of childhood, panic disorder, and OCD.

ASD is characterized by symptoms of dissociation, re-experiencing, arousal, and avoidance occurring within 30 days of the trauma. Often it emerges as a conditioned phobic response to painful procedures [118]. PTSD is similar except dissociative symptoms are not required and the diagnosis is made after 30 days. Young children often exhibit many, but not all, PTSD symptoms, especially avoidance. PTSD symptom scores may give an early opportunity to intervene to reduce the emergence of posttraumatic stress symptomatology. The symptoms of stress disorders in critical care often include insomnia and may include brief episodes of psychotic symptomatology, including agitation and hallucinations.

The mainstays of intervention to reduce acute stress and treat ASD and PTSD in pediatric critical care are benzodiazepines (Table 8), SSRIs, and, to a lesser degree, antipsychotics. In children under 8, benzodiazepines are the principal agents used because of the occurrence of adverse effects, such as hypotension and cardiac arrhythmias, with other agents. Opiates also can be effective for stress symptomatology when anxiety is the result of painful

Table 8
Selected benzodiazepines used in pediatric critical care

Drug	Routes of administration	Onset (minutes)	Half-life (hours)	Metabolism
Clonazepam	PO	30–60	Adult data (20–80 [123])	CYP3A
Diazepam	IV (painful), IM, PO, PR (gel)	IV (1–3) PR (7–15) PO (30–60)	Child data (15–21 [124])	CYP2C19[a] CYP3A
Lorazepam	IV, IM, PO	IV (1–5) IM (10–20) PO (30–60)	Child data (10.5 +/− 2.9 [125])	Phase II glucuronidation only
Midazolam	V, IM, PO, PR	IV (1–3) IM (5–10) PO/PR (10–30)	Child data (0.8–1.8 [126])	CYP3A

[a] 15%–20% of Asians and 3%–5% of whites are poor metabolizers of 2C19 substrates.

stimuli. TCAs, in particular imipramine, have a place but can be administered only enterally. Of the benzodiazepines, midazolam is preferred because it is administered parenterally, it is short acting and effective in reducing procedurally related anxiety and acute stress for brief periods, and it has amnestic properties, which may lessen conditioned aversive responses. Lorazepam is used widely. More potent IV agents that reduce anxiety for major procedures include propofol; for adolescents who have severe injuries, bolusing of IV haloperidol can be helpful; both agents should be used in collaboration with pediatric intensivists. Once patients are able to receive medications enterally, severe stress symptoms may respond to atypical antipsychotics, in particular risperidone, olanzapine, or quetiapine.

Affective disorders: depression and bipolar disorder

Depressive symptomatology resulting from an injury, illness, or medication is common in children in critical care and often is transient. Consulting child psychiatrists need to assure patients' safety while differentiating this from an emergent psychiatric disorder. Affective syndromes, including major depressive disorder, dysthymic disorder, and, increasingly, bipolar disorder, may be seen in hospitalized children. In children who appear markedly sad or psychomotorically retarded or agitated children who have manic-like symptoms, it is first important to make certain they are not suffering from drug side effects, are not delirious, are not intoxicated, or do not have another primary, treatable cause of these symptoms. For example, young children in a PICU who are quiet, sluggish, and tearful may be suffering a hypoactive delirium secondary to CNS infection or be maintaining stillness resulting from inadequately treated, overwhelming pain.

The diagnostic criteria for childhood depressive disorders are the same as those for adults. Making a diagnosis of a mood disorder in children who are medically ill can be challenging for several reasons. First, many have the misconception that sick children are "supposed to be sad" given their medical condition. Instead, it is important to recognize that the stress of hospitalization and medical illness make it more likely that children suffer a treatable depressive disorder. Children young and old who have medical illness may minimize or deny their depressive symptoms [120]. Nevertheless, recent studies demonstrate that even preschool children display the symptoms of adult depression, in particular anhedonia [121]. The criteria for depression include many somatic symptoms (eg, changes in appetite and energy), which typically are low in children who are critically ill. Whether or not children's symptoms are transient features of a medical illness or of a depressive illness is a dilemma. Therefore, in medical settings, cognitive rather than neurovegetative symptoms of depression are particularly important in diagnosis. Children and adolescents who have cancer often have somatic symptoms secondary to their treatment that are consistent with depressive symptoms. As a result, it is challenging to make the diagnosis of depression. This is an important diagnosis to consider, however, as these symptoms are treatable. A recent study by Gothelf and colleagues demonstrates that fluvoxamine reduces the symptoms of depression and anxiety significantly in small sample of young cancer patients [122].

Major depressive disorder

The *DSM-IV* defines a major depressive episode as either anhedonia or depressed mood plus at least five of the following symptoms over the same 2-week period: sleep disturbance, weight or appetite change, decreased concentration or indecision, suicidal ideation or thoughts of death, psychomotor agitation or retardation, loss of energy, and feelings of worthlessness or inappropriate guilt. Child-specific criteria include irritable as opposed to depressed mood and failure to make expected weight gains. Risk factors for depression include family history of depression, worsening illness, severe physical trauma, chronic medical illness, and adverse effects of drugs commonly administered in critical care (eg, morphine).

Dysthymic disorder

Childhood dysthymic disorder is defined as a persistently depressed or irritable mood with at least two symptoms of major depressive disorder that last at least 1 year; with the child never free of these symptoms for more than 2 months. It is not diagnosed if a major depressive episode occurred during the past year.

Bipolar disorder

Bipolar disorder quickly may lead to crises and risk of self-destructive behavior [123]. In a critical care setting, it is commonly, but not always, "secondary" mania or hypomania, not true bipolar disorder. Alcohol, benzodiazepines, steroids, lysergic acid diethylamide (LSD), amphetamines or methylphenidate, drug withdrawal, hyperthyroidism, HIV and other infections, and traumatic brain injury are among the causes [124]. The symptoms according to *DSM-IV-TR*, usually in adolescents but occasionally in prepubertal children, include a persistently elevated or irritable mood, with three of the following seven symptoms: grandiosity, decreased sleep, pressured speech, racing thoughts, distractibility, psychomotor agitation or increased goal-directed activity, and excessive involvement in pleasurable activities [102]. Additional causes of a manic or hypomanic episode include discontinuation of mood stabilizers, the natural onset of bipolar illness, antidepressants, and many other causes. Because patients may be vulnerable to fluid and electrolyte shifts in critical care, lithium may be contraindicated because of risk for lithium intoxication and cardiac arrthymias, and other mood stabilizers cause fewer risks. Antipsychotic agents, generally atypical antipsychotics or mood stabilizers (eg, valproate), or benzodiazepines likely relieve an acute episode rapidly in children or adolescents in critical care.

Adjustment disorders

Adjustment disorders are among the most common psychiatric diagnoses in critical care and on the pediatric ward. The criteria for adjustment disorder include (1) physical or psychologic stressors within the previous 3 months occurring in a family, community, or medical setting which patient or clinician views as responsible for symptoms; (2) symptoms severe enough to impair functioning; (3) excess of a normal and expected reaction to stressors; and (4) acute form remitting within 6 months of the stressor, whereas chronic form lasts more than than 6 months with chronic stressors. These disorders of adjustment occur in 3% to 10% of children in general medical settings and their implications are not benign. Chess and Thomas, in a study of a normal population, found adjustment disorder mainly in the 3- to 5-year-old age group, and it was the primary diagnosis in 40 out of 45 children under 13 who later developed mental illness [125]. Kovacs and colleagues note that 33% of newly diagnosed childhood diabetics develop an adjustment disoder [126]. Also, more than 10% of children who recovered from burns and were readmitted for surgery had an adjustment disorder [127].

Management of disruptive behavior disorders

The most common neurobehavioral disorder of childhood is ADHD (4%–12%) [128]. Other disruptive behavior disorders include ODD and CD. Children who have disruptive behavior disorders (specifically ADHD and ODD) represent a higher percentage of critical care patients than the general population because their high-risk behaviors and impulsivity seem to predispose them to accidents, overdoses, and burns [129]. In a critical care setting, children who have disruptive behavior disorders often present as more difficult to manage medically because their underlying psychiatric illness usually is untreated. As a result, children may present as more irritable and frustrated. Their symptoms of hyperactivity, restlessness, and fidgetiness can interfere with medical care. Uncontrolled hyperactive or impulsive children or angry children who have ODD or CD are at high risk for pulling out lines, refusing medications and procedures, and interfering with medical care. Acutely, inattention symptoms are not problematic. These symptoms do have an impact on children's ability to understand and interpret medical treatment, however, making it more difficult for them to comply. Children who have ODD and CD and who are defiant and disagreeable find their lack of control increasingly distressing and, therefore, are at greater risk for acting out. In the authors' experience, these children, when on steroids, seem to be at high risk for developing behavior and mood symptoms. Given the increased likelihood of accidents and injuries in this population, critical care patients should be screened and treated for ADHD [130]. The mainstay of treatment for ADHD is pharmacotherapy, and psychostimulants should be restarted if children's ADHD symptoms are interfering with care. Stimulants often can be administered safely with most other medications used in a critical care setting, except MAOIs, where concomitant use can result in a hypertensive crisis. Concurrent use with sympathomimetic agents may increase the effect of both medications. The effect on heart rate and blood pressure is mild and usually not clinically significant [131].

Developmental disorders

Development disorders include mental retardation [132], pervasive developmental disorders [133], and specific learning disorders.

Many children in critical care have prior diagnoses of developmental disorders, or they first are diagnosed in critical care. Recognition of special communication and treatment needs for these children and their families is essential to good care. Awareness of the range of possible medications (eg, stimulants, antidepressants, and antipsychotics), their evidence base to help these children, and potential adverse effects during critical care is essential for consulting psychiatrists.

Substance abuse disorders

A significant number of adolescents uses drugs and alcohol on an "experimental basis" [134]. In a 2004 National Institute on Drug Abuse survey, 18.6% of eighth graders reported having had a drink in the past month compared with 35.2% of tenth graders and 48% of high school seniors. For most teens, drugs and alcohol do not cause major problems [135]. The leading causes of death among teenagers, however, which include accidents, homicide, and suicide, often are related to drug and alcohol use [136].

In a critical care setting, psychiatrists typically are called on to evaluate and guide treatment of adolescents who are intoxicated or experiencing a withdrawal syndrome. Distinguishing intoxication and withdrawal from other medical disorders sometimes is difficult. Serum and urine toxicology screens and liver function studies should be performed on anyone suspected of drug use or children and teenagers involved in traumatic accidents. It is important to ask which drugs have been used and to determine quantity and frequency. For example, ruling out psychosis may be needed for a patient who is experiencing the sensation that "bugs are crawling all over him" (formication). A thorough history, however, may make apparent that cocaine intoxication is responsible for these symptoms, in which case comfort measures alone are warranted in the acute treatment phase. Given the focus of this article, only opiates and alcohol are discussed.

Excessive use of alcohol over an extended period of time causes CNS changes, including down-regulation of the number and sensitivity of GABA receptors, decreased GABA concentration, and increased levels of catecholamines. These changes place patients at risk for withdrawal, including seizures, delirium tremens, and even death in some cases. The hallmarks of alcohol withdrawal include nausea and vomiting, tremor, sweating, anxiety and irritability, increased blood pressure and heart rate, and, in some cases, auditory, visual, and tactile disturbances. Benzodiazepines given in tapering doses, IV hydration, and comfort measures, such as NSAIDS for pain, are standard for treating alcohol-withdrawal. Adult studies demonstrate that using rating scales, such as the Clinical Institute Withdrawal Assessment, and providing symptom-triggered benzodiazepine treatment reduce the total dose of benzodiazepines used, shorten length of hospital stay, and maintain patient comfort [137]. Lorazepam in particular is useful as it can be administered IV or orally, is metabolized renally, and is relatively short acting in case oversedation occurs.

Opiate withdrawal may occur in a pediatric critical care setting. Familiarity with local slang terminology is helpful in assessing the degree to which patients may withdraw from opiates. For example, patients often talk about "OCs" and "percs," meaning oxycodone (OxyContin) and acetaminophen with oxycodone (Percocet) tablets, respectively. Furthermore, asking about the amount, frequency, and route of administration of drugs used is important. Patients who use IV heroin and share "works," which include needles, spoons, and other paraphernalia, are at increased risk for hepatitis, HIV, and other infections for which they should be screened. In terms of in-hospital treatment, comfort measures, including NSAIDs for pain, clonidine for hypertension and autonomic lability, benzodiazepines for anxiety, and bismuth salicylate for gastrointestinal upset, may be useful. Clinical experience and a recent study suggest that buprenorphine may be useful particularly in treating adolescent opiate withdrawal on a general pediatric ward or on an outpatient basis [138]. As buprenorphine is a partial opiate antagonist with high opiate receptor affinity, however, it can precipitate withdrawal in patients taking long-acting opiates and may block the analgesic effect of opiates administered to patients who have severe pain. Also, because of hospital formulary restrictions and because a specific license is required to continue treatment of patients who have buprenorphine on an outpatient basis, this is a drug rarely, if ever, used in a PICU setting.

Disorders secondary to neglect and abuse

Children who are neglected or abused may be seen in a critical care setting. It is important to identify and report any cases of neglect or abuse to the appropriate departments and services. More children die from neglect than from abuse. Psychotropic drugs should not be used when they might interfere with children reporting their history of neglect or abuse. Because stress disorders, depression, and mental retardation commonly are diagnosed in children who are neglected or abused, however, a critical care setting likely is where some children are treated first for these or associated disorders, and the treatments often include medications [139,140].

Management of patients after suicide attempt

After suicide attempts, children, primarily adolescents, are admitted and sometimes die in critical care units. Among the causes of suicide attempts are overdoses, shootings, hangings, and self-immolation [141]. The possibility of attempted homicide rather than suicide should be ruled out. The clinical management of patients is shared by an attending pediatrician or surgeon and a child psychiatrist.

Early and thorough history taking, diagnostic evaluation, and institution of protective and therapeutic measures are essential. Usually, once medically stable, adolescents are transferred to an inpatient psychiatric facility. Critical care teams often find caring for these patients challenging. Psychopharmacologic management of patients who are post suicide may be life saving and lessen the overall stress in a critical care setting. It is important to educate critical care teams about underlying illnesses, such as depression or substance abuse, in adolescents that may have precipitated the suicide attempt. When a team has a better understanding of severity of children's illness, they are better able to provide excellent medical and compassionate care.

Palliative care in the critical care setting

Many children who have life-threatening illnesses die in the hospital. For example, recent studies show that up to 49% of children who have terminal cancer die in a hospital [142]. Most children who die in a hospital are in an intensive care setting (neonatal ICU or PICU) [143]. Up to 60% of deaths occurring in a critical care setting follow the withdrawal of life-sustaining treatment [144]. During the past 5 years, more attention has been paid to the symptoms and suffering at end of life. The use of medications to alleviate pain and suffering at end of life now is the standard of care. Aggressive pain management is the mainstay of palliative care. As discussed elsewhere in this issue, the treatment of pain, dyspnea, nausea, and vomiting can reduce significantly the distress of children who are dying. Suffering is not limited to physical symptoms; it includes the emotional and spiritual spheres of life addressed elsewhere in this issue. This type of suffering not only is treatable but also may manifest as physical symptoms or exacerbate physical symptoms already present.

As discussed previously, a thorough evaluation of children and their families is necessary to understand children's experiences and wishes. It is important to consider whether or not this dying process was unexpected, such as after a motor vehicle accident, or expected, as with relapsed cancer. Although no death of a child is anticipated fully, children who are suffering from a terminal illness may present with a different set of issues from children who are acutely and unexpectedly ill. This is the case particularly for parents and siblings. Children who have a terminal illness (eg, relapsed cancer) likely have a team of providers who know them and their families well.

The history obtained from children is invaluable as it is they who are being assessed. In particular, it is important to keep in mind children's and families' wishes, beliefs, worries, and fears.

Depression and anxiety are seen in children at the end of life. Although *DSM-IV-TR* criteria still are considered in this setting, it is difficult to apply them to children who are dying. Depression may present as increased lethargy, insomnia, agitation, sad mood, and irritability. Most children who are in a critical care setting at the end of life experience some symptoms of fatigue or lethargy, appetite loss, psychomotor retardation or agitation, or sleep disturbances, all of which are symptoms of depression. Not all children at the end of life feel sad, hopeless, or suicidal, however. Depression may be indicated by children's behavior. For example, children may not engage in activities (watching videos or listening to music) that they enjoyed previously or interact as much with family members even when medically able. Anxiety also is present at the end of life. This may manifest itself as agitation, separation anxiety, general nervousness, or withdrawal. Pragmatically, differentiating "depression" and "anxiety" from acute stress symptoms at the end of life is less important than responding to presenting symptoms and seeking to relieve children's distress. For those who are experiencing sadness, hopelessness, or anxiety, the first approach is to address these symptoms with psychologic and behavioral interventions. Improving communication by listening to children and families about their concerns; supporting children in expressing their thoughts, feelings, and fears; and offering spiritual counseling and prayer can alleviate much of children's and families' worries. In addition, it is important to consider pharmacologic interventions that not only can be helpful but also are essential adjuncts in the management of distressing symptoms at end of life.

As discussed previously, SSRIs are used to treat depression in children. These medications take at least 2 weeks to remit symptoms; therefore, although SSRIs are used for children who have depression at the end of life, they usually are not initiated during children's last days to alleviate symptoms of depression and anxiety. TCAs, which are not found to treat mood disorders in children, are helpful in alleviating specific symptoms at the end of life, including insomnia and pain [145,146].

Benzodiazepines are used judiciously in end-of-life settings. Many children receive benzodiazepines in critical care settings because of their sedating properties. They may be effective in managing agitation, anxiety, and nausea. The determination of benzodiazepine dose for new-onset agitation and anxiety depends on whether or not children already are receiving benzodiazepines or whether or not this is a new medication intervention. When using benzodiazepines for the first time, it is recommended to start with a relatively low dose to determine tolerance and minimize side effects. Short-acting benzodiazepines (eg, lorazepam) frequently are used on an as-needed basis and converted to standing doses. Standing doses minimize the need for children or parents to ask for medication and minimize the likelihood of a rebound effect. Therefore, standard dosing often is more effective in symptom remission. Route of administration and half-life are the determining factors in choosing a benzodiazepine. Most commonly, lorazepam is used. The initial dose for lorazepam, a short-acting benzodiazepine, is 0.25 mg to 0.5 mg every 4 to 6 hours. Diazepam, a longer-acting medication, is initiated at 0.07 to 0.5 mg/kg/d but is used less often because it is metabolized slowly [146]. Both of these medications can be administered by multiple routes (orally, sublingually; intravenously, rectally, or transdermally). Dougherty and DeBaun, in a retrospective study, report an increase in morphine and benzodiazepine use in the last 3 days of life in children who have cancer [147]. In particular, the increased use of medication is related to neuropathic pain. The use of benzodiazepines does not treat pain (except clonazepam for neuropathic pain) and, therefore, the increased use may have been treating underlying agitation and anxiety in these children or inadequate pain management. In the terminal phase of care, benzodiazepine doses may be titrated to high doses or administered as a continuous infusion to provide comfort.

Although benzodiazepines are useful in critical care settings, the development of paradoxic reactions (ie, children who become disinhibited and more agitated on benzodiazepines) must be monitored. Also, benzodiazepines may exacerbate symptoms of delirium that can be present at the end of life.

Agitation may not respond sufficiently to benzodiazepines or be exacerbated by benzodiazepines. Case reports and experience indicate that antipsychotics decrease agitation and improve sleep [148]. This is important particularly in the management of refractory symptoms and in the terminal phase of care, as agitation may be a manifestation of delirium secondary to metabolic derangements, organ failure, CNS disease, and narcotic use. Pain management should not be minimized to improve children's agitation and sensorium; rather, the use of antipsychotics may relieve these symptoms. Initially, nonsedating antipsychotics are favored, such as haloperidol or the newer atypical agents, such as risperidone [149]. Haloperidol can be administered by multiple routes (orally, introvenously, rectally, or under the tongue). In a palliative care setting, haloperidol initially is dosed at 0.01 to 0.02 mg/kg every 8 to 12 hours and titrated according to tolerance and effect [150]. The newer antipsychotics, such as risperidone, are not available in IV form. Risperidone usually is initiated at 0.125 to 0.25 mg every 12 hours and titrated up to 1 mg per dose as needed (see previous discussion of side effects). Other atypical antipsychotics used in this setting include olanzapine and quetiapine [131]. As children approach end of his life, more sedating antipsychotics, such as chlorpromazine, may be indicated. Chlorpromazine is dosed initially at 0.5 mg/kg every 6 hours and titrated as needed [146].

Concerns often are raised by family and children, especially teenagers, about the sedating and mental clouding effect of medications used at the end of life. Pain and dyspnea (some of the most common symptoms of suffering) management includes use of medications that are sedating and may impair cognition. Studies indicate that stimulant use may counteract these problems and alleviate fatigue, one of the most common end-of-life symptoms noted by patients and families. Yee and Berde report that 5 of 11 adolescents who received methylphenidate or dextroamphetamine showed decreased somnolence or improved ability to interact with others [151]. Other studies looking at the palliative use of methylphenidate in patients who have cancer have been conducted in adults [152]. The results are promising and support the palliative use of methylphenidate. Methylphenidate generally is well tolerated in this setting and can contribute to the following improvements: decreased sedation, increased alertness and cognition, potentiation of opiates, and diminished acute depression in those who are terminally ill. Methylphenidate usually is used in critical care settings, because it has a quick onset of action and a short half-life. A low starting dose of 2.5 mg in the morning and 4 hours later is recommended. The dose may be titrated up to 1 mg/kg per day.

Children who are dying may become delirious. The assessment and management of delirium in this setting often is complicated by three factors. First, one of the rules of treating delirium is to discover and treat the underlying cause. Yet, in the case of children who have terminal illness, the untreatable disease itself may be responsible for the delirium. Second, administering palliative pharmacologic care, including high-dose opiate analgesia and benzodiazepine sedation, may lead to delirium. Third, determine whether or not the delirium is causing harm and should be treated or whether or not it is preventing further suffering at the end of a child's life and does not require aggressive treatment. It is important to find the right balance when considering these three dilemmas.

As the terminal phase of care approaches, children may require heroic doses of medications to alleviate their pain and suffering. Continuous infusions of pain and sedating medications may be needed. Combinations of pain medications, anxiolytics, and neuroleptics may be indicated. Again, during this time, it is essential to keep in mind the wishes of children and parents and to provide as much comfort and caring as possible to children and families.

The family

PICUs inherently are stressful environments not only for children who are critically ill but also for their families. The role of child psychiatrists is to provide care for children who are medically ill and to gain a better understanding of children in the context of their families. Parents often report feeling like their ICU experience is surreal. They frequently lose track of time and are reluctant to leave a child's side and take care of their own needs. In this regard, it is important to have social work services available to provide additional support to family members. The family benefits from useful information about psychopharmacologic treatment. They often provide knowledge about prior responses to medications, questions or requests about medications or dosing, and helpful observations about drug effects or adverse effects.

Psychopharmacology consultation to the critical care team

Child psychiatric consultants bring valuable expertise to teams that are expert in critical care of injury and disease but untrained in psychiatric diagnosis and treatment. Psychiatric skills allow evaluation of risk factors from the history, such as risk-taking, abuse, mental illness, or prior emotional impairment resulting from disease. In addition, when consulting with a bedside care team, much is learned about the changes in mental status of children 24 hours per day and their responses to medications and stress. Using psychiatric and neuropsychiatric skills and collaborating with critical care medical and nursing teams, using established medications judiciously, and using newer drugs in novel ways may be of major benefit in enhancing children's quality of life, pain control, and state of alertness, even at the end of life.

Continuation or discontinuation of psychopharmacologic treatment

Decisions to treat or to discontinue treatment take on new meaning in pediatric critical care. Psychopharmacologic treatments may provide another essential medical intervention for patients suffering from a complex disease or severe injury, even as they survive or during palliative care. Discontinuation of treatment should be done carefully, generally by tapering rather than rapid discontinuation, and with evaluation of the results with reinstitution of treatment as approrropriate. When patients are discharged, it is essential to consider the value of continuation of medication in enhancing continued recovery and preventing relapse versus potential benefits of discontinuation and later reevaluation.

Summary

Psychopharmacologic treatment in pediatric critical care requires a careful child or adolescent psychiatric evaluation, including a thorough review of the history of present illness or injury, any current or pre-existing psychiatric disorder, past history, and laboratory studies. Although there is limited evidence to guide psychopharmacologic practice in this setting, psychopharmacologic treatment is increasing in critical care, with known indications for treatment, benefits, and risks; initial dosing guidelines; and best practices. Treatment is guided by the knowledge bases in pediatric physiology, psychopharmacology, and treatment of critically ill adults. Pharmacologic considerations include pharmacokinetic and pharmcodynamic aspects of specific drugs and drug classes, in particular elimination half-life, developmental considerations, drug interactions, and adverse effects. Evaluation and management of pain is a key initial step, as pain may mimic psychiatric symptoms and its effective treatment can ameliorate them. Patient comfort and safety are primary objectives for children who are acutely ill and who will survive and for those who will not. Judicious use of psychopharmacologic agents in pediatric critical care using the limited but growing evidence base and a clinical best practices collaborative approach can reduce anxiety, sadness, disorientation, and agitation; improve analgesia; and save lives of children who are suicidal or delirious. In addition to pain, other disorders or indications for psychopharmacologic treatment are affective disorders; PTSD; post–suicide attempt patients; disruptive behavior disorders (especially ADHD); and adjustment, developmental, and substance use disorders. Treating children who are critically ill with psychotropic drugs is an integral component of comprehensive pediatric critical care in relieving pain and delirium; reducing inattention or agitation or aggressive behavior; relieving acute stress, anxiety, or depression; and improving sleep and nutrition. In palliative care, psychopharmacology is integrated with psychologic approaches to enhance children's comfort at the end of life. Defining how best to prevent the adverse consequences of suffering and stress in pediatric critical care is a goal for protocols and for new psychopharmacologic research [23,153].

References

[1] Cooper WO, Hickson GB, Fuchs C, et al. New users of antipsychotic medications among children enrolled in TennCare. Arch Pediatr Adolesc Med 2004;158:753–9.

[2] Patel NC, Crismon ML, Hoagwood K, et al. Trends in the use of typical and atypical antipsychotics in children and adolescents. J Am Acad Child Adolesc Psychiatry 2005;44:548–56.

[3] Stoddard FJ, Saxe G. Ten-year research review of physical injuries. J Am Acad Child Adolesc Psychiatry 2001;40:1128–45.

[4] Lubit R. Eth S. Children, Disasters, and the September 11th World Trade Center Attack. In: Ursano RJ, Norwood AE, editors. Trauma and Disaster. Responses and Management. Washington DC: Am Psychiatric Press Inc, Review of Psychiatry; 2003. p. 63–96.

[5] Zatzick D. Collaborative care for injured victims of individual and mass trauma: a health services research approach to developing early intervention. In: Ursano RJ, Fullerton CS, Norwood AE, editors. Terrorism and disaster: individual and Community Mental Health Interventions. Cambridge (UK): Cambridge University Press; 2003. p. 189–208.

[6] Zito JM, Safer DJ, dosReis S, et al. Trends in the prescribing of medications to preschoolers. JAMA 2000;283:1025–30.

[7] Federal Drug Administration. Center for Drug Evaluation and Research. List of drugs receiving a boxed warning pertaining to pediatric suicidality. Available at: www.fda.gov/cder/foi/label/2005/20031s045,20936s020lbl.pdf. Accessed March 22, 2006.

[8] Coyle JT. Psychotropic drug use in very young children. JAMA 2000;283:1059–60.

[9] Coghill D. Evidence-based psychopharmacology for children and adolescents. Curr Opin Psychiatry 2002;15:361–8.

[10] Alpert JE, Fava M, Rosenbaum JF. Psychopharmacologic issues in the medical setting. In: Stern TA, Fricchione GL, Cassem NH, editors. Massachusetts General Hospital handbook of general hospital psychiatry. 5th edition. St. Louis: Mosby; 2004. p. 231–68.

[11] American Academy of Child and Adolescent Psychiatry: Practice parameters for PTSD, ADHD, depressive disorders, bipolar, substance use, suicidal behavior, and other disorders. Available at: www.aacap.org/clinical/. Accessed March 22, 2006.

[12] Clein PD, Riddle MA. Pharmacokinetics in children and adolescents. Child Adolesc Psychiatr Clin North Am 1995;4:59–76.

[13] Slater JA. The medically ill child or adolescent. Pediatric psychopharmacology: principles and practice. In: Martin A, Scahil Ll, Charney DS, et al, editors. New York: Oxford University Press; 2003. p. 631–41.

[14] March JS, Silva SG, Compton S, et al. The child and adolescent psychiatry trials network (CAPTN). J Am Acad Child Adolesc Psychiatry 2003;43:515–8.

[15] Fitzgerald M, Howard RF. The neurobiologic basis of pediatric pain. In: Schechter NS, Berde CB, Yaster M, editors. Pain in infants, children and adolescents. 2nd edition. Philadelphia: Williams and Wilkins; 2003. p. 19–42.

[16] DeBellis MD, Keshavan MS, Clark DB, et al. Developmental traumatology part II: brain development. Biol Psych 1999;45:1271–84.

[17] Goodyer I. Developmental neurobiology and the childhood onset of psychiatric disorders. In: Charney DS, Nestler EJ, editors. Neurobiology of mental illness. 2nd edition. New York: Oxford University Press; 2004. p. 921–9.

[18] Stoddard FJ, Levine JB, Lund K. Psychiatric care of the burn patient. In: Blumenfield M, Strain J, editors. Psychosomatic medicine in the 21st century. Philadelphia: Lippincott/ Williams and Wilkins; in press.

[19] Heckers S, Konradi C. Anatomic and molecular principles of psychopharmacology: a primer for psychiatrists. Child Adolesc Psychiatr Clin North Am 2000;9:1–22.

[20] Hyman SE, Nestler EJ. Initiation and adaptation: a paradigm for understanding psychotropic drug action. Am J Psychiatry 1996;153:151–62.

[21] McEwen BS. UPDATE protective and damaging effects of stress mediators. N Engl J Med 1998;338:171–9.

[22] Stoddard FJ, Sheridan RL, Saxe G, et al. Treatment of pain in acutely burned children. J Burn Care Rehabil 2002;23:135–56.

[23] Stoddard FJ, Todres ID. A new frontier: posttraumatic stress and prevention, diagnosis and treatment. Crit Care Med 2001;29:687–8.

[24] Alpert JE. Drug-drug interactions: the interface between psychotropics and other agents. In: Stern T, Herman J, Slavin P, editors. The MGH guide to psychiatry in primary care. New York: McGraw Hill; 1998. p. 519–34.

[25] Sheridan R, McEttrick M, Bacha G, et al. Midazolam infusion in pediatric patients with burns who are undergoing mechanical ventilation. J Burn Care Rehabil 1994;15: 515–8.

[26] Ziegler VE, Biggs JT, Ardekani AB, et al. Contribution to the pharmacokinetics of amitriptyline. J Clin Pharmacol 1978;18:462–7.

[27] Mallikaarjun S, Salazar DE, Bramer SL. Pharmacokinetics, tolerability, and safety of aripiprazole following multiple oral dosing in normal healthy volunteers. J Clin Pharmacol 2004;44:179–87.

[28] Greenblatt DJ, Wright CE. Clinical pharmacokinetics of alprazolam. Therapeutic implications. Clin Pharmacokinet 1993;24:453–71.

[29] Leppik IE. Metabolism of antiepileptic medication: newborn to elderly. Epilepsia 1992; 33(Suppl):S32–40.

[30] Witcher JW, Long A, Smith B, et al. Atomoxetine pharmacokinetics in children and adolescents with attention deficit hyperactivity disorder. J Child Adolesc Psychopharmacol 2003;13:53–63.

[31] Daviss WB, Perel JM, Rudolph GR, et al. Steady-state pharmacokinetics of bupropion SR in juvenile patients. J Am Acad Child Adolesc Psychiatry 2005;44:349–57.

[32] Furlanut M, Benetello P, Baraldo M, et al. Chlorpromazine disposition in relation to age in children. Clin Pharmacokinet 1990;18:329–31.

[33] Greenblatt DJ, Miller LG, Sharder RI. Clonazepam pharmacokinetics, brain uptake, and receptor interactions. J Clin Psychiatry 1987;48(Suppl):4–11.

[34] Tallian KB, Nahata MC, Lo W, et al. Pharmacokinetics of gabapentin in paediatric patients with uncontrolled seizures. J Clin Pharm Ther 2004;29:511–5.

[35] Hunt RD, Capper L, O'Connell P. Clonidine in child and adolescent psychiatry. J Child Adolesc Psychopharmacol 1990;1:87–102.

[36] Milne RJ, Goa KL. Citalopram. A review of its pharmacodynamic and pharmacokinetic properties, and therapeutic potential in depressive illness. Drugs 1991;41:450–77.

[37] Guitton C, Kinowski JM, Abbar M, et al. Clozapine and metabolite concentrations during treatment of patients with chronic schizophrenia. J Clin Pharmacol 1999;39:721–8.

[38] Morselli PL, Cuche H, Zarifian E. Pharmacokinetics of psychoteropic drugs in the pediatric patient. In: Mendlewicz J, van Praag HM, Karg S, editors. Childhood psychopharmacology: current concepts. Advances in biological psychiatry. Basel (Switzerland): S. Karger; 1978. p. 70–86.

[39] Chen C, Casale EJ, Duncan B, et al. Pharmacokinetics of lamotrigine in children in the absence of other antiepileptic drugs. Pharmacotherapy 1999;19:437–41.

[40] Brown GL, Hunt RD, Ebert MH, et al. Plasma levels of d-amphetamine in hyperactive children. Psychopharmacology (Berl) 1979;62:133–40.

[41] Wilens TE, Cohen L, Biederman J, et al. Fluoxetine pharmacokinetics in pediatric patients. J Clin Psychopharmacol 2002;22:568–75.

[42] Harvey AT, Preskorn SH. Fluoxetine pharmacokinetics and effect on CYP2C19 in young and elderly volunteers. J Clin Psychopharmacol 2001;21:161–6.

[43] Yoshida I, Sakaguchi Y, Matsuishi T, et al. Acute accidental overdosage of haloperidol in children. Acta Pediatr 1993;82:877–80.

[44] Relling MV, Mulhern RK, Dodge RK, et al. Lorazepam pharmacodynamics and pharmacokinetics in children. J Pediatr 1989;114(4 Pt 1):641–6.

[45] Spencer T, Wilens T, Biederman J. Pychotropic medication for children and adolescents. Child Adolesc Psychiatr Clin North Am 1995;4:97–121.

[46] Simons KJ, Watson WTA, Martin TJ, et al. Diphenhydramine: pharmacokinetics and pharmacodynamics in elderly adults, young adults and children. J Clin Pharmacol 1990; 30:665–71.

[47] Spina E, Pollicino AM, Avenoso A, et al. Effect of fluvoxamine on the pharmacokinetics of imipramine and desipramine in healthy subjects. Ther Drug Monit 1993;15:243–6.

[48] Grothe DR, Calis KA, Jacobsen L, et al. Olanzapine pharmacokinetics in pediatric and adolescent inpatients with childhood-onset schizophrenia. J Clin Psychpharmacol 2000; 20:220–5.

[49] Blumer JL. Clinical pharmacology of midazolam in infants and children. Clin Pharmacokinet 1998;35:37–47.

[50] Lloyd P, Flesch G, Dieterle W. Clinical pharmacology and pharmacokinetics of oxcarbazepine. Epilepsia 1994;35(Suppl 3):S10–3.

[51] Gualtieri CT, Hicks RE, Patrick K, et al. Clinical correlates of methylphenidate blood levels. Ther Drug Monit 1984;6:379–92.

[52] Timmer CJ, Sitsen JM, Delbressine LP. Clinical pharmacokinetics of mirtazapine. Clin Pharmacokinet 2000;38:461–74.

[53] Devane CL, Nemeroff CB. Clinical pharmacokinetics of quetiapine: an atypical antipsychotic. Clin Pharmacokinet 2001;40:509–22.

[54] Greenblatt DJ. Clinical pharmacokinetics of oxazepam and lorazepam. Clin Pharmacokinet 1981;6:89–105.

[55] Bialer M, Doose DR, Murthy B, et al. Pharmacokinetic interactions of topiramate. Clin Pharmacokinet 2004;43:763–80.

[56] Sallee F, Stiller R, Perel J, et al. Oral pemoline kinetics in hyperactive children. Clin Pharmacol Ther 1985;37:606–9.

[57] Geller B, Cooper TB, Chestnut EC, et al. Nortriptyline pharmacokinetic parameters in depressed children and adolescents: preliminary data. J Clin Psychpharmacol 1984;4: 265–9.

[58] Green WH. Child & adolescent clinical psychopharmacology. Philadelphia: Lippincott Williams & Wilkins; 2001.

[59] Findling RL, Reed MD, Myers C, et al. Paroxetine pharmacokinetics in depressed children and adolescents. J Am Acad Child Adolesc Psychiatry 1999;38:952–9.

[60] Caley CF, Cooper CK. Ziprasidone: the fifth atypical antipsychotic. Ann Pharmacother 2002;36:839–51.

[61] Preskorn SH. Pharmacokinetics and therapeutics of acute intramuscular ziprasidone. Clin Pharmacokinet 2005;44:1117–33.

[62] Axelson DA, Perel JM, Birmaher B, et al. Sertraline pharmacokinetics and dynamics in adolescents. J Am Acad Child Adolesc Psychiatry 2002;41:1037–44.

[63] Morton WA, Sonne SC, Verga MA. Venlafaxine: a structurally unique and novel antidepressant. Ann Pharmacother 1995;29:387–95.

[64] Gidal BE, Sheth R, Parnell J, et al. Evaluation of VPA dose and concentration effects on lamotrigine pharmacokinetics: implications for conversion to lamotrigine monotherapy. Epilepsy Res 2003;57:85–93.

[65] Fetner HH, Geller B. Lithium and tricyclic antidepressants. Psychiatr Clin North Am 1992; 15:223–4.

[66] Cozza KL, Armstrong SC, Oesterheld JR. Concise guide to drug interaction principles for medical practice. 2nd edition. Washington, DC: American Psychiatric Press; 2000.

[67] Boyer EW, Shannon M. The serotonin syndrome. N Engl J Med 2005;352:1112–20.

[68] Bergeron L, Boule M, Perreault S. Serotonin toxicity associated with concomitant use of linezolid. Ann Pharmacother 2005;39:956–61.

[69] Hammerness P, Parada H, Abrams A. Linezolid: MAOI activity and potential drug interaction. Psychosomatics 2002;43:248–9.

[70] Oesterheld JR, Armstrong SC, Cozza KL. Ecstasy: pharmacodynamic and pharmacokinetic interactions. Psychosomatics 2005;46:189.

[71] Sheridan R, Stoddard F, Querzoli E. Management of background pain and anxiety in critically burned children requiring protracted mechanical ventilation. J Burn Care Rehabil 2001;22:150–3.

[72] Sheridan RL, McEttrick M, Bacha G, et al. Midazolam infusion in pediatric patients with burns who are undergoing mechanical ventilation. J Burn Care Rehabil 1994;15:515–8.

[73] Himmelscher S, Durleux ME. Ketamine for perioperative pain management. Anesthesiology 2005;102:211–20.

[74] Newcomer JW, Farber NB, Jertovic-Todorovic V, et al. Ketamine-induced NMDA receptor hypofunction as a model of memory impairment and psychosis. Neuropsychopharmacology 1999;20:106–18.

[75] Gardner DM, Baldessarini RJ, Waraich P. Modern antipsychotic drugs: a critical overview. CMAJ 2005;172:1703–11.

[76] Blair J, Scahill L, State M, et al. Electrocardiographic changes in children and adolescents treated ziprasidone: a prospective study. J Am Acad Child Adolesc Psychiatry 2005;44: 73–9.

[77] Leonard HL, March J, Rickler KC, et al. Pharmacology of the selective serotonin reuptake inhibitors in children and adolescents. J Am Acad Child Adolesc Psychiatry 1997;36: 725–36.

[78] Emslie GJ, Hughes CW, Crismon ML, et al. A feasibility study of the childhood depression medication algorithm: the Texas Children's Medication Algorithm Project (CMAP). J Am Acad Child Adolesc Psychiatry 2004;45:519–27.

[79] Rynn MA, Siqueland L, Rickels K. Placebo-controlled trial of sertraline in the treatment of children with generalized anxiety disorder. Am J Psychiatry 2001;158:2008–14.

[80] March JS, Biederman J, Wolkow R, et al. Sertraline in children and adolescents with obsessive compulsive behavior: a multicenter randomized controlled trial. JAMA 1998;280: 1752–6.

[81] Alderman J, Wolkow R, Chung M, et al. Sertraline treatment of children and adolescents with obsessive-compulsive disorder or depression: pharmacokinetics, tolerability, and efficacy. J Am Acad Child Adolesc Psychiatry 1998;37:386–94.

[82] Increase in the risk of birth defects. Available at: http://www.fda.gov/cder/drug/advisory/paroxetine200512.htm. Accessed January 29, 2006.

[83] Robert R, Blakeney PE, Villarreal C, et al. Imipramine treatment in pediatric burn patients with symptoms of acute stress disorder: a pilot study. J Am Acad Child Adolesc Psychiatry 1999;38:873–82.

[84] Ryan ND. Treatment of depression in children and adolescents. Lancet 2005;366:933–40.

[85] Steiner H, Saxena K, Chang K. Psychopharmacologic strategies for the treatment of aggression in juveniles. CNS Spectr 2003;8:298–308.

[86] Tobias JD, Berkenbosch JW. Sedation during mechanical ventilation in infants and children: dexmedetomidine versus midazolam. South Med J 2004;97:451–5.

[87] Serlin S. Dexmedetomidine in pediatrics: controlled studies needed [letter]. Anesth Analg 2004;98:1814.

[88] Boyd RD. Neuroleptic malignant syndrome and mental retardation: review and analysis of 29 cases. Am Assoc Ment Retard 1993;98:143–55.

[89] Kumra S, Herion D, Jacobsen LK, et al. Case study: risperidone-induced hepatotoxicity in pediatric patients. J Am Acad Child Adolesc Psychiatry 1997;36:701–5.

[90] Landau J, Martin A. Is liver function monitoring warranted during risperidone treatment? [letter] J Child Adolesc Psychiatry 1998;37:1007–8.

[91] Hanft A, Bourgeois J. Risperidone and pancreatitis [letter]. J Child Adolesc Psychiatry 2004;43:1458–9.

[92] Straus SM, Bleumink GS, Dieleman JP, et al. Antipsychotics and the risk of sudden cardiac death. Arch Intern Med 2004;164:1293–7.

[93] Liperti R, Gambassi G, Lapane KL, et al. Conventional and atypical antipsychotics and the risk of hospitalization for ventricular arrhythmias or cardiac arrest. Arch Intern Med 2005; 165:696–701.

[94] Labellarte MJ, Crosson JE, Riddle MA. The relevance of prolonged QTc measurement to pediatric psychopharmacology. J Am Acad Child Adolesc Psychiatry 2003;42:642–50.

[95] Asch DA, Parker RM. The Libby Zion case: one step forward, two steps backward. N Engl J Med 1988;318:771–5.

[96] Watson WA, Litovitz TL, Rogers GC Jr, et al. 2002 annual report of the American Association of Poison Control Centers Toxic Surveillance System. Am J Emerg Med 2003;21: 353–421.

[97] Gill M, LoVecchio F, Selden B. Serotonin syndrome in a child after a single dose of fluvoxamine. Ann Emerg Med 1999;33:457–9.

[98] Greenhill L, Vitiello B, Riddle MA, et al. Review of safety assessment methods used in pediatric psychopharmacology. J Am Acad Child Adolesc Psychiatry 2003;42:627–33.

[99] Biederman J, Spencer T, Wilens T. Psychopharmacology. In: Wiener JM, Dulcan MK, editors. The textbook of Child and Adolescent Psychiatry. Philadelphia: American Psychiatric Press; 2004. p. 931–73.

[100] Abrams AN, Muriel AC, Rauch PK. Consultation with children. In: Stern TA, Fricchione GL, Cassem NH, et al, editors. Massachusetts General Hospital handbook of general hospital psychiatry. 5th edition. St. Louis: Mosby; 2004. p. 641–70.

[101] American Psychiatric Association. Diagnostic and statistical manual of mental disorders, fourth edition, text revision (IV-TR). Washington, DC: American Psychiatric Press; 2000.

[102] Folstein MF, Folstein SE, McHugh PR. "Mini-mental state". A practical method for grading the cognitive state of patients for the clinician. J Psychiatr Res 1975;12:189–98.

[103] Ouvrier RA, Goldsmith RF, Ouvrier S, et al. The value of the mini-mental status examination in childhood: a preliminary study. J Child Neurol 1993;8:145–8.

[104] Knapp PK, Harris ES. Consultation-liaison in child psychiatry: a review of the past 10 years. Part I: clinical findings. J Am Acad Child Adolesc Psychiatry 1998;37: 139–46.

[105] Anand KS. Long-term consequences of pain in neonates In: Schechter NS, Berde CB, Yaster M, editors. Pain in infants, children and adolescents. 2nd edition. Philadelphia: Wilkins and Williams; 2003. p. 58–70.

[106] Gaffney A, McGrath PJ, Dick B. Measuring pain in children: developmental and instrument issues. In: Schechter N, Berde CB, Yaster M, editors. Pain in infants, children and adolescents. Baltimore: Williams & Wilkins; 2003. p. 128–41.

[107] Heiligenstein E, Steif BL. Tricyclics for pain. J Am Acad Child Adolesc Psychiatry 1989;28: 804–5.

[108] Rogers AG. Use of Amitriptyline for phantom limb pain in younger children. J Pain Symptom Manage 1989;4:96.

[109] Sikich NM, Lerman J. Development and psychometric evaluation of the pediatric anesthesia emergence delirium scale. Anesthesiology 2004;100:1138–45.

[110] Turkel SB, Braslow K, Tavare CJ, et al. The delirium rating scale in children and adolescents. Psychosomatics 2003;44:126–9.

[111] Cassem NH, Murray GB, Lafayette JM, et al. Delirious patients. In: Stern TA, Fricchione GL, Cassem NH, et al, editors. Massachusetts General Hospital handbook of general hospital psychiatry. 5th edition. St. Louis: Mosby; 2004. p. 119–34.

[112] Przbylo HJ, Martini DR, Mazurek AJ, et al. Assessing behavior in children emerging from anesthesia: can we apply psychiatric diagnostic techniques? Paediatr Anaesth 2003;13: 609–16.

[113] Turkel SB, Tavare CJ. Delirium in children and adolescents. J Neuropsychiatry Clin Neurosci 2003;15:431–5.

[114] Stoddard FJ, Wilens T. Delirium. In: Jellinek M, Herzog D, editors. Psychiatric aspects of general hospital pediatrics. Chicago: Yearbook Medical Publishers; 1990. p. 254–9.

[115] Stoddard FJ. Care of infants, children and adolescents with burn injuries. In: Lewis M, editor. Child and adolescent psychiatry. 3rd edition. Philadelphia: Lippincott Williams & Wilkins; 2002. p. 1188–208.

[116] Stoddard FJ, Levine JB, Lund K. Psychiatric care of the burn patient. In: Blumenfield M, Strain J, editors. Psychosomatic medicine in the 21st century. Lippincott Williams and Wilkins; in press.

[117] Ratliff SL, Meyer WJ, Cuervo LJ, et al. The use of haloperidol and associated complications in the agitated, acutely ill pediatric burn patient. J Burn Care Rehab 2004;25: 472–8.

[118] Kavanaugh CK, Lasoff E, Eide Y, et al. Learned helplessness and the pediatric burn patient: Dressing change behavior and serum cortisol and beta endorphin. J Pain Symptom Manage 1991;6:106–77.

[119] Stoddard FJ, Sheridan R, Selter L, et al. General surgery: basic principles. In: Stoudemire A, Fogel BS, Greenberg DB, editors. Psychiatric care of the medical patient. 2nd edition. Oxford University Press; 2000. p. 969–87.

[120] Canning EH, Canning RD, Boyce WT. Depressive symptoms and adaptive style in children with cancer. J Am Acad Child Adolesc Psychiatry 1992;31:1120–4.

[121] Luby JL, Heffelfinger A, Mrakotsky C. The clinical picture of depression in preschool children. J Am Acad Child Adolesc Psychiatry 2003;42:340–8.

[122] Gothelf D, Rubinstein M, Shemesh E, et al. Pilot study: fluvoxamine treatment for depression and anxiety in children and adolescents with cancer. J Am Acad Child Adolesc Psychiatry 2005;44:1258–62.

[123] Wozniak J, Biederman J, Richards JA. Diagnostic and therapeutic dilemmas in the management of pediatric bipolar disorder. J Clin Psychiatry 2001;62:10–5.

[124] Cassem NH, Papakostas GI, Fava M, et al. Mood-disordered patients. In: Stern TA, Fricchione GL, Cassem NH, et al, editors. Massachusetts General Hospital handbook of general hospital psychiatry. 5th edition. Philadelphia: Mosby; 2004. p. 69–92.

[125] Chess S, Thomas A. Origins and evolution of behavior disorders: from infancy to adult life. Cambridge (MA): Harvard University Press; 1984.

[126] Kovacs M. The natural history and course of depressive disorders in childhood. Psychiatr Ann 1985;15:387–9.

[127] Stoddard FJ, Norman DK, Murphy JM, et al. Psychiatric outcome of burned children and adolescents. J Am Acad Child Psychiatry 1989;4:589–95.

[128] Clinical Practice Guideline. Diagnosis and evaluation of the child with attention-deficit hyperactivity disorder. Pediatrics 2000;105:1158–70.

[129] Rowe R, Maughan B, Goodman R. Childhood psychiatric disorder and unintentional injury: findings from a national cohort study. J Pediatr Psychol 2004;29:119–30.

[130] Lam LT. Attention deficit disorder and hospitalization due to injury among older adolescents in New South Wales, Australia. J Atten Disord 2002;6:77–82.

[131] Prince JB, Wilens TE, Biederman J, et al. Psychopharmacology for children and adolescents. In: Stern TA, Fricchione GL, Cassem NH, et al, editors. Handbook of general hospital psychiatry. Philadelphia: Mosby; 2004. p. 411–5.

[132] Madrid AL, State MW, King BH. Pharmacologic management of psychiatric and behavioral symptoms in mental retardation. Child Adolesc Psychiatr Clin North Am 2000;9:225–44.

[133] McDougle CJ, Scahill L, McCracken JT, et al. Research units on pediatric psychopharmacology (RUPP) autism network: background and rationale for an initial controlled study of risperidone. Child Adolesc Psychiatr Clin North Am 2000;9:201–24.

[134] Jaffe SL, Simkin DR. Alcohol and drug abuse in children and adolescents. In: Lewis M, editor. Child and adolescent psychiatry: a comprehensive textbook. 2nd edition. Baltimore: Williams & Wilkins; 2002. p. 895–911.

[135] National Institute on Drug Abuse. Monitoring the future study: trends in prevalence of various drugs for 8th-graders, 10th-graders, and 12th-Graders. Available at: http://www.drugabuse.gov/infofacts/HSYouthtrends.html. Accessed November 5, 2005.

[136] Soderstrom CA, Dearing-Stuck BA. Substance misuse and trauma: clinical issue and injury prevention. Adolesc Med 1993;4:423–38.

[137] Gastfriend DR, Elman I, Sohkhah R. Psychotherapy of substance abuse and dependence. Psychatr Clin North Am 1998;5:211–9.

[138] Marsch LA, Bickel WK, Badger GJ, et al. Comparison of pharmacological treatments for opioid-dependent adolescents: a randomized controlled trial. Arch Gen Psychiatry 2005;62: 1157–64.

[139] Kaplan SJ. Child sexual abuse. In: Lewis M, editor. Child and adolescent psychiatry: a comprehensive textbook. 3rd edition. Baltimore: Williams & Wilkins; 2002. p. 1217–22.

[140] Kaplan SJ. Physical abuse and neglect. In: Lewis M, editor. Child and adolescent psychiatry: a comprehensive textbook. 2nd edition. Baltimore: Williams & Wilkins; 2001. p. 1208–16.

[141] Stoddard FJ. A psychiatric perspective on self-inflicted burns. J Burn Care Rehabil 1993;14: 480–2.

[142] Wolfe J, Grier HE, Klar N, et al. Symptoms and suffering at the end of life in children with cancer. N Engl J Med 2000;342:326–33.

[143] Carter BS, Howenstein M, Gilmer MJ, et al. Circumstances surrounding the deaths of hospitalized children: opportunities for pediatric palliative care. Pediatrics 2004;114:361–6.

[144] Garros D, Rosychuk RJ, Cox PN. Circumstances surrounding end of life in a pediatric intensive care unit. Pediatrics 2003;112:371.

[145] Frager G, Shapiro B. Pediatric palliative care and pain management. In: Holland JC, editor. Psycho-oncology. New York: Oxford University Press; 1998. p. 907–22.

[146] Spiegel L. Pediatric psychopharmacology. In: Holland JC, editor. Psycho-oncology. New York: Oxford University Press; 1998. p. 954–61.

[147] Dougherty M, DeBaun MR. Rapid increase of morphine and benzodiazepine usage in the last three days of life in children with cancer is related to neuropathic pain. J Pediatr 2003; 142:373–6.

[148] Bealke JM, Meighen KG. Risperidone treatment of three seriously medically ill children with secondary mood disorders. Psychosomatics 2005;46:254–8.

[149] Shiveld J, Leentjens AF. Delirium in severely ill young children in the pediatric intensive care unit (PICU). J Child Adolescent Psychiatry 2005;44:392–4.

[150] Himelstein BP, Hilden J, Boldt A, et al. Medical progress: pediatric palliative care. N Engl J Med 2004;350:1752–62.

[151] Yee JD, Berde C. Dextroamphetamine or methylphenidate as adjuvants to opioid analgesia for adolescents with cancer. J Pain Symptom Manage 1994;9:122–5.

[152] Rozans M, Dreisbach A, Lertora JJL, et al. Palliatve uses of methylphendate in patients with cancer: a review. J Clin Oncol 2002;20:335–9.

[153] Saxe G, Stoddard F, Courtney D, et al. Relationship between acute morphine and course of PTSD in children with burns: a pilot study. J Am Acad Child Adoles Psychiatry 2001;40: 915–21.

ELSEVIER
SAUNDERS

Child Adolesc Psychiatric Clin N Am
15 (2006) 657–682

CHILD AND
ADOLESCENT
PSYCHIATRIC CLINICS
OF NORTH AMERICA

Pain in Children Who Have Life-Limiting Conditions

Renée McCulloch, BMBS, MRCPaeds (UK),
Dip Pall Med (Paeds)*,
John J. Collins, MBBS, PhD, FFPMANZCA, FRACP

*The Children's Hospital at Westmead, Corner Hawksbury Road and Hainsworth Road,
Locked Bag 4001, Westmead, New South Wales 2145, Australia*

According to the World Health Organization (WHO) and the International Association for the Study of Pain [1], *pain* is "an unpleasant sensory and emotional experience associated with actual or potential tissue damage, or described in terms of such damage. In other words pain is a somatopsychic phenomenon."

The treatment of pain and alleviation of suffering should be the priority of every health care professional. Pain is a subjective, complicated phenomenon. It encompasses an enmeshment of conscious and subconscious factors: physical, psychologic, social, and spiritual. Each of these factors must be identified and evaluated if pain is to be understood and managed appropriately in any individual.

Over the last decade, increasing attention has been drawn toward the field of pediatric palliative care. An emerging body of experienced professionals are committed to developing a high standard of care accessible to all children and adolescents who have life-limiting illnesses. In addition, a significant proportion of time and effort has been dedicated to the investigation and management of pain in children and adolescents. Some of this knowledge may be directly related to the management of pain in those who have life-limiting illnesses. The complexity and questions of ethical validity of pain research in this particular pediatric population are fraught with difficulties. These are reflected in the paucity of available literature [2].

Palliative care for children is a broad discipline. Originally, in adults, the term "palliative care" was synonymous with end-of-life care. However, with

* Corresponding author.
E-mail address: reneem4@chw.edu.au (R. McCulloch).

doi:10.1016/j.chc.2006.02.001
childpsych.theclinics.com

improvement in health care and modern medical intervention, a small but significant number of children now live with complex chronic health needs associated with considerable morbidity. This large cohort of children who have life-limiting conditions may potentially receive "palliative care" over many years. This holistic care is focused on supporting the children and their families or caregivers in an appropriate environment (home, hospital, or hospice), providing symptom control and emotional support within a seamless individualized framework.

Pain is a prevalent symptom in this clinically diverse group of infants, children, and young people. The aforementioned definition of pain from the International Association for the Study of Pain implies a conscious awareness of pain. It is the interpretation of this "awareness" that challenges the health professional caring for the child or adolescent in pain. This interpretation can become even more complex in the neonate, preverbal, or neurocognitively impaired patient.

Epidemiology

It is impossible to be precise about epidemiologic data for children and young people living with life-limiting illness; there are no comprehensive registries. Studies generally involve small numbers of patients, and the huge variation and scope in morbidity are difficult to measure.

The following information, produced by the Association of Children with Life Threatening Conditions/Royal College of Physicians United Kingdom [3], is a helpful resource when considering the number and variable pathologic conditions of children requiring palliative care management:

> District-based data indicates the prevalence of severely ill children with life-limiting conditions in need of palliative care is at least 12 per 10,000. In practice it is suggested therefore that in a health district of 250,000 people, with a child population of approximately 50,000, in one year:
> Mortality: Eight are likely to die of a life-threatening condition, three of these from cancer, two of heart disease and three of other life-limiting conditions.
> Prevalence: Between 60-85 children are likely to have a life-limiting condition about half of whom will need active palliative care at any one time.
> In the United States, the Institute of Medicine reported that more than 50,000 children die each year, and hundreds of thousands more experience a life-limiting condition [4].

Pain in children who have cancer

The high prevalence of pain in pediatric patients who have cancer has been recognized for many years. It is well documented that children who have cancer experience pain related not only to disease but also to treatment and procedures. In 1987, Miser and colleagues [5] assessed the prevalence of pain in the pediatric and young adult cancer population. They found that 50% of inpatients and 25% of outpatients reported pain at the time of interview. Most pain was treatment related; tumor-related pain was reported in one third of hospital inpatients and 20% of outpatients. Treatment-related pain problems include mucositis, abdominal pain, pain associated with infection, and neuropathic pain [6,7]. Van Cleve and colleagues [8] reported similar patterns using a longitudinal descriptive study to collect data from 95 children (aged 4 to 17 years) who had leukemia during the first year of treatment. Most children in this study experienced intermittent moderate to severe pain at each of the seven data collection points over the year.

A further study by Miser and colleagues [9] showed that pain was the presenting symptom in 62% of children newly diagnosed with cancer. They also found that pain in this context had been persistent for a median of 74 days before treatment. One third of the patients reporting moderate to severe pain in this study were receiving no analgesia at all.

Children who have cancer pain often experience multiple symptoms that cause them significant distress and suffering. Collins and colleagues [10] measured symptom prevalence, characteristics, and distress in 160 children aged 10 to 18 years who had cancer. They found that symptom distress is relatively higher among inpatients, children who have solid tumors, and those undergoing chemotherapy treatments. The most common symptoms (prevalence greater than 35%) were lack of energy, pain, drowsiness, nausea, cough, lack of appetite, and psychologic symptoms (feeling sad, feeling nervous, worrying, feeling irritable). Of these, the symptoms that caused high distress in more than one third of patients were feeling sad, pain, nausea, lack of appetite, and feeling irritable.

Symptom experience in younger children has also been evaluated by Collins and colleagues [10], who assessed 149 children (aged 7 to 12 years) undergoing treatment for cancer. Approximately one third of this group had experienced lethargy, pain, and/or insomnia. The relationship between pain and suffering in children and young people must be acknowledged and addressed if care is to be truly holistic.

Pain in children who have noncancer diagnoses

Many causes of pain exist in children who have life-limiting conditions such as neuromuscular disorders, cystic fibrosis, and HIV/AIDS. Often these children suffer from chronic disease-related pain problems, with acute exacerbations of pain during intercurrent illnesses.

Pain may be underrecognized and underreported in children who have chronic conditions. A cross-sectional study over a 13-month period performed by Lolekha and colleagues [11] in 61 Thai children (aged 4 to 15 years) who had HIV/AIDS showed that 44% reported pain compared with 13% in the control group (age-matched controls with no chronic condition). Of those in pain, only 44% received analgesic treatment.

Historically, aggressive treatment of pain with opioid analgesia has not been part of the routine management plan in children who have cystic fibrosis, possibly because of fears of respiratory compromise. Koh and colleagues [12] published a survey assessing acute and chronic pain symptoms in 46 children (mean age 12.9 years) who had cystic fibrosis (CF). This outpatient group reported low-intensity frequent pain (occurring at least once a week), mainly localized to the abdomen, chest, and head/neck regions. A small subset of the group (15%) experienced pain lasting half a day or longer, and 11% had moderately intense pain. In this group, frequency and intensity of pain did not correlate with disease severity.

Chronic pain in patients who have CF has been reported in other studies. A retrospective review at a tertiary center evaluated pain in young adults who had advanced CF and found that chest pain and headaches were the most prevalent pain complaints; abdominal, back, and limb pain also occurred regularly. Successful analgesia without adverse effects was achieved using opioids in those who were referred for pain management [13].

The end-of-life treatment pathway for children and young people who have CF often involves significant disease-related treatments that are provided in parallel with palliative care and comfort measures. Pain seems to be a significant symptom in this population. Of 44 patient charts reviewed at the Children's Hospital in Boston, 38 patients (86%) received opiates for severe dyspnea and pain at the end of life. The duration of treatment varied between 1 month and 1 hour before death [14].

Pain in the neurocognitively impaired child

Children with special needs, including those who have significant physical disability and cognitive impairment, are at risk for poor pain management [15]. Over the last 10 years there has been increasing awareness of the pain experiences of these vulnerable children. A qualitative study that interviewed 15 parents and caregivers of 12 children with profound special needs found that all parents believed that their children had suffered with pain all of their lives and had simply been required to "learn to live with it" [16].

Breau and colleagues [17] studied episodes of pain in 94 children (aged 3 to 18 years) who had moderate to profound learning difficulties. Data was collected at four specific weekly points over 1 year from the main caregivers. This study found that 78% of children experienced pain during the studied time points. Pain related to accidents was the most frequent type (30%); other causes included gastrointestinal pain (22%), infection (20%), and musculoskeletal pain (19%). Pain intensity scores were higher in those with nonaccidental pain, which occurred more frequently in children who had the most severe cognitive impairment. Other studies have highlighted dislocated hips, back pain secondary to scoliosis and facet joint arthritis, muscle spasm, and gastroesophageal reflux as causes of pain in children who have developmental disability [18–20].

In a recent study by Houlihan and colleagues [21], pain was evaluated in 198 children who had various degrees of cerebral palsy. Pain was related to severity of motor impairment and the presence of a gastrostomy; 11% of parents reported pain experiences on a daily basis. Pain was correlated with the number of absences from school and days spent in bed. Pain frequency was greatest in the more severely affected children. The authors concluded that "Pain was more prevalent with more severe impairment and was associated with educational and social consequences." This conclusion coincides with data from a group of 34 verbally limited, cognitively impaired children whose parents collected information regarding pain experience over a 2-week period. The majority of children suffered from pain experiences; four experienced moderate or severe pain on 5 or more days. No child in the study group was receiving active pain management [22].

The available literature supports the notion that those children with the most complex impairment suffer from a considerable burden of pain. This pain is multifactorial and significantly affects the children and their families.

Pain in children at the end of life

Pain is a common symptom in children and adolescents at the end of life. A review of deaths in a children's hospice reported that more than 80% of patients had pain recorded as a symptom in the last month of life [23]. A recent retrospective study examined assessment and treatment of symptoms during end-of-life care over a 1-year period in a children's hospital. Of the 105 children who died in the hospital, 90% received analgesics in the 72 hours before death [24].

The number of children who die with inadequately treated pain is not known. In 1998, a Finnish study retrospectively recorded the analgesic requirements of 70 children who died from cancer-related diseases and interviewed the children's parents. Eighty-nine percent of patients required regular analgesics at the end of life. Those who had brain tumors and solid tumors required a longer duration of treatment than those who had leukemia (66, 58, and 17 days, respectively). Significantly, in 19% of the children, analgesia was thought to have been suboptimal [25]. Inadequately treated pain appears to be a recurring feature when parents are asked to recall the symptoms of their dying children [26,27].

Assessment and measurement of pain in children

Successful pain management involves comprehensive, age-appropriate assessment, an individual treatment plan, and regular review. It is imperative that the cause and mechanism of pain be identified. Factors influencing the pain experience and pain-related behaviors must also receive consideration.

For pediatric pain to be managed well, a thorough assessment must include appropriate measurement of pain. Measurement relies on a metric dimension applied to a specific aspect of pain, traditionally considered in terms of pain severity. Assessment involves considering all the factors that may be affecting a child's pain experience: developmental stage, intelligence, personality, temperament, previous pain experience, expectation and acceptance of pain, child and parent coping strategies, fear and anxieties, cultural background, and prognosis.

Pain assessment includes collecting factual information: the history of illness and disease pathology; the quantity, type, and frequency of medication given; dose-limiting side effects; and the nursing staff's impression of the child's pain. Although any particular piece is potentially unreliable, gathering all available information is an important part of the assessment process. Preferentially, children are asked about their pain using their own usual descriptive language. Often the parent or caregiver is relied on for a proxy measure of pain on the child's behalf. This is valuable information, but care must be taken to maintain the patient as the primary source if possible. Listening and paying attention to the child or adolescent helps the patient and family to develop trust and confidence in the health professional; it also validates the pain experience.

Assessment should include all the standard parameters: location, radiation, duration, associated sensation, exacerbating and relieving factors, previous pain experience, impact on emotions, and degree of impairment of usual activities.

Most children older than 2 years can report the presence and location of pain, but the cognitive skills required to describe pain intensity do not develop until the age of 3 or 4 years [28–30]. This ability to describe and quantify pain follows developmental age progression with much variability. Children who are 5 years or older can usually rate and score pain, whereas 8-year-olds are able to describe the quality of the pain experience. Describing how pain affects emotion requires more abstract concepts [31–33].

Practical pain measurement tools

Pain measurement tools of variable reliability and validity are available for use in pediatrics. Many have been developed in the context of postoperative care or pain research or for use in specific clinical situations. Measures are classified into self-report, behavioral, or physiologic measures.

Self-report measures are considered the "gold standard" measurement tool for patients who have sufficient cognitive and language ability to understand the concepts and deliver an accurate response [31,34]. They exist in verbal and nonverbal formats. Visual analogue scales with various facial expressions have excellent practical utility and validity, especially in young children. They consist of a series of faces with a range of expressions, from neutral or smiling to crying and distress [28,29,31,34]. Quantitative self-report scales, such as the 0 to 10 Likert-type scale, require a more complex understanding of proportionality that generally emerges between the ages of 5 and 7. The concept that pain severity occurs between anchors, within a scale from 0 to 10, must be understood for a patient to self-report pain intensity.

Changes in physiologic parameters, such as in blood pressure or heart rate, are occasionally helpful, especially in intensive care units when one is assessing the sedated patient. They are usually used in conjunction with other measures of acute pain. However, they are neither consistent nor reliable correlates of pain, especially in the setting of chronic pain.

It may be impossible to use self-report methods in some children, for instance in infants, the preverbal or cognitively impaired child, or the very ill. Formal behavior measurement scales that use body posture, movement, facial expression, and crying have been developed and show good reliability [35,36]. Ramelet and colleagues [37] comment that behavioral measurement scales may not be suitable for evaluating pain in the critically ill child, because the items included were derived from relatively healthy children and may not reflect pain behavior in the seriously ill.

The measurement of pain in the cognitively impaired has received greater attention in recent years. A substantial number of children in this population die prematurely and are thought to suffer from frequent pain episodes. Existing verbal communication skills obviously limit the use of self-report measures in this group. Variable facial expressions and body movements (abnormal posturing, contractures, paralysis, involuntary posturing) preclude standardized coding. In addition, manifestation of disability, such as spasm, crying out, or grimacing, can mimic behaviors commonly attributed to pain. Biersdorff [38] has described paradoxical pain behaviors in which individuals have learned to mimic pain behavior while not in pain. In the same vein, the cognitively impaired child who laughs during a painful procedure may use laughter as a signal for pain. A study of the pain cues reported by caregivers of noncommunicative children (aged 2 to 12 years) who had life-limiting conditions revealed a common "core" of six behavioral pain cues, including screaming or yelling, crying, showing distressed facial expression, becoming difficult to comfort, flinching when touched, and tensing the body [39].

The Non Communicating Children's Pain Check list was originally validated for use in the home by parents and caregivers and then modified for use postoperatively [40–42]. In the third study, 24 children were observed by one caregiver and one researcher pre- and postoperatively and each child's pain intensity rated. Breau and colleagues [42] concluded that familiarity with an individual child was not necessary for pain assessment. This result contrasts with that of a study involving 15 parents of children with profound special needs who believed that the assessment of pain in their children was a complex process requiring in-depth knowledge and skills developed over years. In this qualitative study, all the parents based their pain assessments on a change in behavioral pattern and individual mood of the child. The parents believed that they were underutilized by professionals as a resource and that they had to act as "strident advocates" for alleviation of their child's pain [16].

The Gauvain-Piquard Scale [43] is a behavioral observation tool that has been specifically developed for the measurement of chronic pain in children aged 2 to 6 years who have cancer. The revised edition contains 15 items: nine specific to pain assessment, six indicative of "psychomotor retardation," and four relating to anxiety. It specifically acknowledges the psychologic effects of chronic pain in this population.

The Memorial Assessment Scale is a multidimensional symptom assessment tool that has been modified from an adult version and developed for children who have cancer. Two available scales have been validated in different age groups. They evaluate pain as well as other symptoms. Children reported on how frequent, distressing, and severe they found their symptoms, thus producing some insight into the impact of symptoms on level of functioning [10,44].

No specific scales exist for measuring pain in the palliative care situation or at the end of life in children. In fact, retrospective studies have shown inadequate pain assessment in this cohort [24,45]. A Canadian study revealed that only 5 out of 77 charts (6%) of children who had died in the hospital contained specific pain assessment and treatment records [45]. The Joint Commission on Accreditation and Health care Organizations in the United States has mandated pain assessment in charting of hospitalized patients. The standardization of documentation and implementation of improved treatment planning are the necessary next steps for improvement of pain management.

Therapeutics

The management of pain in children and adolescents who have life-limiting illness pivots on continuing evaluation, assessment, measurement, and treatment. This process requires commitment from a dedicated team who can follow the pain trajectory over time. Addressing the impact of pain or treatments on function and feelings is central to this process. It has been well documented that physicians underestimate patients' pain and discomfort and tend to misunderstand quality of life issues, particularly with regard to subjective attributes in chronic disease [46,47]. An awareness of this discrepancy is essential to a functioning relationship between the physician, patient, and family.

It is clear that parents and caregivers value consistent input from someone who knows their child well. Contro and colleagues [26] interviewed 68 bereaved family members and found that, despite describing the torment of seeing their child in pain, they believed that their child's pain was "well managed." These comments may reflect parents' difficulty in acknowledging suboptimal care or belief that their child's pain was resistant to medical management. The authors quote parents who expressed gratitude toward clinicians who sought advice, gave honest information, and made trials of different options for analgesia, thus endorsing care and attention as paramount.

Nonpharmacologic management of pain

Growing evidence supports the valuable contribution of nonpharmacologic intervention to pain management in children and adolescents. Nonpharmacologic techniques include psychologic intervention, acupuncture, transcutaneous electrical nerve stimulation, and physical therapies such as massage and heat therapy. In-depth discussion of these techniques is beyond the scope of this article. Cognitive-behavioral psychologic interventions for pain management are discussed in detail elsewhere in this volume, in the article by Yaldoo-Poltorak and Benore.

Pharmacologic management of pain

A wealth of analgesic studies is now available to the clinician. The challenge is to interpret these data with regard to the various pediatric populations (neonate, infant, young child, and older) and in the setting of serious illness. The pharmacokinetics and pharmacodynamics of drugs vary with the physical development of a child. Age-related differences in renal blood flow, protein binding of drugs, maturity of the hepatic-enzyme systems, and many other factors contribute to the effects and metabolism of analgesic medication [48].

Historically, therapeutic trials in children have been difficult to perform. Pediatrics is fraught with practical and ethical dilemmas. This problem is heightened in the field of pediatric palliative care, where there are a wide range of pathologic conditions and statistically small numbers of children. The very nature of the pediatric treatment pathway and the often sudden switch to palliation are also limiting. For instance, parents and physicians of children who have advanced cancer attempt curative treatment even at a late stage in the disease trajectory. Consequently, there is a limited cohort of children with a chronic pain model available for evaluation.

When prescribing analgesics, it is beneficial to distinguish the mechanism or mechanisms of pain. Pain mechanisms are generally described in terms of nociceptive pain and neuropathic pain:

Nociceptive pain: tissue damage or inflammation detected by a normally functioning nervous system. This may also be described as somatic or visceral pain.

Neuropathic pain: discomfort that arises because of an abnormal excitability in the peripheral or central nervous system.

Nonopioid analgesics
Acetaminophen (paracetamol). Acetaminophen is the most widely used analgesic agent in pediatrics. It has both analgesic and antipyretic properties.

It is useful for mild to moderate pain and has a good safety margin when used in appropriate doses. It has a synergistic effect when used in combination with an opioid [49].

Acetaminophen is now available in the intravenous preparation in some countries (not including the United States) and has been shown to be effective in infants and children [50]. This preparation may prove to be particularly beneficial to those at the end of life when the oral route is not suitable. Rectal dosing has been frequently used in this population but has variable, slow absorption; larger doses are therefore recommended [51].

Nonsteroidal anti-inflammatory drugs. Nonsteroidal anti-inflammatory drugs (NSAIDs) are also widely used in infants and children. They have anti-inflammatory effects in addition to analgesic and antipyretic properties. They are often used as adjuncts to opioid therapy and have been shown to reduce postoperative opioid requirements [52]. No proven benefit of the intravenous route over the oral route exists, nor is there evidence to suggest that one NSAID has more analgesic effect than another [53]. Caution should be exercised with prolonged exposure to NSAIDs, because they can cause gastrointestinal bleeding, nephropathy, and bleeding secondary to platelet dysfunction [54].

The newer selective cyclo-oxygenase–2 (COX-2) inhibitors have less of an effect than the classical NSAIDs on in-vitro platelet function and have been shown to reduce gastric side effects in short-term use [55,56]. Recent studies in adults showing cardiovascular complications with short-term use have led to prompt international withdrawal of some of these drugs. Little conclusive evidence exists concerning the use of COX-2 inhibitors in children, with postoperative studies reporting variable results. It may be appropriate to prescribe this class of drug in the pediatric palliative care setting, because the analgesic benefit may outweigh potential risks.

Adjuvants. Adjuvant analgesics are defined as drugs with a primary indication other than pain that have analgesic properties in some situations. They are primarily used in patients who have chronic pain either as a first-line medication or as a coanalgesic. Adjuvant analgesics consist of a varied group of medications with considerable diversity of primary indications. Some adjuvants have broad analgesic properties (eg, corticosteroids, antidepressants, neuroleptics), whereas others have more specific indications, for instance, neuropathic pain (anticonvulsants, N-methyl-D-aspartate receptor antagonists), bone pain (bisphosphonates, calcitonin), musculoskeletal pain (benzodiazepines, botulinum toxin A), and pain from bowel spasm or obstruction (anticholinergics, octreotide). A paucity of data support the use of adjuvants in acute pain, although N-methyl-D-aspartate receptor antagonists (eg, ketamine) and membrane stabilizers (eg, lidocaine) have been used with success in acute pain crises.

Many children who have life-limiting conditions experience chronic pain. Simple opioid regimes are often adequate for relieving pain. Seventy percent of adult patients who have cancer achieve good pain control with straightforward opioid management [57]. In some situations, such as when there is a significant element of neuropathic pain, an adjuvant may provide analgesic benefit. Adult studies have shown that as much as 40% to 50% of cancer pain may be classified as neuropathic [58]. Because young children are often unable to report the quality of pain, the presence of neuropathic pain may go unrecognized in this group.

Randomized controlled trials have shown the efficacy of both antidepressants and anticonvulsants in a variety of chronic neuropathic pain states in adults. Evidence suggests that antidepressant treatment (ie, amitriptyline) may be better as a first-line adjuvant analgesic than an anticonvulsant [59,60]. A single night-time dose of amitriptyline is the usual starting point for children who have neuropathic pain (after an initial electrocardiogram to exclude underlying arrhythmias). However, gabapentin is also frequently used in children because of its safety and tolerability profile.

Although clinical trials describing the use of adjuvants as analgesics exist, there are few comparative studies. The use of these medications in the palliative care setting is usually based on the nature of the pain complaint and knowledge of the pharmacologic characteristics and actions of the adjunct. The doses required for children have evolved from anecdotal report, extrapolation from adult data, and knowledge of the doses and side-effect profile of the drug in its primary indication. Initially low doses are titrated upward depending on effect and tolerability.

Opioids

Opioids are prescribed for moderate to severe pain in children and infants. They provide the cornerstone for pain management in children who have life-limiting illnesses. Historically, children have received inadequate doses of morphine, presumably because of fears of potential respiratory depression or addiction. Adult studies have shown that the risk for addiction is negligible [61]. No evidence suggests that the risk is any different in the pediatric population. In fact, a Brazilian study examining the clinical aspects and treatment of pain in children and adolescents who had cancer found psychologic dependence on morphine in 2% (2/111) of patients, with one of these already suffering from underlying drug dependence [62]. Unfortunately, fears regarding dependence still persist: a recent Canadian survey of pain practices in pediatric oncology centers cited fear of addiction as a barrier to optimal pain management [63]. This fear mirrors the worries often expressed by parents and caregivers to clinicians when discussing the prescribing of opioids in children.

Guidelines for pediatric pain management now exist in many hospitals, focusing generally on procedural, postoperative, or acute pain. Few if any guidelines exist for pediatric pain management in patients with complex chronic conditions at the end of life. Guidelines are available for children who have cancer, but it is difficult to establish adherence by and efficacy to clinicians [1,64,65]. A survey of 47 pediatric departments in Sweden, with a 100% response rate, showed that 63% of respondents followed the WHO "analgesic ladder," but 72% believed that pain could have been treated more effectively [66].

Initial dose recommendations for opioid prescription are outlined in Table 1.

Codeine. WHO guidelines recommend the use of codeine, a weak opioid, for moderate pain. Codeine must be extensively metabolized by the liver to produce an active morphine metabolite. A large proportion of children have inefficient hepatic conversion of codeine (as large as 36% in a recent pediatric study), resulting in inadequate analgesia and an increased requirement for rescue analgesia [67]. Generally, the use of codeine is limited to short-term treatment of mild pain.

Morphine. Despite limitations, over the past decade, a greater understanding of the pharmacokinetics and pharmacodynamics of opioids has encouraged more confident and appropriate prescribing. This is especially true for morphine. Morphine is typically the first-choice opioid for moderate to severe pain in pediatric palliative care worldwide. This popularity is due to its cost, accessibility, familiarity, effectiveness, and convenience. It is also the only opioid that has been extensively studied in children. Doses must be adjusted according to age, weight, and individual response. It is important to be aware that neonates and young infants have significant differences in morphine metabolism compared with older children [68,69]. For example, the elimination half-life of parenteral morphine is 6 to 8 hours in a neonate, compared with 2 hours in older children [70]. Because the clearance and half-life of morphine are shorter in children than adults, a smaller dosing interval may be required to achieve good pain control, particularly with slow-release medication [71,72]. Immediate-release morphine should be prescribed at an appropriate interval of every 2 to 4 hours, in some cases hourly in a supervised environment when titrating doses.

Historically, clinicians have been reluctant to use opioids in children with nonmalignant disease on a long-term basis. Once again, this reluctance was probably due to fears of addiction and escalating doses secondary to tolerance. Over the last decade, these concerns have been rationalized, and opioids are now being judiciously prescribed in children with nonmalignant chronic pain.

It is usual to consider alternative opioids when there are undesirable side effects of morphine or reduced renal function. However, there are also occasions when alternative opioids offer specific advantages over morphine.

Oxycodone. Oxycodone is a semisynthetic opioid with agonist activity at both the kappa and mu receptors. Its analgesic and side-effect profiles are

Table 1
Starting doses of commonly used opioids in pediatric patients according to body weight

Drug	Usual IV starting dose		Usual po starting dose	
	<50 kg	>50 kg	<50 kg	>50 kg
Morphine	0.1 mg/kg q 3–4 h	5–10 mg q 3–4 h	0.3 mg/kg q 3–4 h	30 mg q 3–4 h
Hydromorphone	0.015 mg/kg q 3–4 h	1–1.5 mg q 3–4 h	0.06 mg/kg q 3–4 h	6 mg q 3–4 h
Oxycodone	Not available	Not available	0.3 mg/kg q 3–4 h[a]	10 mg q 3–4 h
Fentanyl	0.5–1.5 mcg/kg q 1–2 h	25–75 mcg q 1–2 h	Not available	Not available

[a] Smallest tablet size is 5 mg.

Data from Berde CB, Collins JJ. Analgesic therapy and palliative care in children. In: Wall and Melzack's Textbook of Pain. 5th edition. Philadelphia: Elsevier; 2006. p. 1133.

similar to those of morphine, to which it is an effective alternative [73]. The equianalgesic dose of oral oxycodone is between one half and two thirds that of oral morphine, but it has a systemic bioavailability of as much as 90% [74]. Oxycodone has been administered by the buccal, nasal, and rectal routes [74–76]. A long-acting preparation of oxycodone is available for use. The importance and clinical relevance of oxycodone in the management of pediatric pain are still emerging.

Hydromorphone. Hydromorphone is a morphine analogue with similar pharmacokinetic and pharmacodynamic properties, but it is approximately 5 to 7.5 times more potent than morphine and has higher bioavailability [77,78]. It is generally used as an alternative to morphine when an opioid switch is required or, practically, when the volume of morphine solution becomes excessive.

Collins and colleagues [79] compared the safety and efficacy of hydromorphone with morphine in the treatment of mucositis in children following bone marrow transplant. Although the numbers in this study were small (10 patients participated), the authors concluded that hydromorphone was not superior to morphine in terms of analgesic efficacy and side effect profile and that hydromorphone may be less potent in children than the adult equipotency tables indicate. Systematic reviews in the adult literature have found no difference between hydromorphone and other opioids in terms of analgesia, side effects, and patient preference [80].

Fentanyl. Fentanyl is a synthetic opioid with several useful properties. It is highly lipophilic and is 80 to 100 times more potent than morphine. Fentanyl is available in a transdermal "patch" preparation, bypassing the need for intravenous or subcutaneous administration. This property is especially useful in palliative care when oral or intravenous administration is difficult, limiting, or causing distress or when compliance is an issue. The patch is most useful in the context of chronic pain and has been evaluated in the pediatric cancer and palliative populations [81–83]. It is not suitable in circumstances where rapid-dose adjustments are anticipated or as a first-line opioid. It does not appear to culminate in renal failure and may offer a better side-effect profile, with reduced constipation, itching, and urinary retention [83,84].

In a small study using a clinical protocol, feasibility, tolerability, and utility of transdermal fentanyl were demonstrated in 11 children with cancer pain. The mean clearance and volume of distribution of transdermal fentanyl were the same in children and adults, but the variability was higher in adults [81]. A larger study is required to confirm these findings.

A recent international study by Finkel and colleagues [85] has assessed the safety and tolerability profile of transdermal fentanyl, in addition to titration and conversion schedules, in a single-arm, nonrandomized, multicenter trial. In 173 patients (malignant n = 132; nonmalignant n = 67) aged 2 to 16 years who completed an initial 15-day treatment period, pain intensity scores and treatment satisfaction improved from baseline. Stable analgesic requirements were reached after 6 days (ie, two patch changes) in most patients.

Until recently, the dosage of the lowest-strength fentanyl patch was often too high as an initial starting dose for infants and small children. A 12-µg per hour fentanyl patch is now available in some countries. This will facilitate the use of the transdermal patch in younger age groups.

A transmucosal form of fentanyl is also available for breakthrough pain. It is absorbed quickly from the oral mucosa and acts within minutes [86]. It is particularly useful in mechanical pain. Again, the available preparations are in relatively large doses for young children but may be appropriate for the older age group. Obviously, a degree of understanding and compliance is required for successful use.

Methadone. Methadone is a synthetic opioid agonist with N-methyl-D-aspartate antagonist (NMDA) properties. It is therefore of potential benefit in those patients who have neuropathic or mixed pain problems. Over the last decade there has been increasing use of methadone as a second-line opioid in adult patients who have cancer. It is well absorbed and has no known active metabolites [87]. Methadone may be administered by the oral, rectal, intravenous, and nasal routes [88,89]. Anecdotally, methadone has been used successfully by the buccal/nasal route in children at the end of life when the oral route is no longer available.

Concerns exist about the prescribing of methadone; it has a long, unpredictable half-life (as long as 120 hours) and consequent potential for delayed toxicity. These concerns are heightened in children because minimal published evidence exists, other than limited reports of the use of methadone in small patient numbers [90–92]. Methadone is used frequently worldwide, because in some countries it is one of the cheaper, most available opioids.

N-methyl-D-aspartate receptor antagonists

Ketamine. Ketamine is widely used in children as an anesthetic agent. In subanesthetic doses, it is analgesic. In children there is concern that it may cause unpleasant psychomimetic side effects, such as hallucinations and excessive sedation [93].

Ketamine is a noncompetitive antagonist of the NMDA receptor [94]. Extensive research into the role of the NMDA receptor in pain pathophysiology has renewed clinical interest in ketamine as a potentially valuable analgesic, specifically in the context of nociceptive and neuropathic pain. Strong pain stimuli activate NMDA receptors, inducing central sensitization (spinal cord neuronal excitability), wind-up phenomenon (an acute form of pain amplification), and pain memory by means of dorsal horn neurones [94]. Ketamine has a role in blocking these actions.

Ketamine has been shown to improve analgesia in patients who have severe pain that is poorly responsive to opioids and to reduce opioid requirements in opioid-tolerant patients [95,96]. In postoperative patients, ketamine has an opioid-sparing effect [97]. Its use as an adjunct to opioids has been limited, because clinical trials have shown contradictory results [98].

Insufficient data exist to advocate the use of ketamine as a standard analgesic in pediatric pain. Occasionally, ketamine is useful in complex pain situations when standard pharmacotherapies have failed. Clinical usage in pediatrics is increasing in the setting of rapid opioid dose escalation, perceived tolerance, and severe neuropathic pain.

Routes of administration

Opioids may be administered by many different routes: oral, parenteral, rectal, intravenous, subcutaneous, intramuscular, topical, intraspinal, intrathecal, nebulized, buccal, and intranasal. This flexibility is often advantageous in the end-of-life situation when the oral route is no longer feasible.

Many children do not have central venous access available for intravenous administration of drugs at the end of life. The subcutaneous route of administration can be useful in this situation. It offers a constant delivery of medication that may be easily titrated. Several drugs may be administered at the same time by means of a portable infusion pump. Most pumps also offer the option of delivering a bolus dose of medication. This route offers simplicity with relatively little medical or nursing input. Subcutaneous infusion rates should rarely exceed 1 to 3 mL/h [99]. Subcutaneous cannulas are placed after application of topical local anesthetic and can be patent for several days.

Rectal administration of medication can be useful in the infant and young child, although there is significant variability of rectal drug absorption. It is not recommended in children who have cancer because of increased risk for infection.

Opioids such as diamorphine, methadone, fentanyl, and oxycodone are increasingly being administered by the buccal or sublingual route. The buccal route is more tolerable than the nasal route and offers rapid absorption, bypassing the first-pass hepatic mechanism [100]. Symptoms are relieved quickly and effectively. Parents often describe the difficulty of "waiting" for enteral opioids to take effect. Hence there is huge benefit in a fast-acting, easily administered, effective analgesic in the pediatric population.

Intraspinal analgesia is used rarely as a means of analgesia in pediatric terminal malignancy [101]. Collins and colleagues [102,103] have described three groups of patients in whom this approach may be beneficial: (1) children who have dose-limiting side effects despite adjunctive treatment; (2) children whose pain is poorly responsive to huge opioid infusions; and (3) children who have depressed mental status secondary to opioids and in whom sedation is not desirable.

Other physical approaches to analgesia

Although modalities such as radiotherapy, radiologic guided nerve blocks, transcutaneous nerve stimulation, and radiopharmaceuticals are prominent in clinical practice, little published evidence supports their use in pediatrics.

The use of strontium-89 has been reported to be beneficial in children who have metastatic cancer, but the numbers studied were too small to draw clinical conclusions [104]. Palliative radiotherapy is frequently requested for relief from bone pain caused by metastatic disease. A case series of 29 children with metastatic neuroblastoma reported some benefit after radiotherapy to painful sites [105].

The pediatric pain crisis

A pain crisis in any child must be addressed quickly and effectively. The pain crisis in a child at the end of life is an emergency. It may involve multiple pathologic conditions or be due to escalating pain symptoms from a single cause. It is preferable that a specific diagnosis is made in this situation, because treating the primary cause of the pain will ultimately yield the most effective outcome.

The management of severe, intractable pain involves incremental intravenous or subcutaneous doses at regular 10- to 15-minute intervals until effective analgesia or somnolence occurs. This process requires a confident and familiar approach to opioid administration and may require the physician to be present at the bedside orchestrating this management. The "opioid loading dose" is the total amount of opioid needed to achieve a reduction in pain intensity. In most patients, a continuous infusion of opioid is then required to maintain analgesia. The infusion rate is calculated from the loading dose required. This is often significantly more than the "standard" doses quoted in pediatric prescribing reference manuals. In other circumstances, intermittent parenteral opioid may be an alternative to an intravenous infusion if pain is unpredictable and sporadic.

When a child is particularly at risk for a pain crisis at home, appropriate arrangements must be made in order for the family to administer medication safely and effectively. The buccal route is an efficient and effective mode of delivery either with or without additional intravenous or subcutaneous access.

Episodic (breakthrough) pain

Episodic pain is a "transitory exacerbation of pain that occurs in addition to otherwise stable persistent pain" [106]. Historically, episodic pain has been associated with malignant disease. In children who have complex, non-malignant conditions, episodic pain can be a frequent complaint secondary to a multitude of pathologic conditions, such as muscle spasm, reflux esophagitis, or orthopedic problems. Episodic pain may occur in any condition when baseline analgesia is inadequate and simply "wears off." Classic cancer-related episodic or "incident" pain is associated with more severe pathologic conditions and consequent functional and psychologic distress [107].

The incidence and prevalence of episodic pain have been studied in adult patients who have cancer, and morbidity is significant [108]. No such data exist in the pediatric population.

Treatment is aimed at the cause of pain, but "breakthrough" or "rescue" doses of analgesia are often required for the alleviation of episodic pain. These are additional intravenous, oral, or buccal doses of opioid that are incorporated into the analgesic regimen. The dose is calculated as one tenth to one sixth of the total daily oral opioid requirement and may be given hourly or more often if necessary.

When children have severe pain for which they require frequent doses of additional analgesia, a patient-controlled analgesia (PCA) device may offer more convenient and effective pain relief. This device can deliver bolus doses of intravenous or subcutaneous drugs as necessary. Children from the age of 7 are able to use a PCA effectively [109].

Opioid dose escalation

When pain can be controlled by the opioid loading technique described earlier, subsequent opioid dose escalation may be calculated as follows:

If greater than approximately four to six breakthrough doses of opioid are required in a 24-hour period, then the hourly average of this total daily rescue opioid should be added to the baseline opioid infusion. An alternative is to increase the baseline infusion by 50% [110].

Breakthrough doses are kept as a proportion of the baseline opioid infusion rate and, with dose titration, are recalculated as between 50% and 200% of the hourly basal infusion [110].

Opioid switching

Although most patients receive effective analgesia with morphine, a small number (approximately 10% to 30% of adult patients who have cancer pain) may suffer from inadequate pain relief, intolerable side effects, or both [111]. In these circumstances it is now becoming standard clinical practice to switch to an alternative opioid. The evidence to support this practice is largely anecdotal or based on uncontrolled or observational studies [112]. Data regarding opioid switching in pediatrics are emerging. A recent study reviewing opioid prescriptions in a large children's hospital showed that opioid switching was employed in 9% of all opioid prescriptions. This practice resulted in an improved side-effect profile without a significant change in pain scores. Itching was the most common indication for switching the opioid [113].

Frequently, following a period of single opioid use, equivalent analgesia may be attained with a second opioid at a dose that is markedly less than the corresponding equianalgesic quantity (approximately 50% for short half-life opioids). Similarly, the dose of methadone (which has a prolonged half-life) required for a switch from a short half-life opioid is on the order of 10% to

20%. No protocol for opioid switch doses or equianalgesic tables exist that are specific to pediatrics. Usually the doses are extrapolated using available adult data. Protocols for methadone dose conversion and titration have been documented in the adult literature [114,115].

Opioid side effects

Evaluation of opioid side effects should be included in the assessment of analgesic effectiveness. All opioids produce a range of side effects, including constipation, nausea and vomiting, pruritis, sedation, vivid dreams, urinary retention, and respiratory depression. Itching and constipation are common problems. Administration of a laxative should be commenced on initiation of opioid treatment. Children rarely volunteer information about side effects, so inquiries should be made directly to the child and his or her caregiver. Adverse effects may confer greater weight in children than adults. Children may not "tolerate" side effects as adults would. This ability to acknowledge cause and effect evolves with maturity. Children may be unable to rationalize with themselves about the benefits of continuing an opioid that provides good pain relief but makes them itchy. Side effects must therefore be anticipated and managed aggressively. Left untreated, the side effects may be as distressing as the pain for which the medication is being prescribed, if not more.

New evidence exists regarding the use of naloxone, an opioid receptor antagonist, to counteract opioid-induced side effects. In a double-blind prospective randomized, controlled study, Maxwell and colleagues [116] studied 46 postoperative children and adolescents. They found that a parallel small-dose naloxone infusion significantly reduced the incidence of opioid-induced side effects without affecting opioid-induced analgesia. This practice may be advantageous when there are dose-limiting side effects despite opioid switching.

Confusion and agitation are symptoms that are not only distressing for the child or adolescent but also profoundly upsetting to their caregivers. The memory of the symptomatology of the dying child remains with parents and caregivers forever and can drastically affect the bereavement process [117]. Generally, judicious titration of opioids and the use of adjuvant medication can broaden the therapeutic approach and mitigate or prevent drug-induced toxicity.

A strong possibility that symptoms are attributable to opioid therapy may support changing to an alternative opioid. This clinical decision is related to proximity to the child's death and the anticipated time required for titration of the alternative opioid to achieve effective pain relief. An alternative in the end-of-life situation would be to initiate and maintain sedation. This option must only be considered when other reversible causes of agitation and distress (such as urinary retention, constipation, pain, and discomfort) have been ruled out.

Intractable pain

Pain that is resistant to standard treatments is intractable. Intractable pain that does not respond to alternative treatment modalities is refractory. Intractable pain in children usually occurs in patients who have cancer as treatments fail to contain the disease process. A retrospective study performed in 1995 evaluated the opioid requirements of 199 children who had terminal malignancy. Twelve patients (6%) required excessive opioid doses, and eight of these needed "extraordinary measures," such as sedation or subarachnoid infusion or both, to alleviate their pain. Eleven of these patients had neuropathic pain due to tumor invasion as the overriding feature of their intractable pain [102].

Over the last 10 years, pediatric pain management has evolved and developed. A greater understanding of the use and manipulation of opioids in conjunction with concurrent treatment options has enabled complex pain management in children to become more sophisticated. The increasing use in pediatrics of drugs familiar to adult pain services has facilitated this evolution. Radiologically guided therapeutics and the use of invasive procedures have also made progress. It is perhaps less often that sedation is required for the management of intractable pain.

Sedation for refractory pain

Palliative sedation therapy is the use of sedative medication to relieve intolerable and refractory distress by reduction in patient consciousness. The degree of sedation may vary; mild sedation maintains a degree of consciousness, whereas deep sedation renders the person almost or completely unconscious. Although sedation may be intermittent in some circumstances, in the context of intractable pain, sedation is expected to continue to alter patient consciousness until death. The wishes of the child (if appropriate) and family must be considered and openly discussed. Complex ethical issues regarding continual sedation and the principle of the double effect have been discussed extensively in the literature. Specific reference to pediatric practice is again lacking.

No consensus exists on the most appropriate medication for sedation. A variety of drugs have been used in this situation, including barbiturates, benzodiazepines (primarily midazolam), and phenothiazines. When sedation is employed, there is a clear imperative to maintain adequate opioid analgesia at an optimal level.

Summary

Children and adolescents who have life-limiting conditions are vulnerable to acute and chronic pain problems. Many compounding and complicating factors often need to be explored in this setting. Barriers to effective pain management include poor assessment and measurement of pain and a lack of specialist knowledge. Fears regarding the use of opioids and their association with the end of life must be addressed openly and with clarity. Day-to-day management should include continual appraisal of pain issues if quality of life is to be maximized.

Pain is a complicated phenomenon. The impact of pain and the complicated dynamic of suffering in children and young people who have life-limiting conditions must not be underestimated. The clinician must be vigilant and take responsibility for all aspects of pain management in these patients.

References

[1] The world health report [pamphlet]. Geneva (Switzerland): World Health Organization; 1995.
[2] Cooley C, Adeodu S, Aldred H, et al. Paediatric palliative care: a lack of research-based evidence. Int J Palliat Nurs 2000;6(7):346–51.
[3] The Association for Children with Life-Threatening or Terminal Conditions and Their Families and the Royal College of Paediatrics and Child Health. A guide to the development of children's palliative care services. Bristol, Great Britain: The Association for Children with Life-Threatening or Terminal Conditions and Their Families; 2003.
[4] Field MJ, Behman RE. When children die: improving palliative and end-of-life care for children and their families. Washington, DC: National Academic Press; 2003.
[5] Miser AW, Dothage P, Wesley RA, et al. The prevalence of pain in a pediatric and young adult population. Pain 1987;29:265–6.
[6] Ljungman G, Gordh T, Sorensen S, et al. Pain in paediatric oncology: interviews with children, adolescents and their parents. Acta Paediatr 1999;88(6):623–30.
[7] Ljungman G, Gordh T, Sorensen S, et al. Pain variations during cancer treatment in children: a descriptive survey. Pediatr Hematol Oncol 2000;17(3):211–21.
[8] Van Cleve L, Bossert E, Beecroft P, et al. The pain experience of children with leukemia during the first year after diagnosis. Nurs Res 2004;53(1):1–10.
[9] Miser AW, McCalla J, Dothage JA, et al. Pain as a presenting symptom in children and young adults with newly diagnosed malignancy. Pain 1987;29(1):85–90.
[10] Collins JJ, Devine TD, Dick GS, et al. The measurement of symptoms in young children with cancer: the validation of the Memorial Symptom Assessment Scale in children aged 7–12. J Pain Symptom Manage 2002;23(1):10–6.
[11] Lolekha R, Chanthavanich P, Limkittikul K, et al. Pain: a common symptom in human immunodeficiency virus–infected Thai children. Acta Paediatr 2004;93(7):891–8.
[12] Koh JL, Harrison D, Palermo TM, et al. Assessment of acute and chronic pain symptoms in children with cystic fibrosis. Pediatric Pulmonol 2005;40(4):330–5.
[13] Ravilly S, Robinson W, Suresh S, et al. Chronic pain in cystic fibrosis. Pediatrics 1996;98(4): 741–7.
[14] Robinson WM, Ravilly S, Berde C, et al. End-of-life care in cystic fibrosis. Pediatrics 1997; 100(2):205–9.
[15] Anand KJS, Craig KD. New perspectives on the definition of pain. Pain 1996;67(1):3–6.
[16] Carter B, McArthur E, Cunliffe M. Dealing with uncertainty: parental assessment of pain in their children with profound special needs. J Adv Nurs 2002;38(5):449–57.
[17] Breau LM, Camfield CS, McGrath PJ, et al. Risk factors for pain in children with severe cognitive impairments. Dev Med Child Neurol 2004;46(6):364–71.
[18] Nolan J, Chalkiadis GA, Low J, et al. Anaesthesia and pain management in cerebral palsy. Anaesthesia 2000;55(1):32–41.
[19] Hunt AM, Burne R. Medical and nursing problems of children with neurodegenerative disease. Palliat Med 1995;9:19–26.

[20] Spencer JD. Reconstruction of dislocated hips in children with cerebral palsy. Br Med J 1999;318(7190):1021–2.

[21] Houlihan CM, O'Donnell M, Conaway M, et al. Bodily pain and health-related quality of life in children with cerebral palsy. Dev Med Child Neurol 2004;46(5):305–10.

[22] Stallard P, Williams L, Lenton S, et al. Pain in cognitively impaired, non-communicating children. Arch Dis Child 2001;85(6):460–2.

[23] Hunt AM. A survey of signs, symptoms and symptom control in 30 terminally ill children. Dev Med Child Neurol 1990;32(4):341–6.

[24] Carter BS, Howenstein M, Gilmer MJ, et al. Circumstances surrounding the deaths of hospitalized children: opportunities for pediatric palliative care. Pediatrics 2004;114(3):361–6.

[25] Eccleston C, Morley S, Williams A, et al. Review: psychological interventions reduce the severity and frequency of chronic pain in children and adolescents. Evid Based Med 2003;8(3):89.

[26] Contro N, Larson J, Scofield S, et al. Family perspectives on the quality of pediatric palliative care. Arch Pediatr Adolesc Med 2002;156(1):14–9.

[27] Wolfe J. Suffering in children at the end of life: recognizing an ethical duty to palliate. J Clin Ethics 2000;11(2):157–63.

[28] Champion GD, Goodenough B, von Baeyer C, et al. Measurement of pain by self-report. In: Finley GA, McGrath PJ, editors. Measurement of pain in infants and children. Seattle (WA): IASP Press; 1998. p. 5–20.

[29] Hicks CL, von Baeyer CL, Spafford PA, et al. The Faces Pain Scale revised: toward a common metric in pediatric pain measurement. Pain 2001;93(2):173–83.

[30] Hunter M, McDowell L, Hennessy R, et al. An evaluation of the Faces Pain Scale with young children. J Pain Symptom Manage 2000;20(2):122–9.

[31] McGrath PA, Gillespie J. Pain assessment in children and adolescents. In: Turck DC, Melzack R, editors. Handbook of pain assessment. 2nd edition. New York: Guildford Press; 2001. p. 97–119.

[32] Shih AR, von Baeyer CL. Preschool children's seriation of pain faces and happy faces in the Affective Facial Scale. Psychol Rep 1994;74(2):659–65.

[33] St-Laurent-Gagnon T, Bernard-Bonnin AC, Villeneuve E. Pain evaluation in preschool children and their parents. Acta Paediatr 1999;88(4):422–7.

[34] McGrath PJ, Unruh AM. Measurement and assessment of paediatric pain. In: Wall PD, Melzack R, editors. Textbook of pain. 4th edition. New York: Churchill Livingstone; 1999. p. 371–84.

[35] Grunau RVE, Craig KD. Pain expression in neonates: facial action and cry. Pain 1987; 28(3):395–410.

[36] Merkel SI, Voepel-Lewis T, Shayevitz JR, et al. The FLACC a behavioral scale for scoring postoperative pain in young children. Pediatr Nurs 1997;23(3):293–7.

[37] Ramelet AS, Abu-Saad HH, Rees N, et al. The challenges of pain measurement in critically ill young children: a comprehensive review. Aust Crit Care 2004;17(1):33–45.

[38] Biersdorff KK. Incidence of significantly altered pain experience among individuals with developmental disabilities. Am J Ment Retard 1994;98(5):619–31.

[39] Stallard P, Williams L, Velleman R, et al. Brief report: behaviors identified by caregivers to detect pain in noncommunicating children. J Pediatr Psychol 2002;27(2):209–14.

[40] Breau LM, McGrath PJ, Camfield C, et al. Preliminary validation of an observational pain checklist for persons with cognitive impairments and inability to communicate verbally. Dev Med Child Neurol 2000;42(9):609–16.

[41] Breau LM, Camfield C, McGrath PJ, et al. Measuring pain accurately in children with cognitive impairments: refinement of a caregiver scale. J Pediatr 2001;138(5):721–7.

[42] Breau LM, Finley GA, McGrath PJ, et al. Validation of the Non-communicating Children's Pain Checklist—postoperative version. Anesthesiology 2002;96(3):528–35. [Erratum appears in Anesthesiology 2002;97(3):769.]

[43] Gauvain-Piquard A, Rodary C, Rezvani A, et al. The development of the DEGR(R): a scale to assess pain in young children with cancer. Eur J Pain 1999;3(2):165–76.

[44] Collins JJ, Byrnes ME, Dunkel IJ, et al. The measurement of symptoms in children with cancer. J Pain Symptom Manage 2000;19(5):363–77.

[45] McCallum DE, Byrne P, Bruera E. How children die in hospital. J Pain Symptom Manage 1920;20:417–23.

[46] Hodgkins M, Albert D, Daltroy L. Comparing patients' and their physicians' assessments of pain. Pain 1985;23(3):273–7.

[47] Janse AJ, Sinnema G, Uiterwaal CSPM, et al. Quality of life in chronic illness: perceptions of parents and paediatricians. Arch Dis Child 2005;90(5):486–91.

[48] Berde CB, Sethna NF. Analgesics for the treatment of pain in children. N Engl J Med 2002; 347(14):1094–103.

[49] Korpela R, Korvenoja P, Meretoja OA. Morphine-sparing effect of acetaminophen in pediatric day-case surgery. Anesthesiology 1999;91(2):442–7.

[50] Murat I, Baujard C, Foussat C, et al. Tolerance and analgesic efficacy of a new i.v. paracetamol solution in children after inguinal hernia repair. Paediatr Anaesth 2005;15(8): 663–70.

[51] Birmingham PK, Tobin MJ, Fisher DM, et al. Initial and subsequent dosing of rectal acetaminophen in children: a 24-hour pharmacokinetic study of new dose recommendations. Anesthesiology 2001;94(3):385–9.

[52] Vetter TR, Heiner EJ. Intravenous ketorolac as an adjuvant to pediatric patient-controlled analgesia with morphine. J Clin Anesth 1994;6(2):110–3.

[53] Tramer MR, Williams JE, Carroll D, et al. Comparing analgesic efficacy of non-steroidal anti-inflammatory drugs given by different routes in acute and chronic pain: a qualitative systematic review. Acta Anaesth Scand 1998;42(1):71–9.

[54] Tramer MR, Moore RA, Reynolds DJ, et al. Quantitative estimation of rare adverse events which follow a biological progression: a new model applied to chronic NSAID use. Pain 2000;85(1–2):169–82.

[55] Goldstein JL, Silverstein FE, Agrawal NM, et al. Reduced risk of upper gastrointestinal ulcer complications with celecoxib, a novel COX-2 inhibitor. Am J Gastroenterol 2000;95(7): 1681–90.

[56] Leese PT, Hubbard RC, Karim A, et al. Effects of celecoxib, a novel cyclooxygenase-2 inhibitor, on platelet function in healthy adults: a randomized, controlled trial. J Clin Pharmacol 2000;40(2):124–32.

[57] Vielhaber A, Portenoy RK. Advances in cancer pain management. Hematol Oncol Clin North Am 2002;16(3):527–41.

[58] Caraceni A, Portenoy RK, Ashby MA, et al. An international survey of cancer pain characteristics and syndromes. Pain 1999;82(3):263–74.

[59] Wiffen P, Collins S, McQuay H, et al. Anticonvulsant drugs for acute and chronic pain. Cochrane Database Syst Rev 2005;20:CD001133.

[60] Saarto T, Wiffen PJ. Antidepressants for neuropathic pain. Cochrane Database Syst Rev 2005.

[61] Joranson DE, Ryan KM, Gilson AM, et al. Trends in medical use and abuse of opioid analgesics. JAMA 2000;283(13):1710–4.

[62] Caran EMM, Dias CG, Seber A, et al. Clinical aspects and treatment of pain in children and adolescents with cancer. Pediatr Blood Cancer 2005;45(7):925–32.

[63] Ellis JA, McCarthy P, Hershon L, et al. Pain practices: a cross-Canada survey of pediatric oncology centers. J Pediatr Oncol Nurs 2003;1:26–35.

[64] Berde CB, Ablin AR, Glazer J, et al. American Academy of Pediatrics: report of the subcommittee on disease-related pain in childhood cancer. Pediatrics 1990;86:818–25.

[65] McGrath PA. Development of the World Health Organization Guidelines on Cancer Pain Relief and Palliative Care in Children. J Pain Symptom Manage 1996;12:87–92.

[66] Ljungman G, Kreuger A, Gordh T, et al. Treatment of pain in pediatric oncology: a Swedish nationwide survey. Pain 1996;68(2–3):385–94.

[67] Williams DG, Patel A, Howard RF. Pharmacogenetics of codeine metabolism in an urban population of children and its implications for analgesic reliability. Br J Anaesth 2002; 89(6):839–45.

[68] Bouwmeester NJ, Anderson BJ, Tibboel D, et al. Developmental pharmacokinetics of morphine and its metabolites in neonates, infants and young children. Br J Anaesth 2004;92(2): 208–17.

[69] Kart T, Christrup LL, Rasmussen M. Recommended use of morphine in neonates, infants and children based on a literature review: part 2—clinical use. Paediatr Anaesth 1997;7(2): 93–101.

[70] Bhat R, bu-Harb M, Chari G, et al. Morphine metabolism in acutely ill preterm newborn infants. J Pediatr 1992;120(5):795–9.

[71] Hunt A, Joel S, Dick G, et al. Population pharmacokinetics of oral morphine and its glucuronides in children receiving morphine as immediate-release liquid or sustained-release tablets for cancer pain. J Pediatr 1999;135(1):47–55.

[72] Hain RD, Hardcastle A, Pinkerton CR, et al. Morphine and morphine-6-glucuronide in the plasma and cerebrospinal fluid of children. Br J Clin Pharmacol 1999;48(1):37–42.

[73] Bruera EB. Randomized, double-blind, cross-over trial comparing safety and efficacy of oral controlled-release oxycodone with controlled-release morphine in patients with cancer pain. J Clin Oncol 1998;16(10):3222–9.

[74] Lugo RA, Kern SE. The pharmacokinetics of oxycodone. J Pain Palliat Care Pharmacother 2004;18(4):17–30.

[75] Attia MW. Buccal oxycodone reduced pain more than placebo in children with acute undifferentiated abdominal pain: commentary. Evid Based Med 2005;10(5):147.

[76] Kokki H, Lintula H, Vanamo K, et al. Oxycodone vs placebo in children with undifferentiated abdominal pain: a randomized, double-blind clinical trial of the effect of analgesia on diagnostic accuracy. Arch Pediatr Adolesc Med 2005;159(4):320–5.

[77] Lawlor P, Turner K, Hanson J, et al. Dose ratio between morphine and hydromorphone in patients with cancer pain: a retrospective study. Pain 1997;72(1–2):79–85.

[78] Moriarty M, McDonald CJ, Miller AJ. A randomised crossover comparison of controlled release hydromorphone tablets with controlled release morphine tablets in patients with cancer pain. Journal of Clinical Research 1999;2:1–8.

[79] Collins JJ, Geake J, Grier HE, et al. Patient-controlled analgesia for mucositis pain in children: a three-period crossover study comparing morphine and hydromorphone. J Pediatr 1996;129(5):722–8.

[80] Quigley C. Hydromorphone for acute and chronic pain. Cochrane Database Syst Rev 2005.

[81] Collins JJ, Dunkel IJ, Gupta SK, et al. Transdermal fentanyl in children with cancer pain: feasibility, tolerability, and pharmacokinetic correlates. J Pediatr 1999;134(3):319–23.

[82] Noyes M, Irving H. The use of transdermal fentanyl in pediatric oncology palliative care. Am J Hosp Palliat Care 2001;18(6):411–6.

[83] Hunt IS, Goldman A, Devine TB, et al. Transdermal fentanyl for pain relief in a paediatric palliative care population. Palliat Med 2001;15:405–12.

[84] Koren G, Crean P, Goresky GV. Pharmacokinetics of fentanyl in children with renal disease. Res Commun Chem Pathol Pharmacol 1984;46(3):371–9.

[85] Finkel JC, Finley A, Greco C, et al. Transdermal fentanyl in the management of children with chronic severe pain: results from an international study. Cancer 2005; 104(12):2847–57.

[86] Hanks GW, Nugent M, Higgs CMB, et al. Oral transmucosal fentanyl citrate in the management of breakthrough pain in cancer: an open, multicentre, dose-titration and long-term use study. Palliat Med 2004;18(8):698–704.

[87] Bruera E, Sweeney C. Methadone use in cancer patients with pain: a review. J Palliat Med 2002;5(1):127–38.

[88] Dale O, Hoffer C, Sheffels P, et al. Disposition of nasal, intravenous, and oral methadone in healthy volunteers. Clin Pharmacol Ther 2002;72(5):536–45.

[89] Dale O, Sheffels P, Kharasch ED. Bioavailabilities of rectal and oral methadone in healthy subjects. Br J Clin Pharmacol 2004;58(2):156–62.

[90] Shir Y, Shenkman Z, Shavelson V, et al. Oral methadone for the treatment of severe pain in hospitalized children: a report of five cases. Clin J Pain 1998;14(4):350–3.

[91] Sabatowski R, Kasper SM, Radbruch L. Patient-controlled analgesia with intravenous L-methadone in a child with cancer pain refractory to high-dose morphine. J Pain Symptom Manage 2002;23(1):3–5.

[92] Miser AW, Miser JS. The use of oral methadone to control moderate and severe pain in children and young adults with malignancy. Clin J Pain 1985;1(4):243–8.

[93] Dix P, Martindale S, Stoddart PA. Double-blind randomized placebo-controlled trial of the effect of ketamine on postoperative morphine consumption in children following appendicectomy. Paediatr Anaesth 2003;13(5):422–6.

[94] Klepstad P, Maurset A, Moberg ER, et al. Evidence of a role for NMDA receptors in pain perception. Eur J Pharmacol 1990;187(3):513–8.

[95] Fitzgibbon EJ, Viola R. Parenteral ketamine as an analgesic adjuvant for severe pain: development and retrospective audit of a protocol for a palliative care unit. J Palliat Med 2005;8(1):49–57.

[96] Mercadante S, Arcuri E, Tirelli W, et al. Analgesic effect of intravenous ketamine in cancer patients on morphine therapy: a randomized, controlled, double-blind, crossover, double-dose study. J Pain Symptom Manage 2000;20(4):246–52.

[97] Weinbroum AA. A single small dose of postoperative ketamine provides rapid and sustained improvement in morphine analgesia in the presence of morphine-resistant pain. Anesth Analg 2003;96(3):789–95.

[98] Bell R, Eccleston C, Kalso E. Ketamine as an adjuvant to opioids for cancer pain. Cochrane Database Syst Rev 2003;1:CD003351.

[99] Bruera E, Brenneis C, Michaud M, et al. Use of the subcutaneous route for the administration of narcotics in patients with cancer pain. Cancer 1988;62:407–11.

[100] Geldner G, Hubmann M, Knoll R, et al. Comparison between three transmucosal routes of administration of midazolam in children. Paediatr Anaesth 1997;7(2):103–9.

[101] Saroyan JM, Schechter WS, Tresgallo ME, et al. Role of intraspinal analgesia in terminal pediatric malignancy. J Clin Oncol 2005;23(6):1318–21.

[102] Collins JJ, Grier HE, Kinney HC, et al. Control of severe pain in children with terminal malignancy. J Pediatr 1995;126(4):653–7.

[103] Collins JJ, Grier HE, Sethna NF, et al. Regional anesthesia for pain associated with terminal pediatric malignancy. Pain 1996;65(1):63–9.

[104] Charron M, Brown M, Rowland P, et al. Pain palliation with strontium-89 in children with metastatic disease. Med Pediatr Oncol 1996;26(6):393–6.

[105] Paulino AC. Palliative radiotherapy in children with neuroblastoma. Pediatr Hematol Oncol 2003;20(2):111–7.

[106] Mercadante S, Radbruch L, Caraceni A, et al. Episodic (breakthrough) pain: consensus conference of an expert working group of the European Association for Palliative Care. Cancer 2002;94(3):832–9.

[107] Portenoy RK, Payne D, Jacobsen P. Breakthrough pain: characteristics and impact in patients with cancer pain. Pain 1999;81(1–2):129–34.

[108] Caraceni A, Martini C, Zecca E, et al. Breakthrough pain characteristics and syndromes in patients with cancer pain. An international survey. Palliat Med 2004;18(3):177–83.

[109] Berde CB, Lehn BM, Yee JD, et al. Patient-controlled analgesia in children and adolescents: a randomized, prospective comparison with intramuscular administration of morphine for postoperative analgesia. J Pediatr 1991;118(3):460–6.

[110] Cherney NI, Foley KM. Nonopioid and opioid analgesics in pharmacotherapy. Hematol Oncol Clin North Am 1996;10(1):79–102.

[111] Indelicato RA, Portenoy RK. Opioid rotation in the management of refractory cancer pain. J Clin Oncol 2003;21:87–91.

[112] Quigley C. Opioid switching to improve pain relief and drug tolerability. Cochrane Database Syst Rev 2004;(3):CD004847.

[113] Drake R, Longworth J, Collins JJ. Opioid rotation in children with cancer. J Palliat Med 2004;7(3):419–22.

[114] Inturrisi CE, Portenoy RK, Max MB, et al. Pharmacokinetic-pharmacodynamic relationships of methadone infusions in patients with cancer pain. Clin Pharmacol Ther 1990;47(5): 565–77.

[115] Manfredi PL, Houde RW. Prescribing methadonea unique analgesic. J Support Oncol 2003;1(3):216–20.

[116] Maxwell LG, Kaufmann SC, Bitzer S, et al. The effects of a small-dose naloxone infusion on opioid-induced side effects and analgesia in children and adolescents treated with intravenous patient-controlled analgesia: a double-blind, prospective, randomized, controlled study. Anesth Analg 2005;100(4):953–8.

[117] Kenny NP, Frager G. Refractory symptoms and terminal sedation of children: ethical issues and practical management. J Palliat Care 1996;12(3):40–5.

ELSEVIER
SAUNDERS

Child Adolesc Psychiatric Clin N Am
15 (2006) 683–691

CHILD AND
ADOLESCENT
PSYCHIATRIC CLINICS
OF NORTH AMERICA

Cognitive-Behavioral Interventions for Physical Symptom Management in Pediatric Palliative Medicine

Dunya Yaldoo Poltorak, PhD[a],*, Ethan Benore, PhD[b]

[a]Section of Behavioral Medicine, Children's Hospital, Cleveland Clinic,
9500 Euclid Avenue/A120, Cleveland, OH 44195, USA
[b]NeuroDevelopmental Center, Akron Children's Hospital, One Perkins Square,
Akron, OH 44308, USA

The prevalence and management of physical symptoms in children with progressive diseases have garnered increasing interest over the last several years [1–3]. Symptoms vary relative to diagnosis, stage of disease, and which therapeutic interventions have been attempted. The alleviation of symptoms, with the ultimate intention of improvement of quality of life, is a fundamental component of pediatric palliative medicine. Although symptoms in individuals who are dying often are divided into physical and psychological, it is evident that there is an interaction between the physical and psychological determinants of symptoms. Factors such as anxiety, depression, symptom preoccupation, cognitive appraisal, and perceived control can exacerbate physical symptoms or influence perceptions of symptoms [4]. Developmentally sensitive assessment of physiologic and psychological contributors to symptoms is indicated.

Common physical symptoms in dying children include pain, fatigue, insomnia, and nutritional concerns (eg, anorexia, nausea/emesis, feeding difficulties). Cognitive-behavioral interventions for the management of these symptoms have been widely researched in various chronic illness populations. There is a paucity of research specific to the pediatric palliative population, and this area is ripe for further investigation. Overall, clinical and empirical evidence suggests good promise for the application of cognitive-behavioral principles and interventions, at least as an adjunct to pharmacologic or surgical interventions, if not as the primary intervention, for the amelioration of symptoms in pediatric palliation. The ultimate goal when

* Corresponding author.
E-mail address: yaldood@ccf.org (D.Y. Poltorak).

using these interventions in palliative patients is to promote healthy cognitions and behaviors that facilitate coping with physical and psychological discomfort and improve quality of life.

Overview of cognitive-behavioral interventions

The focus of cognitive-behavioral interventions for symptom management is multifaceted and includes (1) alteration of maladaptive behaviors; (2) alteration of self-statements, images, and feelings that interfere with adaptive functioning; (3) alteration of assumptions and beliefs that contribute to habitual perceptions and reactions [4]; and (4) training in new behaviors and ways of thinking that promote healthier functioning. Symptoms that might be perceived as vague and overwhelming are translated into identifiable difficulties that can be actively addressed.

Cognitive restructuring can be taught as a method for identifying and changing thoughts and feelings that might exacerbate physical symptoms. In an empathetic manner, the palliative patient can be encouraged to self-monitor maladaptive thoughts and emotions that precede, accompany, or follow the exacerbation of symptoms. Awareness of increased emotional distress and muscle tension that might surround the exacerbation of symptoms is encouraged. The pediatric palliative patient also can be guided in the use of *positive self-statements* for symptom management (eg, "I have been able to cope with this symptom before, and I can do it again").

Cognitive distraction is a particularly useful technique, because the child with an advanced disease is likely to overattend to bodily sensations that otherwise might have been ignored if the child were healthy. The child might perceive each new sensation as a symptom of physical decline. Because it is difficult to attend fully to more than one thing at any given time, simply encouraging a child to distract himself or herself with activities, such as reading a book, watching television, playing a game, or talking with a friend, can be useful for symptom management.

Activity-rest cycling, an activity pacing method, also can be helpful in managing discomfort. Activities that might be encouraged to some degree, but also might be difficult for a child with an advanced disease to tolerate (eg, walking), can be broken up into periods of activity followed by rest (eg, 10 minutes of activity followed by 5 minutes of rest), with cycling repeated as appropriate.

Decreasing distress associated with various components of medical management can be useful in managing a child's overall distress, which can have an impact on physical symptoms. Several behavioral strategies using applied behavioral analysis can facilitate medication administrations. Walco [5] developed a behavioral protocol for pill swallowing, and various adaptations of this treatment have been applied to several pediatric populations [6,7]. As with other medical procedures, it is beneficial to make medication administration predictable, brief, and rewarding.

Numerous specific relaxation exercises can be implemented in anticipation of a stressful event or as a response to stress and physical discomfort. Examples of these techniques include *diaphragmatic breathing, guided imagery,* and *progressive muscle relaxation.* Each of these techniques is easy to teach and simple for children to learn. Use of these techniques can facilitate adaptive coping and be an effective means of symptom management. It is generally recommended that these techniques be taught to patients as early in the illness as possible. Patients initially should be encouraged to practice these techniques as frequently as possible, including during times when symptoms are less overwhelming, to gain mastery of the techniques and appreciate greater benefit from their use.

Diaphragmatic breathing can be used in any situation with no behavioral indication in which the child is doing anything different from "normal." This technique can be especially appealing for children and adolescents. Diaphragmatic breathing can be used alone or in combination with other techniques. Guidelines for instructing patients on the use of this technique are presented in Box 1. Instructions can be adapted and modified for children at various developmental levels. *Guided imagery* involves the use of one's imagination for visualization of a relaxing scene or experience. This technique is typically most effective when the child chooses the specific image to visualize. *Progressive muscle relaxation* involves the systematic tensing and relaxing of specific muscle groups. The child can be taught to begin with the muscles in the feet, tensing all of these muscles and holding the tension for 10 seconds, followed by relaxation of these same muscles for 10 seconds. The child is taught to repeat this process with the next set of muscles (eg, legs, stomach) until every area of the body has been relaxed. In clinical practice, this technique is most useful for managing insomnia or anticipatory anxiety associated with uncomfortable procedures. Because muscle tensing can exacerbate pain in some patients, this technique is less often recommended for the specific management of pain.

It is useful to guide parents and other members of the medical team in the use of various cognitive-behavioral strategies. Parents can practice these techniques with their children. Parents and other members of the care team can prompt and encourage children to use effective coping strategies that they have learned. These individuals, along with the psychologist, can model healthy coping behaviors for the child and encourage their practice. Positive reinforcement can be used to reward healthy coping behaviors and promote their continued use.

Symptom-specific recommendations

Pain

Pain is among the most common and distressing symptoms in patients with advanced disease. Pain can be related to the illness itself or to

---

Box 1. Guidelines for teaching diaphragmatic breathing to children

1. Instruct the child to sit or lie down in a comfortable position. Further instructions should be reviewed with the child first and the technique should be modeled before requiring the child's participation.
2. Help the child to locate his or her diaphragm muscle (eg, "the soft spot right underneath the middle of your ribcage and on top of your belly").
3. Instruct the child to take a slow, gentle breath in through the nose. The child should be guided to keep the upper body (eg, shoulders) relaxed. Using the metaphor of having a balloon in the belly that the child will attempt to fill slowly, just as much as feels comfortable, is often useful in helping the child to focus on the diaphragm muscle and keep the upper body relaxed.
4. Instruct the child to hold the breath for a few seconds or as long as feels comfortable and natural.
5. Instruct the child to exhale slowly and gently through the mouth, slowly releasing the air from the balloon. Children can be encouraged to blow out in the same way as they would if they were trying to blow a very large bubble with a bubble wand.
6. The cycle can be repeated several times.

---

treatments and procedures. Muscular tension and psychological distress can exacerbate pain, and anxiety in anticipation of or during painful medical procedures can exacerbate perceptions of procedural pain [8]. Several cognitive-behavioral interventions have been found to be useful in reducing pain, including modeling, use of diaphragmatic breathing, imagery, distraction, offering of positive incentives, and behavioral rehearsal [9–11]. Children who have significant anxiety in anticipation of painful procedures benefit from developmentally appropriate explanation of procedures, information regarding what any given procedure might sound or feel like from the child's perspective, and explanation of what benefits might be expected. Children should be encouraged to ask questions. Allowing children to have some control over procedures (eg, permission to choose which arm will be used for a needle stick) also can help reduce anxiety. Children also might benefit from instruction and practice in behaviors that promote a successful procedure (eg, lying still). Telling children when procedures are over can help to facilitate a return from heightened physiologic arousal to a more calm state.

In an adult population, systematic training of partners in cognitive-behavioral pain management techniques (specifically relaxation training, imagery, and activity-rest cycling) was found to increase partner self-efficacy and to be beneficial for management of cancer pain and other end-of-life symptoms [12]. Similar findings have been observed in clinical practice in parents and their dying children.

Fatigue

Fatigue is common to many advanced diseases and can be attributed to inactivity, poor nutrition, dehydration, anemia, pain, depression, insomnia, medication side effects, and radiation side effects [13]. Increasing fatigue is often the first sign of deterioration in a patient with advanced disease [14], however, and it is common for patients to infer that fatigue indicates physical decline. Patients should be educated or reminded about possible alternative explanations for fatigue. Several nonpharmacologic strategies for management of fatigue have been shown to be beneficial, including performing essential functions in the morning, scheduling a regular afternoon nap, avoiding complete inactivity, and engaging in even very mild exercise if possible [15]. Psychologists can be instrumental in assisting children and their families in implementing these strategies. Because depression can contribute to fatigue, assessment of emotional functioning, with psychological or pharmacologic intervention as indicated, is essential.

Insomnia

Children with advanced illness also may experience insomnia. Several factors contribute to insomnia, including pain, lack of physical activity during the day, multiple medications that affect arousal, anxiety, and depression [13,14]. It is important to emphasize the distinction between day (time to be awake) and night (time to be asleep) [16]. To regulate sleep-wake patterns and induce relatively greater fatigue at night, children should be encouraged to be physically or mentally active (as able) during the day. Activities should be rotated throughout the child's day to maintain high levels of motivation and activity. Curtains should remain open, and although the child might require comfortable clothing, changing out of pajamas during the day is helpful. Activity should be kept to a minimum at night. The National Sleep Foundation [17] has provided basic recommendations for sleep hygiene, which include having a quiet room with dim lighting and minimal interruptions from others. To the extent that is possible, these recommendations should be encouraged in inpatients and outpatients. It may be helpful to postpone or alter nonurgent medical care during nighttime hours to promote better sleep hygiene.

Assessment and treatment of depressive and anxious symptoms, which might be contributing to insomnia, is essential. Relaxation exercises, particularly progressive muscle relaxation, can assist children in achieving sleep and in returning to sleep with repeated nighttime awakenings. Children who spend a frequent amount of time awake in their beds have particular difficulty maintaining good sleep habits. In this situation, the classically conditioned drowsiness linked to lying in bed is disrupted or extinguished. The bed no longer provides a cue to promote sleep. To re-establish this conditioned response, children should be encouraged to leave their beds (or modify their position in bed by moving to a seated position) when they are unable to fall asleep after 20 to 30 minutes and to engage in a boring or repetitive activity to promote drowsiness. When they begin to feel drowsy, they are to return to bed (or return to a lying-down position) and attempt to fall asleep again.

Nutritional concerns

Children with advanced illness may show reduced caloric intake, food refusal, changes in food preference, nausea, and emesis. Nutritional concerns can have a negative impact on medical care and present as primary concerns for the child and family. Anorexia can result from altered taste and smell, pain, mouth sores, swallowing difficulties, nausea and vomiting, medication side effects, constipation, and depression [13]. Nausea and emesis may be secondary to treatment (eg, chemotherapy, opioids), metabolic disturbances, or constipation and might reflect a conditioned response [15].

Feeding difficulties have been addressed from a behavioral perspective across several disease populations. In a systematic review of the literature, Kerwin [18] found contingency management (with planned ignoring and positive reinforcement) to be an efficacious intervention. Linscheid et al [19] described four components of behavioral procedures to increase caloric intake. First, social attention can be made contingent on eating, whereas behaviors associated with food avoidance or refusal are blocked or ignored. Second, desirable and undesirable consequences can be used to increase compliance with eating demands and reduce food refusal or avoidance. Third, food intake can be controlled to increase appetite during mealtimes. Snacks may be refused between meals with the intention of increasing the chance that a child would be willing to eat during meals. Finally, adults can modify cues or prompts to eat or use additional shaping and prompt fading to promote a more complex or wider range of eating behaviors. In palliative patients, parents may be reluctant to employ certain behavioral procedures, however, which they might view as "forcing" children to eat or ignoring children. Education, guidance, and reassurance often are indicated.

Modifying situational factors (ie, antecedent management) also may provide benefit for children. Children may develop less appetite because of the frequency and duration that food is presented. Meal presentation may be altered to promote appetite. Smaller meals may be presented to avoid overwhelming a child with the demand to eat, allowing for the successful completion of a meal. In the hospital, food may be visually presented only during certain times of the day, as opposed to food trays and snack foods frequently being present [16]. Children can be praised for eating even when they do not feel hungry. Verbal praise can be paired with rewarding activities (eg, a parent can play a favorite game with a child), to enhance the reinforcement of eating despite the absence of appetite. Additionally, stimuli may be present in the room that can limit one's appetite. Emesis buckets may prompt feelings of nausea instead of hunger. These stimuli should be placed out of sight, while remaining readily available. Measurable outcomes should be provided. Children may respond better to the demand to eat when they are striving for identified goals (eg, 3 cans of Pediasure before 2 PM or 50% of tray eaten). Parents and medical staff can limit the frequency of discussing a child's food avoidance and need to eat, to reduce cognitive focus on food and increase a child's self-efficacy regarding eating [20–22].

Additional research has focused on cognitive-behavioral interventions for management of nausea and emesis specifically among pediatric cancer patients. Research has suggested that children with cancer do not automatically engage in effective coping strategies for management of nausea and emesis [23]. Training children in the use of cognitive-behavioral interventions for the management of nausea and emesis yields promise as an adjunctive intervention. In a systematic review of empirically evaluated treatments [24], use of guided imagery combined with suggestion was considered a well-established treatment for management of nausea and emesis. This intervention was found to be effective for management of symptoms that occurred in anticipation of receiving chemotherapy and symptoms that occurred after chemotherapy had been administered. Cognitive distraction combined with relaxation was found to be a probably efficacious treatment, and use of other types of distraction (eg, playing video games) showed good promise.

Summary

The alleviation of symptoms, with the ultimate intention of improvement of quality of life, is a fundamental component of pediatric palliative medicine. Psychological factors can exacerbate physical symptoms or influence the perception of symptoms in children with advanced disease. Cognitive-behavioral interventions have yielded positive outcomes for the management of symptoms across various disease populations. There is a paucity of evidence specific to the application of these interventions in pediatric palliation, although evidence-based treatments developed through investigation of other disease populations can be applied in pediatric palliation. Children tend to be receptive to these noninvasive interventions, which can decrease fear and anxiety, increase self-efficacy and sense of control, and improve overall coping. Continued investigation into the use of these interventions in pediatric palliation is encouraged.

References

[1] Hunt AM. A survey of signs, symptoms and symptom control in 30 terminally ill children. Dev Med Child Neurol 1990;32:341–6.

[2] Mallinson J, Jones PD. A 7-year review of deaths on the general paediatric wards at John Hunter Children's Hospital, 1991–97. J Paediatr Child Health 2000;36:252–5.

[3] Wolfe J, Grier HE, Klar N, et al. Symptoms and suffering at the end of life in children with cancer. N Engl J Med 2000;342:326–33.

[4] Turk DC, Feldman CS. A cognitive-behavioral approach to symptom management in palliative care: augmenting somatic interventions. In: Chochinov HM, Breitbart W, editors. Handbook of psychiatry in palliative medicine. New York: Oxford University Press; 2000. p. 223–40.

[5] Walco GA. A behavioral treatment for difficulty in swallowing pills. J Behav Ther Exp Psychiatry 1986;17:127–8.

[6] LaGrone RG. Hypnobehavioral therapy to reduce gag and emesis with a 10-year-old pill swallower. Am J Clin Hypn 1993;36:132–6.

[7] Beck MH, Cataldo M, Slifer KJ, et al. Teaching children with attention deficit hyperactivity disorder (ADHD) and autistic disorder (AD) how to swallow pills. Clin Pediatr 2005;44:515–26.

[8] Turk D, Fernandez E. On the putative uniqueness of cancer pain: do psychological principles apply? Behav Res Ther 1990;28:1–13.

[9] Jay SM, Elliot CH, Katz E, Siegal SE. Cognitive-behavioral and pharmacologic interventions for children's distress during painful medical procedures. J Consult Clin Psychol 1987;55:860–5.

[10] Bauchner H, Vinci R, Bak S, et al. Parents and procedures: a randomized controlled trial. Pediatrics 1996;98:861–7.

[11] Carlson KL, Broome M, Vessey JA. Using distraction to reduce reported pain, fear, and behavioral distress in children and adolescents: a multisite study. J Soc Pediatr Nurs 2000;5:75–85.

[12] Keefe FJ, Ahles TA, Sutton L, et al. Partner-guided cancer pain management at the end of life: a preliminary study. J Pain Symptom Manage 2005;29:263–72.

[13] Stuber ML, Bursch B. Psychiatric care of the terminally ill child. In: Chochinov HM, Breitbart W, editors. Handbook of psychiatry in palliative medicine. New York: Oxford University Press; 2000. p. 255–64.

[14] Levy MH, Catalano RB. Control of common physical symptoms other than pain in patients with terminal disease. Semin Oncol 1985;12:411–30.

[15] Portenoy RK. Physical symptom management in the terminally ill: an overview for mental health professionals. In: Chochinov HM, Breitbart W, editors. Handbook of psychiatry in palliative medicine. New York: Oxford University Press; 2000. p. 99–130.

[16] Hain R, Weinstein S, Oleske J, et al. Holistic management of symptoms. In: Carter BS, Levetown M, editors. Palliative care for infants, children, and adolescents: a practical handbook. Baltimore: The Johns Hopkins University Press; 2004. p. 163–95.

[17] National Sleep Foundation. Sleep for kids—teaching kids the importance of sleep: sleep tips. Available at: http://www.sleepforkids.org/html/tips.html. Accessed November 14, 2005.

[18] Kerwin ME. Empirically supported treatments in pediatric psychology: severe feeding problems. J Pediatr Psychol 1999;24:193–214.

[19] Linscheid TR, Budd KS, Rasnake LK. Pediatric feeding disorders. In: Roberts MC, editor. Handbook of pediatric psychology. 3rd edition. New York: Guilford Press; 2003. p. 481–98.

[20] Chatoor I. Feeding disorders in infants and toddlers: diagnosis and treatment. Child Adolesc Psychiatric Clin N Am 2002;11:163–83.

[21] Stark LJ, Opipari LC, Jelalian E, et al. Child behavior and parent management strategies at mealtimes in families with a school-age child with cystic fibrosis. Health Psychol 2005;24:274–80.

[22] de Moor J, Didden R, Tolboom J. Severe feeding problems secondary to anatomical disorders: effectiveness of behavioural treatment in three school-aged children. Educ Psychol 2005;25:325–40.

[23] Tyc VL, Mulhern RK, Jayawardene D, Fairclough D. Chemotherapy-induced nausea and emesis in pediatric cancer patients: an analysis of coping strategies. J Pain Symptom Manage 1995;10:338–47.

[24] McQuaid EL, Nassau JH. Empirically supported treatments of disease-related symptoms in pediatric psychology: asthma, diabetes, and cancer. J Pediatr Psychol 1999;24:305–28.

ELSEVIER
SAUNDERS

Child Adolesc Psychiatric Clin N Am
15 (2006) 693–715

CHILD AND
ADOLESCENT
PSYCHIATRIC CLINICS
OF NORTH AMERICA

Multidisciplinary Care
of the Dying Adolescent

David R. Freyer, DO[a,b,]*, Aura Kuperberg, PhD,
LCSW[c,e], David J. Sterken, MN, CPNP[a],
Steven L. Pastyrnak, PhD[d], Dan Hudson,
MDiv, BCC[c,e], Tom Richards, BA, CCLS[f]

[a]*Division of Hematology/Oncology/Bone Marrow Transplantation,
DeVos Children's Hospital, 100 Michigan NE, Mailcode 85, Grand Rapids, MI 49503, USA*
[b]*Michigan State University College of Human Medicine, East Lansing, MI, USA*
[c]*Teen Impact Program, Children's Center for Cancer and Blood Diseases,
Children's Hospital Los Angeles, 4650 Sunset Boulevard, Mailstop 99,
Los Angeles, CA 90027, USA*
[d]*Division of Psychology/Psychiatry, DeVos Children's Hospital, 100 Michigan NE,
Mailcode 61, Grand Rapids, MI 49503, USA*
[e]*Spiritual Care Department, Children's Hospital Los Angeles, 4650 Sunset Boulevard,
Mailstop 38, Los Angeles, CA 90027, USA*
[f]*Department of Pediatric Hematology/Oncology,
The Children's Hospital at The Cleveland Clinic, 9500 Euclid Avenue,
Cleveland, OH 44195, USA*

Every year in the United States, nearly 3000 adolescents die from chronic disease, such as cancer, cystic fibrosis, renal failure, congenital heart disease, or acquired immunodeficiency syndrome [1]. Optimum palliative care for dying adolescents exceeds what may be provided by any single clinician, owing to the diversity of developmental tasks and correlative needs that arise in the physical, intellectual, emotional, social, and spiritual realms [2]. In adolescents, life-limiting illness may result in severe alterations in appearance, stamina, self-image, psychosexual maturation, peer and family relationships, educational achievement, and acquisition of independence [3]. To assist in the care of this challenging population, this article describes the

Supported in part by Grant No. CA98543-03 (Subcontract No. 14180) from the National Cancer Institute and National Childhood Cancer Foundation (DRF).

* Corresponding author. Division of Hematology/Oncology/Bone Marrow Transplantation, DeVos Children's Hospital, 100 Michigan NE, Mailcode 85, Grand Rapids, MI 49503.

E-mail address: david.freyer@spectrum-health.org (D.R. Freyer).

distinct but interrelated roles of a multidisciplinary palliative care team comprising the physician, nurse, clinical psychologist, medical social worker, chaplain, and child life specialist (Table 1). As presented here, the unifying theme for the functioning of these team members is respect for the developmental tasks of adolescence.

Medical and nursing considerations: managing care and advocating for the patient

The physician and nurse play several complementary roles in caring for the adolescent with life-threatening illness. These include (1) initiating

Table 1
Multidisciplinary team members: their roles and key functions in caring for dying adolescents

Team member	General role	Key functions
Physician	Management of overall medical care	1. Initiate and coordinate palliative care 2. Manage symptoms
Nurse	Patient advocacy	1. Support autonomy 2. Address family needs 3. Reduce suffering through clinical interventions 4. Manage environment at time of death
Clinical psychologist	Promotion of positive emotional adjustment	1. Assess emotional and cognitive status 2. Assist team in addressing underlying psychologic issues 3. Manage behavioral crises 4. Recommend psychiatric referral as indicated
Medical social worker	Enhancement of support networks	1. Assess baseline quality of social networks 2. Evaluate and manage "network stress" 3. Support strong social ties with family and peers 4. Provide peer-based intervention, if available
Chaplain	Spiritual support	1. Assess religious beliefs and practices of patient and family 2. Evaluate level of spiritual-emotional-cognitive development 3. Support teen in discovering personal meaning of illness 4. Provide rituals as desired
Child life specialist	Assistance with communication and adjustment	1. Assess knowledge and coping style 2. Use child life "tools" to facilitate knowledge, coping, self-understanding, and self-expression

Care of the dying adolescent requires a holistic and multidisciplinary approach that involves considerable overlap of some services provided by individual team members. The key functions highlighted here are not to imply exclusivity but to indicate prominent opportunities for certain disciplines. Assistance from other team members in carrying out those key functions is implied.

palliative care services, (2) identifying and managing symptoms, (3) coordinating multidisciplinary care, and (4) advocating for the adolescent.

Initiating palliative care services

A critical function for the physician and nurse is promptly initiating palliative care when indicated. Delaying palliative care results in a cascade of negative effects, including difficulty gaining control of symptoms, reliance on crisis-oriented management, heightened patient and parental fear and anxiety, and absence of a framework for preventive interventions and sound decision making [4–6].

One fundamental barrier to instituting palliative care is uncertainty as to when it should start. It has been suggested that palliative care should begin at the point when alleviation of symptoms becomes more important to the patient than other treatment-related end points, such as disease control [7]. The preferred care paradigm is one that selectively integrates specific palliative interventions as they become necessary. Gradually, the proportion of care that is "palliative" increases as disease-directed treatment decreases [4]. This "blended" approach ensures that early symptoms will not be neglected and also protects teenagers and families from having to choose between curative efforts and palliation. Other barriers to initiating palliative care include teen and family resistance due to inaccurate information, psychologic issues, or cultural and religious beliefs (summarized in [7]).

Identifying and managing symptoms

As a continuation of their conventional roles in treating the underlying disease, physicians and nurses are responsible for managing symptoms due to the disease or its treatment. Palliative care has been defined as the active, total care of patients who have life-threatening illness, focused on controlling pain and other symptoms and addressing psychologic, social, and spiritual concerns [4]. Consistent with this definition, the primary clinical goal for dying adolescents is to relieve suffering and maximize quality of life. In general, the appropriateness of any intervention is judged in relation to that goal. Interventions worthy of consideration are those that enhance comfort, satisfaction, dignity, and personal fulfillment, whereas treatments that are ineffective or overly burdensome (from the adolescent's perspective) should be discontinued [8].

How symptoms are perceived by the adolescent and reported to care providers is highly subjective. Some adolescents may underreport certain symptoms, fearing what they might signify, attempting to reduce dependency on others, or attempting to avoid hospitalization and unwanted interventions. Others may be excessively aware of bodily sensations magnified by underlying anxiety. Drawing on their knowledge of the teenager, physicians and nurses need to interpret symptoms carefully to understand and treat their causes, which may be physical or psychologic [9]. Assessment of comfort should be directed toward "total" pain, which encompasses physical as well as psychosocial and spiritual distress [10]. Common symptoms at the end of life include pain, fatigue, dyspnea, anorexia, nausea, and anxiety [11]. Pain assessment tools suitable for adolescents have been devised [12–14].

Effective symptom management involves reassuring the teen that (1) symptoms will be taken seriously, (2) effective interventions will be made available whenever possible, and (3) the adolescent will be allowed to choose whether and when those interventions are actually used. Choice about use of palliative care interventions is important to adolescents and may contribute to a greater sense of control [15]. Specific information about treating common end-of-life symptoms is available in other articles in this issue and in other recent sources [10,11,16,17].

Coordinating multidisciplinary care

Effective palliative care requires expertise from multiple disciplines, including medicine, nursing, psychology, social work, child life therapy, and chaplaincy [2]. Coordinating the activities of these consultants is crucial to prevent fragmentation of care. Evidence indicates that, when coordination of care is lacking, pain and other symptoms are increased and satisfaction with care is decreased among dying children and their families [18,19].

Coordination of end-of-life care needs to be a priority at multiple levels. The physician and nurse primarily responsible for an adolescent's terminal care are logical choices for the role of ensuring that all medical and other health professionals are consulted as indicated. They should also ensure that good communication takes place among these consultants and with the patient, keeping in mind that there may be variable levels of experience and comfort among consultants in working with dying adolescents.

Advocating for the adolescent: the special role of the nurse

Nursing holds a privileged seat at the bedside of the dying adolescent. This honor is bestowed on nursing as a result of the ongoing relationship that has been forged between nursing staff and the adolescent patient. Nursing care can be invasive, and being allowed to enter into the personal world of the adolescent, who is body conscious and at times suspicious of adults, is an honor that should not be taken lightly. All the hours and months spent with the adolescent caring for physical needs, listening to fears, and sharing in joys prove to be vital steps toward gaining the trust of the adolescent who is now faced with death.

The relationships established by the nurse with the adolescent patient, the patient's family, and other members of the treatment team grant the nurse a unique vantage point from which to act as a patient advocate and care coordinator. The history of the nurse/patient relationship allows for a holistic perspective that proves advantageous to the nurse in advocating for the patient's physical, mental, emotional, and spiritual needs. Being a voice for the dying adolescent patient means having gained his or her trust, not something the adolescent abdicates readily to just any adult. Trust is earned and signifies that the adolescent believes the nurse will keep his or her best interests at heart even while not necessarily agreeing with the adolescent's decision. Advocacy promotes the adolescent's autonomy and right to make choices, by promoting open communication between the adolescent, family members, and the treatment team. Advocacy promotes normalcy through the encouragement of peer interaction and participation in events meaningful to the adolescent (eg, prom or homecoming) and by offering control in the face of uncertainty [20].

One of the greatest rewards of advocating for the dying adolescent is helping the adolescent bring closure to the business of life. The nurse can help to facilitate the completion of the adolescent's life agenda by creating an environment that promotes open communication and closure of relationships that proved valuable in shaping the experience of the adolescent. An atmosphere of honesty and openness allows the parents of the adolescent to disengage from the deep feeling of connectedness during the adolescent's final days of life. The nurse aids the parents in this process by reminding them that the need to disconnect is in no way a reflection on their parenting abilities.

The culture of the death experience and dying process is largely managed by nursing. Although the adolescent appears to have little or no hope of cure, caring for him or her becomes increasingly complex as every attempt is made by the treatment team to provide a transition that is free of unnecessary suffering. As the experience of care shifts from cure to terminal care, the nurse must often put aside technology, trusting instead "gut instinct" and intuition. Nursing interventions are geared toward relieving the physical, mental, emotional, and spiritual distress related to the dying process. At a time when the family could feel abandoned by the treatment team, the nurse provides care that consistently echoes the compassion of each team member. The family and adolescent must be assured that every effort will be made to prevent undue suffering. Preparation for the final transition indicates that the nurse continue to use relationship, careful assessment, and theory to create an environment that promotes spontaneous and thoughtful expression of the feelings associated with the eventual loss of the adolescent.

Psychologic considerations: promoting adaptive coping

The role of the child/adolescent psychologist typically encompasses those of both the neuropsychologist (specialist in brain-behavior function) and the clinical psychologist (specialist in emotional function). Experience suggests that routinely introducing the psychologist to teenagers and their families early in the illness tends to reduce any negative perceptions associated with that role. The psychologist strives for a balance that entails being readily available without being intrusive.

Cognitive-emotional development and the adolescent's concept of death

Emotional development in the healthy adolescent is driven by the need to work toward autonomy and independence [21,22]. During *early adolescence* (approximately 11 to 14 years of age), individuals are searching for identity, establishing meaningful relationships, and developing dreams and long-term goals. Increased conflict with adult authority figures may be common as adolescents formulate their own opinions about right and wrong, following rules, and finding balance among relationships with peers and family. During this stage, adolescents often experiment with various activities as part of their identity formation. Adaptively, this may involve trying out different sports, clubs, clothes, hairstyles, and peer groups. Maladaptively, this may result in experimenting with drugs and engaging in other risky behaviors. During *middle adolescence* (approximately 15 to 17 years of age), individuals become more focused and preoccupied, sometimes at the expense of family and schoolwork. During this period, it is common for adolescents to feel invincible and exempt from death, even as most understand its finality. Mood swings are common, due in part to hormonal surges but also to the battle raging within over being medically dependent on others while developmentally craving independence. In the phase of *late adolescence* (approximately 18 to 20 years of age), adolescents develop their own stable systems of values and faith. Successful transition through this phase results in greater self-confidence, realistic vocational and life goals, and an increased appreciation of the ability to exist within various educational, occupational, societal, and family systems. Greater emotional stability develops along with a heightened sense of concern for others. Increased self-reliance and ability to compromise are displayed. The ultimate success resulting from this phase of adolescence is emergence as a reasonably self-sufficient individual who is capable of handling the responsibilities of adulthood, including good decision making.

An adolescent's concept of death evolves alongside an increasing capacity for complex and abstract thinking. Adolescents approximately 12 years and older generally understand that death is universal, irreversible, and inevitable [23–25]. They also begin to understand their death in terms of its impact on others [26].

Adapting to the reality of death

Facing the possibility of death may alter an adolescent's transition through all phases of emotional development, depending on the individual characteristics of the patient and personal support systems [3]. Feelings of invincibility are replaced by the gross realization of personal mortality.

Unwanted disease-related physical changes occur at an age when individuals are most sensitive to their appearance and evaluation by others. Attainment of independence and privacy is hindered by medical dependence on family and care providers. Adaptive responses to these challenges include communication and sublimation as routes to eventual acceptance. Maladaptive responses can take both internalized or externalized forms [27].

Internalized distress may result in fear, worry, low self-esteem, a sense of hopelessness or helplessness, general depression, irritability, and increased somatic complaints. If the clinician recognizes these symptoms, the psychologist may be useful in determining how they relate to the underlying illness. Adolescents who internalize their distress typically rely on avoidance and withdrawal as their primary emotional defenses. In the short term, these defenses may be adaptive and prevent an individual from being overwhelmed. Over the longer term, however, these defenses used in excess may interfere with the functioning of communication as a means of gaining control and coming to terms with the eventual outcome of the illness.

Externalized distress involves the adolescent's projecting his or her own thoughts and feelings onto other persons. Yelling at parents or refusing treatment may occur out of the need to control a situation and find an outlet for anger and frustration. Often the specific target is an individual or entity the adolescent perceives as "easy," "safe," or more tangible than the underlying cause of the frustration. For example, an adolescent unable to yell at her cancer can express her anger toward a nurse, parent, or sibling. Typically, the most extreme manifestation of externalizing coping defenses is newly defiant or aggressive behavior. Substance abuse and increased sexual activity may also be seen [24]. The dual role of the psychologist is to develop behavioral management strategies to manage crises if they occur while addressing the emotional cause of the behavior.

Intervening effectively to promote adaptive coping

Most adolescents suffering from chronic illness appear to use a combination of internalizing and externalizing defenses that are both adaptive and maladaptive [3]. Experience suggests that adolescents who rely predominantly on externalizing defenses, although more acutely challenging to their parents and staff, are sometimes more amenable to psychologic intervention. Because their emotions and opinions are readily apparent, the psychologist can provide a better understanding of what needs to be addressed. In contrast, adolescents who internalize their feelings provide less useful information. To gain insights, the psychologist may meet with these individuals and also rely on the perspectives of parents or familiar care providers (eg, primary nurses, social workers, child life specialists, and chaplains). If psychologic assessment finds that loss of control is a source of distress, the psychologist can work with other team members to identify areas where the teenager can exert more choice.

Social considerations: optimizing networks of support

In the face of a life-and-death experience, one of the most significant roles of the social worker is to assess the availability of natural social networks, such as family, community, and peers, and to muster these resources to support and assist the adolescent and his or her family at this crucial time. When strong and appropriate social supports are not available, social work has a distinctive contribution within the multidisciplinary team.

Social support and the buffering effect

The ability to cope during periods of suffering depends on the extent and nature of the personal and clinical social network system. To assess the quality of social support networks for the adolescent patient and his or her family, it is important to understand key processes. The *buffering hypothesis* suggests that adequate levels of social support act to reduce the negative effects of stress, enabling the individual to cope more effectively [28]. However, the availability of social support can be seriously affected by stressful life events, especially if those events are stigmatizing in nature. As a result, the structure of social support networks may be altered significantly when previous and potential helpers feel uncomfortable or threatened by the event. Moreover, even individuals who remain in the support network may feel less comfortable, and their uneasiness can contribute to a strained and even harmful relationship [29]. Socially induced stress, such as family distress, loss of cohesion in communities, fragmentation of care, and lack of continuity in the current health care system, may also reduce the buffering effect [30].

Network stress

Having a child who has a terminal illness can lead to emotional instability, uncertainty, and strains on family members [31]. "Network stress" occurs when potential helpers are just as upset as the individual in need of support and are able to offer only limited amounts of support [32]. Many adolescents who have a life-threatening illness experience emotional isolation within their own families [33]. Adolescents may want to express feelings and fears about dying yet be unable to do so because of the distress it might cause in the family [9]. Moreover, parents unintentionally discourage their child from overt expression of normal fears and negative emotions by communicating in an overly optimistic and cheerful fashion. The reluctance of parents to show honest feelings represents their own denial, grief, and struggle to accept their child's death [34]. In one recent study, adolescents report that parents expect them to be strong, upbeat, and pleasant [35]. Because unexpressed fears and concerns may result in adverse effects, it is important for the social worker to help parents acknowledge their own emotional pain so that it does not become an impediment to the adolescent [34].

When network stress is present, adolescents may need to signal their awareness and distress indirectly. In some patients, it may be manifested as a heightened awareness of running out of time to live [34]. Health professionals need to be alert to events that may trigger fears and concerns [34]. It may even take a crisis to begin a therapeutic dialogue with the dying adolescent. One recently encountered terminally ill male adolescent openly expressed a desire to have sexual relations with a teenage girl he had met at a teen group meeting. She made frequent visits to his bedside, and a relationship quickly developed. Soon the young man requested a hospital bed and privacy for the two of them so they could have sex. Separate from the question of social appropriateness, the urgency and demand that characterized his request reflected a profound acknowledgment of his limited time and loss of normalcy. The social worker was able to use the patient's feelings around this event to begin discussion about his own death.

Strong family support

Optimally, strong family support will be available to help the teenager experience autonomy and maintain hope. As discussed later in this article, the most profound choice facing a terminally ill adolescent is whether to continue disease-directed treatment. Such choices are influenced by factors that include pre-existing family dynamics [36]. Adolescents with strong social ties may experience an increased sense of personal control, self-esteem, meaning, and self-concept [30]. Decision making itself is important for the adolescent and has been linked to better coping and adjustment [15]. Families also can help teenagers maintain hope. Hopefulness has been identified as a "protecting mechanism" that is relevant to the care of the seriously ill adolescent [37,38]. Hope can continue even when death is imminent. When an adolescent realizes cure is not possible, he or she may adapt by shifting focus to more immediate goals, like reaching the next holiday or significant event. Significant events in a young person's life can offer hope and be a reminder of normal adolescent activities [34]. One young woman dying of metastatic malignancy was enabled, through the help of family and friends, to realize her hope of dying at home, surrounded by loved ones, in a balloon-filled room on the night of her 21st birthday.

The critical role of peers and peer-based intervention

The importance of the peer group and social acceptance by the peer group in normal adolescent development have been well documented. Woodgate [29] points out that effective adolescent coping is often directly related to receiving the needed support from the peer group. Peer relationships offer the best way for any adolescent to engage in his or her individuation process, formulate an identity, and enhance a sense of independence [3]. For the dying adolescent, anything that fosters socialization and normalcy is the best strategy [9]. The health care team may promote this process by encouraging young persons to stay connected to their informal peer networks or join formal support groups.

Given the challenges facing chronically ill adolescents in finding informal social support, group support programs represent a particularly viable approach for buffering the impact of stress [39,40]. Kuperberg [41] noted that adolescents who have cancer and develop relationships with similarly affected peers have a more positive self-image and use a broader range of coping mechanisms. Other benefits derive from opportunities for role modeling [42] and peer reinforcement [43]. Studies of diagnosis-oriented camp programs suggest that this type of intervention can enhance a cancer patient's self-esteem, as well as improve family communications [44]. Participating actively and engaging in reciprocal relationships may offset the nonreciprocal and passive roles patients play in the medical environment [45].

The Teen Impact Program: an example of successful peer-based intervention

Established in 1988, the Teen Impact Program, based at Childrens Hospital Los Angeles, is a comprehensive, multidimensional psychosocial treatment model that provides age-appropriate activities such as support groups, 3-day retreats, adventure therapy trips, and special events to help adolescents who have cancer navigate the obstacles of their disease and treatment. As a family-based intervention, the program also includes therapy groups for parents and siblings. Since its inception, Teen Impact has served thousands of adolescents and young adults on and off cancer treatment throughout Southern California [41].

The program has developed rituals to help both the dying adolescent and the Teen Impact community. One of these rituals is the "Teen Impact Tree," designed and constructed by group members as a way to remember and memorialize friends who have died. The portable tree can be taken on overnight retreats and to other special events. Members write messages on paper leaves and hang them on the tree. All the leaves have been kept and stored in a safe place. Also, Teen Impact members and staff attend funerals and memorial services and send sympathy cards to families of members who have died. A beautifully engraved plaque paying tribute to teenagers who have "bravely battled cancer" hangs in a special area on the hospital grounds. Teens can congregate in this tranquil space.

Spiritual considerations: building bridges to the beyond

Clinicians caring for adolescents who have life-threatening illnesses typically feel uncomfortable addressing spiritual issues for their patients and families because they lack training and sufficient experience [46]. Chaplains are professionals trained to address these issues and may be of assistance to both the dying adolescent and other health professionals striving to provide comprehensive palliative care.

Spiritual development in adolescents

According to Markstrom [47], the psychosocial development of adolescents readies them to address issues of religion and spirituality. Several theories of faith development through childhood and adolescence have been described [48,49]. Most of these involve spiritual and religious growth that is intertwined with the normal stages of cognitive and emotional development. For example, according to the work of Piaget [50], adolescence marks a shift from concrete operational thinking to formal operations, which supports a greater capacity for abstract religious thought [49]. According to Erikson [51], adolescence is primarily concerned with the consolidation of identity, which alters the adolescent's notions of trust relationships that underpin conceptions of God [49]. Synthesizing the developmental theories of Piaget, Erikson, and others, Fowler and Dell [48] developed a theory of seven stages of faith development. Those most applicable to the adolescent are stages three (synthetic-convention) and four (individuating-reflexive). Together, these encompass the period in which adolescents begin to seek a personal relationship with God, choose and then critically evaluate core spiritual values and beliefs, and develop a more independent sense of self-identity and judgment [48,49,52]. The spiritual potential of this stage has been characterized by Loder [53] as "emerging as each one senses the underlying void that is opening up as each moves out into an unknown future to which she is biologically, socially, and culturally destined." The adolescent thus moves beyond the concrete religious impressions of childhood to reflections on issues and concepts embedded in the existential and transcendental realms [48,49]. Adolescents are now wrestling with existential questions, such as "What is a lifetime?" "Why do I live it?" and "Is there a God?"

Spirituality and the dying adolescent

In the adolescent, impending death provokes profound spiritual questions about meaning, faith, hope, justice, religious belief, and an afterlife [54]. Stuber and Houskamp [54] point out that the search for identity and transcendent meaning, characteristic of this age group, is a familiar theme in adolescent coming-of-age stories (eg, *Siddhartha*) and may be accelerated by imminent death. Traditional concepts of trust (in parents and family) and justice (fairness in life) are challenged by the experience of life-threatening illness. Religious beliefs of an earlier age may be modified or replaced by a new hunger for a more workable spiritual ideology. Now the adolescent's relationship with God may become deeply intimate, with the new God-image incorporating personal qualities of loving acceptance, understanding, loyalty, and support during times of crisis [49,52]. As reviewed by Loder [53], an event with special significance for dying adolescents is what Erikson termed *homo religiosus*. According to this view, the adolescent is open to a transformation that transfigures the life span, creating a type of "religionless faith." The Divine Spirit dramatically and powerfully penetrates and permeates the whole person so that he or she is consumed by the Divine Presence [53]. Dying adolescents have described this experience as an overwhelming sense of the immanent presence of the Divine or of having seen the face of God. The adolescent who has this experience may choose to withdraw from the "standard, mainline socialized solutions to identity, reality, or ideology and insist instead on finding her own roots for ego identity" [53]. The energy involved in discovering "Who am I?" shifts to acceptance of "Why I am." The *homo religiosus* experience of the dying adolescent is the answer to the meaning of his or her entire existence, or, in Erikson's terms, the ability to affirm "life itself in the face of death itself" [53]. For some families and staff, this experience can be challenging to understand.

Role of the chaplain

Too often overlooked and underused as a clinical resource, the chaplain seeks to address the spiritual needs of dying adolescents in ways that are personally respectful, culturally sensitive, and practical [55]. A religious and spiritual assessment is regarded as essential for comprehensive medical care of adolescents [56]. It has been recommended that the starting point for understanding an adolescent's spirituality be an assessment of the family's beliefs and practices [52,56]. In the absence of validated, clinical spiritual assessment scales for children and adolescents, the recommended approach involves active listening, careful behavioral observation, and evaluating the adolescent's level of cognitive and emotional development [56,57].

Spiritual care interventions focus on supporting the adolescent's search for identity and illness-related meaning [52,56]. Based on the adolescent's developmental stage, Hart and Schneider [52] have recommended creating an atmosphere characterized by openness and acceptance. Specific interventions include (1) helping the adolescent derive meaning from personal illness in philosophical or religious terms, (2) supporting peer relationships, using teen groups where available, (3) providing rituals when desired by the adolescent, (4) listening with empathy, (5) taking the necessary time to develop an honest, trusting relationship, and (6) assessing and documenting the teenager's verbalized values and belief [52]. Through a sensitive presence with active listening, the chaplain supports the adolescent's intensely personal development of a relationship with the Higher Power and, regardless of religious belief, the spiritual and deeply human search for meaning, purpose, hope, and value in life [2,52,54]. The chaplain also needs to communicate to other palliative care team members the spiritual context surrounding important medical and psychosocial events.

The chaplain's role is also to bridge the gap to something larger than the adolescent's immediate experience. As Bearison explains [58], "For many children, whether they come from religious families or not, faith in God becomes an important way of dealing with the pain, frustrations, and side effects of treatment. When they are trying to come to grips with the fear of dying and, sometimes, with the inevitability of impending death, many children find solace in putting themselves in the hands of God." A chaplain can serve as a sounding board for the family, talking quietly with parents about their adolescent's need to die and encouraging them to communicate openly in the face of sadness and fear. When young people perceive that parents or members of the treatment team are willing to talk and answer questions honestly, a veil of pretenses is lifted, and teenagers become aware that they do not have to travel their frightening road alone.

Child life intervention: facilitating communication and acceptance

The child life specialist has a unique opportunity to assist the patient approaching the end of life. As stated by the Child Life Council [59], "It is often the child life specialist who is the only member of the team to observe the true potential of the patient, for it is the child life specialist who sees the child under the most 'normal' of circumstances, engaged in the art of being a child. The relationship that develops between the child life specialist and patients during their repeated non-medical encounters fosters a level of trust and comfort which allows the children to express fears, discontents and misconceptions about their care."

Using the tools of child life therapy

The essence of the child life intervention consists of establishing an intimate and therapeutic relationship with the adolescent. In part, this is accomplished through preparation of the patient for medical events and procedures through age-appropriate therapeutic recreational activities [60]. In describing an interventional child life program for patients undergoing endoscopy, Mahajan and colleagues [61] highlight the need children and adolescents have for information to help them control their imaginations and to separate reality from fantasy, which is often more frightening than what will actually happen.

The child life specialist's relationship often allows entry into the teenager's private world of fears and concerns. The effective use of "child life tools," such as visual art, writing, digital technology (video and audio), music, and other contemporary means of communication, assists the teenager in both self-understanding and self-expression. The relationship of trust between the adolescent and the child life specialist empowers the adolescent to use these tools to navigate the journey of chronic illness and approaching death.

Working with the dying adolescent

According to Judd [62], "Adolescents themselves perhaps have the most difficult time of all facing the possibility of death. Adolescence, particularly with its inherent struggle for identity and independence, is totally at odds with death. It is against the grain for adolescents to accept death. Their new-found sexual capacities, steps toward identity and independence, their physical and emotional growth, their ambitions and emphasis on physical attractiveness and the need for privacy and control are all jeopardised by a life-threatening illness."

Adolescents, like adults, take an uneven ride through the five stages from denial to acceptance of impending death, as described by Kübler-Ross [63]. Initially, adolescents are typically private about their feelings. Using the tools of communication noted earlier, the child life specialist helps teenagers navigate this journey. Dealing with sadness is a major goal in using these tools [64]. While struggling to accept the inevitability of death, the adolescent may need to communicate important thoughts, repair damaged relationships with parents and siblings, express gratitude, and say goodbye [62]. Child life specialists can coach teenagers to find the medium best suited to communicate feelings as death approaches. Legacy building is a particularly meaningful activity. With the child life specialist's assistance, one recently encountered young adult mother who had relapsed cancer found peace and acceptance of her death through leaving a video journal behind for her 18-month-old daughter; another adolescent left a music video in which she used sign language to say farewell to her parents.

Decision making by adolescents at the end of life

Nowhere do the normal adolescent developmental tasks of gaining autonomy and finding meaning appear more applicable than in the area of medical decision making. Based on an understanding of relevant developmental, ethical, and legal considerations, the multidisciplinary team can assist the adolescent in becoming an effective decision maker. When successful, this process not only provides for informed choice but also implies respect for the dignity of the adolescent.

The distinction between functional and legal competence

Much of the difficulty encountered in medical decision making by adolescents arises from their status as minors. In the United States, persons less than 18 years of age are not ordinarily considered legally competent to make binding medical decisions [65]. Despite this, clinicians have observed that many minors, especially teenagers who are chronically ill and have acquired considerable medical experience, exhibit significant knowledge and insight about their condition, prognosis, and treatment preferences [66,67]. This observation has led to efforts to define the essential cognitive features of one who has the *functional*, rather than *legal*, competence necessary for making medical decisions. Leiken [68] and King and Cross [69] have asserted that the functional requirements for competency include the abilities to reason, to understand, to choose voluntarily, to appreciate the nature of the decision, and to have a mature conceptualization of death. Accumulating research on decision making suggests that most adolescents do possess these capabilities, similar to competent adults [70].

Based on these considerations, pediatric health professionals, psychologists, ethicists, and lawyers agree that adolescents 14 years and older should be presumed, in the absence of contrary evidence, to possess the functional competence required to make binding medical decisions for themselves concerning discontinuation of life-prolonging therapy and other end-of-life issues [65,70–73]. Some clinicians have noted that adolescents younger than 14 years also may show evidence of functional competence owing to the maturing effects of chronic illness and exposure to death [66,67]. Children approximately 10 to 12 years old may be capable of a mature understanding of death, recognizing that death is universal, unalterable, and permanent [23–25]. These considerations form the basis for the proposal that terminally ill, cognitively intact adolescents aged approximately 10 years and older should be presumed to have functional decision-making capacity unless there is evidence to the contrary [74]. Empiric research in support of this proposal is limited. However, a recent study by Hinds and colleagues [75] of adolescent patients aged 10 to 20 years who had cancer and were making end-of-life decisions found that 18 of 20 subjects demonstrated features characteristic of competent decision making.

In the United States, the legal status of end-of-life decision making by adolescents is inconsistent [65,71,76]. Some states have "emancipated minor statutes" that allow binding medical decisions when the minor is married, a parent, or financially independent. Some states have permitted application of the "mature minor doctrine" through the courts to endow competent adolescents with medical decision-making authority on a case-by-case basis [77]. (A different legal framework is used in the Canadian province of Ontario, where patients are deemed to have capacity not according to age, but based on their ability to understand relevant information and to appreciate reasonably foreseeable consequences of the decision [78].) In the United States, legal intervention should be necessary only when there is serious disagreement between the functionally competent minor and responsible adults about a major treatment decision [65]. In most cases, the responsible adult will be willing to enact the wishes of the minor by making the legally valid treatment decision along the lines of a modified "substituted judgment" standard (the application of a patient's previously expressed values and preferences in a medical decision made on his or her behalf) [67,72]. Evidence that this occurs is found in a recent study, where interviewed parents of dying adolescents indicated that deciding as their child preferred was the most important factor in their end-of-life decisions [75]. For fully competent adolescents, advance treatment directives may be useful for clearly delineating their decisional preferences, but currently these instruments are not legally binding as they are for adults [2,65,71,72].

Fashioning a decisional role for the adolescent: role of the multidisciplinary team

The goal of the multidisciplinary team should be to support the adolescent in functioning at his or her highest level of competency. Because the capacity for good decision making reflects not only cognitive understanding but also experience, insight, and external support, the appropriate decisional role for each adolescent will be different [70]. Members of the multidisciplinary team collaborate in supporting the adolescent in several key areas (Table 2).

Competency assessment

The psychologist may be particularly important in assessing the functional competency of the patient. At present, no strict criteria exist for determining decision-making ability [70]. Previous school evaluations and records may give insight into an adolescent's ability to reason and process information. More helpful may be the use of standardized cognitive measures, such as current editions of the Wechsler Scale of Intelligence or the Stanford Binet Intelligence Scales. In general, age-adjusted scores that are significantly below normal may be suggestive of a learning problem that could limit functional competence. It is essential for the psychologist to rule out coexisting states of delirium, dementia, severe anxiety, and mood disorders that may contribute to errors in judgment, emotional and behavioral impulsivity, and thought disorganization (impaired perception of reality). Adjunctive consultation with a psychiatrist should be pursued when indicated. Practice considerations presented by the American Psychological Association [79] suggest that functional competency assessments include a well-documented mental status examination with specific attention to the patient's ability to (1) understand and remember relevant information, (2) appreciate the consequences (positive and negative) of different decisions, (3) demonstrate a consistent underlying set of values that guide the decision, and (4) communicate the decision and its rationale. These are consistent with other recently published criteria [80].

Communication

Along with promoting independence, providing effective communication is a critical aspect of supporting adolescents as decision makers [80]. Communication is bidirectional and includes *information sharing by care providers* (ie, relevant medical information concerning disease status, treatment options [including their benefits and burdens], and prognosis) and *self-expression by the patient* (ie, thoughts, feelings, and preferences). In a study of end-of-life decision making by adolescent patients who had cancer and their parents, receipt of accurate information about the health and disease status of the patient was rated as the most important factor [36]. When new, potentially decisive medical information becomes available

Table 2
Multidisciplinary team approach for supporting decision making by dying adolescents

Component of support	Key team member(s)	Examples of intervention(s)
Competency assessment	Physician/Nurse	Evaluate clinical consistency of meeting functional criteria for competency (see text)
	Psychologist	Determine adequacy of cognitive function using standardized testing and formal competency assessment, where required. Evaluate for presence of clinically significant psychopathology.
Communication	Physician/Nurse	Provide ongoing, complete, accurate medical information to patient/family. Maintain open communication milieu that encourages questions and expression of opinions.
	Social worker	Facilitate effective communication within family and peer support networks
	Child life specialist	Increase knowledge and facilitate self-expression through use of child life modalities and "tools."
Values clarification	Physician/Nurse	Assist in comprehending options, their consequences, and how values may be embodied in choices
	Psychologist	Through counseling, assist in increasing self-awareness
	Chaplain	Support discovery of core values and spiritual meaning of illness/impending death; facilitate insights relevant to decision making
	Child life specialist	Cultivate insights through journaling and other modalities of self-discovery.
Decision-making experience	Physician/Nurse	Over time, provide opportunities for decision-making experience, beginning with simple care choices and building toward greater complexity. Encourage family to respect teen's emerging decision-making role.
Affirmation, empowerment, and hope	Physician Nurse Psychologist Chaplain Child life specialist	As a team, express value of individual in all interactions; respect privacy and dignity of patient. Help patient to identify and reach important life goals before dying. Facilitate peer networking where possible. Help family respect emerging autonomy of teen.

Care of the dying adolescent requires a holistic and multidisciplinary approach that involves considerable overlap of some services provided by individual team members. The interventions highlighted here are not to imply exclusivity but to indicate prominent opportunities for certain disciplines. Assistance from other team members in carrying out those interventions is implied.

that could alter a patient's choices (eg, worsening cancer despite treatment), a formal conference involving the adolescent, family, other significant support persons, and the care team may be effective. Such a conference involves discussion of current disease status, probable outcome, treatment options, including their risks, and the likely clinical course at the end of life, along with available options for symptom management [66,81]. It may need to be explained to well-intentioned parents that withholding dire information from the adolescent is not only dishonest and disrespectful but usually counterproductive in these astute patients, serving only to alienate them and exacerbate their anxiety. Honest communication between parent and teenager also appears to be beneficial for the parent; a large study of parents who lost children to cancer found that none who had talked with their child about death regretted it, whereas 27% of those who had not discussed death with their child regretted not having done so [82]. From original diagnosis onward, an optimal communication milieu is one characterized by honesty, openness, an adolescent focus, a nonjudgmental approach, receptiveness to questions, and sensitivity to individual communication styles that may include nonverbal forms (eg, music and art).

Values clarification

Effective communication patterns also facilitate conversations in which family and care providers help adolescents explore their developing beliefs and values. An understanding of the adolescent's social networks (family, peers, and community), spiritual beliefs or religious practices, hopes, and dreams will help reveal his or her priorities in life. Guiding adolescents to an awareness of these may help them understand how their choices can embody their deepest convictions and help them achieve self-actualization.

Decision-making experience

Like most other aspects of life, decision making is a skill that is acquired over time and through direct experience. Clinical observation suggests that allowing a dying adolescent to be primary medical decision maker is a notion embraced most readily in families where children are given decision-making experience in other arenas. Most adolescents facing death have a gradual trajectory of illness that allows a sensitive medical team to promote decision-making skills from early on in the course. Whenever possible, even young children should be given guided opportunities to make choices about appropriate aspects of their care. At first, these may be simple choices such as the flavor of a medication; later, the adolescent might perhaps choose the class of analgesic and route of its administration, based on recommended options, weighing side effects and availability of parenteral access. Through this approach, adolescents facing death may be "trained" to face more momentous decisions that await them. As discussed previously, adolescents who demonstrate functional competence can be allowed to have decisive control over major choices, including discontinuation of disease-directed treatment, whereas those who do not can still be given control over less crucial matters. Like palliative care itself, medical decision making for the minor is not an "all or none" phenomenon.

Affirmation, empowerment, and hope

Finally, the dying adolescent needs the help of multidisciplinary team members to develop the sense of personal identity and self-confidence necessary for stepping into the role of mature decision maker. This goal is achieved gradually in myriad ways: by building self-esteem through teenager-oriented child life activities and peer networks; by directing medical conversation primarily toward the adolescent; by providing patient, sensitive explanations to sad parents about the importance of letting go and allowing the teenager to decide; and by helping the teenager achieve important personal life goals before dying. Research has found that hope remains a vital force in the lives of seriously ill adolescents [38]. Even when the hope for cure will not be realized, the palliative care team can encourage hope directed toward meaningful, achievable short-term goals.

Bereavement

Bereavement services address the grief reaction experienced by survivors of the adolescent. Grief affects the adolescent preparing for death, parents, siblings, and clinical staff [24,83,84]. Parental grief after losing a child is deep and long-lasting, and it is particularly complex following the death of an adolescent [85]. This complexity results from normal tension in adolescent family relationships that may lead to several forms of parental guilt, interfering with completion of the normal mourning process [85]. In addition to sadness, siblings often experience both "survivor guilt" and anger over perceived neglect and the stress placed on the family [84]. Being older and more peer-oriented than younger children, adolescents typically leave behind remarkably extensive networks of close friends, often including other adolescent patients. In contrast to sudden death, chronic illness provides an opportunity for preparation that benefits bereavement [85]. During that phase, the multidisciplinary team may promote adaptive coping through involving parents and siblings in care and using traditional discussion, journals, poetry, music, art, and religious rituals of preparation for death [83–86]. Afterward, memorial services and private remembrances for family and peers may be held if desired. Depending on the circumstances, teen support groups to which the adolescent belonged may have a variety of reactions, including sadness, fear, anger, dismay, and admiration. Some teen groups have their own formal rituals of remembrance [41]. Depending on family preferences, follow-up bereavement care from the treatment team may be helpful in the form of notes, phone calls, or other contact, especially at stressful times, including the patient's birthday, date of death, and holidays. Psychologists and specially trained child life specialists may provide grief counseling and other forms of sibling support [60].

Summary

The adolescent at the end of life poses a unique combination of challenges resulting from the collision of failing health with a developmental trajectory meant to lead to attainment of personal independence. Because virtually all spheres of the dying adolescent's life are affected, optimal palliative care for these young persons requires a multidisciplinary team whose members have a good understanding of their complementary roles and a shared commitment to providing well-coordinated care. Members of the team include the physician (to initiate and coordinate palliative care management); the nurse (to work collaboratively with the physician and adolescent, especially through effective patient advocacy); the psychologist (to assess and manage the patient's neurocognitive and emotional status); the social worker (to assess and optimize support networks); the chaplain (to support the adolescent's search for spiritual meaning); and the child life specialist (to facilitate effective communication in preparing for death). A crucial area for dying adolescents is medical decision making, where the full range of combined support is needed. By helping the young person continue to develop personal autonomy, the multidisciplinary team will enable even the dying adolescent to experience dignity and personal fulfillment.

Acknowledgments

Vicki Peterson contributed useful information to the discussion of the chaplain's role.

References

[1] Anderson RN, Smith BL. Deaths: leading causes for 2001. National vital statistics reports. Vol. 52, no. 9. Hyattsville (MD): National Center for Health Statistics; 2003. Available at: http://www.cdc.gov/nchs/data/nvsr/nvsr52/nvsr52_09.pdf. Accessed October 8, 2005.
[2] Himelstein BP, Hilden JM, Boldt AM, et al. Pediatric palliative care. N Engl J Med 2004;350: 1752–62.
[3] Suris JC, Michaud PA, Viner R. The adolescent with a chronic condition. Part I: developmental issues. Arch Dis Child 2004;89:938–42.
[4] Frager G. Pediatric palliative care: building the model, bridging the gaps. J Palliat Care 1996; 12:9–12.
[5] Goldman A. Home care of the dying child. J Palliat Care 1996;12:16–9.
[6] Vickers JL, Carlisle C. Choices and control: parental experiences in pediatric terminal home care. J Pediatr Oncol Nurs 2000;17:12–21.
[7] Hilden JM, Himelstein BP, Freyer DR, et al. End-of-life care: special issues in pediatric oncology. In: Foley KM, Gelband H, editors. Improving palliative care for cancer (report from Institute of Medicine). Washington, DC: National Academy Press; 2001. p. 161–95.
[8] Guidelines on the termination of life-sustaining treatment and care of the dying. Briarcliff Manor: The Hastings Center; 1987.
[9] George R, Hutton S. Palliative care in adolescents. Eur J Cancer 2003;39:2662–8.
[10] Kang T, Hoehn S, Licht DJ, et al. Pediatric palliative, end-of-life and bereavement care. Pediatr Clin North Am 2005;52:1029–46.

[11] Wolfe J, Friebert S, Hilden J. Caring for children with advanced cancer: integrating palliative care. Pediatr Clin North Am 2002;49:1043–62.

[12] Savedra MC, Tesler MD. Assessing children's and adolescents' pain. Paediatrician 1989;16: 24–9.

[13] Beyer JE, Wells N. The assessment of pain in children. Pediatr Clin North Am 1989;36: 837–54.

[14] Crandall M, Savedra M. Multidimensional assessment using the adolescent pediatric pain tool: a case report. J Spec Pediatr Nurs 2005;10:115–23.

[15] Klopfenstein KJ, Hutchison C, Clark C, et al. Variables influencing end-of-life care in children and adolescents with cancer. J Pediatr Hematol Oncol 2001;23:481–6.

[16] Hanks G, Doyle D. Oxford textbook of palliative medicine. 3rd edition. Oxford (UK): Oxford University Press; 2003.

[17] Initiative for pediatric palliative care. Available at: http://www.ippcweb.org. Accessed October 8, 2005.

[18] Collins JJ, Stevens MM, Cousens P. Home care for the dying child: a parent's perception. Aust Fam Physician 1998;27:610–4.

[19] Wolfe J, Grier HE, Klar N, et al. Symptoms and suffering at the end of life in children with cancer. N Engl J Med 2000;342:326–33.

[20] Pazola KJ, Gerberg AK. Privileged communication—talking with a dying adolescent. MCN Am J Matern Child Nurs 1990;15:16–21.

[21] Hamburg BA. Psychosocial development. In: Friedman SB, Fisher MM, Schonberg SK, et al, editors. Comprehensive adolescent health care. 2nd edition. St. Louis (MO): Mosby; 1998. p. 38–49.

[22] Sigel EJ. Adolescent growth and development. In: Greydanus DE, Patel DR, Pratt HD, editors. Essential adolescent medicine. New York: McGraw-Hill; 2006. p. 3–15.

[23] Kenyon BL. Current research in children's conceptions of death: a critical review. Omega: Journal of Death and Dying 2001;43:63–91.

[24] Hinds PS, Oakes LL, Hicks J, et al. End-of-life care for children and adolescents. Semin Oncol Nurs 2005;21:53–62.

[25] Foley GV, Whittam EH. Care of the child dying of cancer: part I. CA Cancer J Clin 1990;40: 327–54.

[26] Klopfenstein KJ. Adolescents, cancer and hospice. Adolesc Med 1999;10:437–43.

[27] Achenbach TM, Rescorla LA. Manual for the ASEBA school-age forms and profiles. Burlington (VT): University of Vermont Research Center for Children, Youth and Families; 2001.

[28] Bloom JR, Kang SH, Romano P. Cancer and stress: the effects of social support on a resource. In: Cooper C, Watson M, editors. Cancer and stress: psychological, biological, and coping studies. New York: John Wiley; 1991. p. 95–124.

[29] Woodgate RL. Social support in children with cancer. A review of the literature. J Pediatr Oncol Nurs 1999;16:201–13.

[30] Kane JR, Hellsten MB, Coldsmith A. Human suffering: the need for relationship-based research in pediatric end-of-life care. J Pediatr Oncol Nurs 2004;21:1–6.

[31] Trask PC, Paterson AG, Trask CL, et al. Parent and adolescent adjustment to pediatric cancer: association with coping, social support, and family function. J Pediatr Oncol Nurs 2003; 20:36–47.

[32] Shinn M, Lehmann S, Wong NW. Social interaction and social support. J Soc Issues 1984; 40:55–76.

[33] Nichols ML. Social support and coping in young adolescents with cancer. Pediatr Nurs 1995; 21:235–40.

[34] Beale EA, Baile WF, Aaron J. Silence is not golden: communicating with children dying from cancer. J Clin Oncol 2005;23:3629–31.

[35] Ettinger RS, Heiney SP. Cancer in adolescents and young adults. Cancer 1993;71(Suppl): 3276–80.

[36] Hinds PS, Oakes L, Furman W, et al. End-of-life decision making by adolescents, parents and healthcare providers in pediatric oncology: research to evidence-based practice guidelines. Cancer Nurs 2001;24:122–36.

[37] Ritchie MA. Sources of emotional support for adolescents with cancer. J Pediatr Oncol Nurs 2001;18:105–10.

[38] Hinds PS. The hopes and wishes of adolescents with cancer and the nursing care that helps. Oncol Nurs Forum 2004;31:927–34.

[39] Plante WA, Lobato D, Engel R. Review of group interventions for pediatric chronic conditions. J Pediatr Psychol 2001;26:435–53.

[40] Roberts CS, Piper L, Denny J, et al. A support group intervention to facilitate young adults' adjustment to cancer. Health Soc Work 1997;22:133–41.

[41] Kuperberg AL. The relationship between perceived social support, family behavior, self-esteem and hope on adolescents' strategies for coping with cancer. Dissertation Abstracts International Section A: Humanities and Social Sciences 1994;56(9-A):3744.

[42] Ell KO, Reardon KK. Psychosocial care for the chronically ill adolescent: challenges and opportunities. Health Soc Work 1990;15:272–82.

[43] Carr-Gregg M, Hampson R. A new approach to the psychosocial care of adolescents with cancer. Med J Aust 1986;145:580–3.

[44] Bluebond M, Perkel D, Goetzel T. Pediatric cancer patients' peer relationships: the impact of an oncology camp experience. J Psychosoc Oncol 1991;9:67–80.

[45] Chesler MA, Yoak M. Difficulties for providing help in a crisis: relationship between parents of children with cancer and their families. In: Kobalk HB, editor. Helping patients and their families. San Francisco (CA): Jossey-Bass; 1984.

[46] Devictor D. Are we ready to discuss spirituality with our patients and their families? Pediatr Crit Care Med 2005;6:492–3.

[47] Markstrom CA. Religious involvement and adolescent psychosocial development. J Adolesc 1999;22:205–21.

[48] Fowler JW, Dell ML. Stages of faith and identity: birth to teens. Child Adolesc Psychiatr Clin N Am 2004;13:17–33.

[49] Brown JD. Body and spirit: religion, spirituality and health among adolescents. Adolesc Med 2001;12:509–23.

[50] Piaget J. The child and reality. New York: Penguin; 1976.

[51] Erikson EH. Childhood and society. 2nd edition. New York: Norton; 1963.

[52] Hart D, Schneider D. Spiritual care for children with cancer. Semin Oncol Nurs 1997;13:263–70.

[53] Loder JE. The logic of the spirit. San Francisco (CA): Jossey-Bass; 1998.

[54] Stuber ML, Houskamp BM. Spirituality in children confronting death. Child Adolesc Psychiatr Clin N Am 2004;13:127–36.

[55] Dell ML. Religious professionals and institutions: untapped resources for clinical care. Child Adolesc Psychiatr Clin N Am 2004;13:85–110.

[56] Sexson SB. Religious and spiritual assessment of the child and adolescent. Child Adolesc Psychiatr Clin N Am 2004;13:35–47.

[57] Houskamp BM, Fisher LA, Stuber ML. Spirituality in children and adolescents: research findings and implications for clinicians and researchers. Child Adolesc Psychiatr Clin N Am 2004;13:221–30.

[58] Bearison DJ. God and prayer. In: They Never Want to Tell You: Children Talk about cancer. Cambridge (MA): Harvard University Press; 1991. p. 129–31.

[59] Child Life Council. Official documents. Rockville (MD): The Child Life Council; 2002.

[60] American Academy of Pediatrics—Committee on Hospital Care. Child life services. Pediatrics 2000;106:1156–9.

[61] Mahajan L, Wyllie R, Steffen R, et al. The effects of a psychological preparation program on anxiety in children and adolescents undergoing gastrointestinal endoscopy. J Pediatr Gastroenterol Nutr 1998;27:161–5.

[62] Judd D. The stages of emotional reactions to life-threatening illness. In: Give sorrow words: working with the dying child. New York: Hayworth Press; 1995. p. 60–1.

[63] Kübler-Ross E. On death and dying: what the dying have to teach doctors, nurses, clergy and their own families. New York: MacMillan; 1969.

[64] Heagarty M. Terminal and life-threatening illness in children. In: Gellert E, editor. Psychosocial aspects of pediatric care. New York: Grune and Stratton; 1978. p. 69–70.

[65] Hartman RG. Dying young: cues from the courts. Arch Pediatr Adolesc Med 2004;158: 615–9.

[66] Nitschke R, Meyer WH, Sexauer CL, et al. Care of terminally ill children with cancer. Med Pediatr Oncol 2000;34:268–70.

[67] Freyer DR. Children with cancer: special considerations in the discontinuation of life-sustaining treatment. Med Pediatr Oncol 1992;20:136–42.

[68] Leiken S. A proposal concerning decisions to forgo life-sustaining treatment for young people. J Pediatr 1989;115:17–22.

[69] King NMP, Cross AW. Children as decision-makers: guidelines for pediatricians. J Pediatr 1989;115:10–6.

[70] Kuther TL. Medical decision-making and minors: issues of consent and assent. Adolescence 2003;38:343–58.

[71] Weir RF, Peters C. Affirming the decisions adolescents make about life and death. Hastings Cent Rep 1997;27:29–40.

[72] American Academy of Pediatrics—Committee on Bioethics. Guidelines on forgoing life-sustaining medical treatment. Pediatrics 1994;93:532–6.

[73] American Academy of Pediatrics—Committee on Bioethics. Informed consent, parental permission, and assent in pediatric practice. Pediatrics 1995;95:314–7.

[74] Freyer DR. Care of the dying adolescent: special considerations. Pediatrics 2004;113:381–8.

[75] Hinds PS, Drew D, Oakes LL, et al. End-of-life care preferences of pediatric patients with cancer. J Clin Oncol 2005;23:1–9 [E-pub version released September 19, 2005.]

[76] Traugott I, Alpers A. In their own hands: adolescents' refusal of medical treatment. Arch Pediatr Adolesc Med 1997;151:922–7.

[77] Sigman GS, O'Connor C. Exploration for physicians of the mature minor doctrine. J Pediatr 1991;119:520–5.

[78] Ontario health care consent act of 1996. Available at: http://192.75.156.68/DBLaws/Statutes/English/96h02_e.htm. Accessed October 9, 2005.

[79] American Psychological Association, Public Interest Directorate. End of life issues and care: issues to consider when exploring end-of-life care. Washington, DC: American Psychological Association; 2001. Available at:. http://www.apa.org/pi/eol/issues.html . Accessed October 31, 2005.

[80] McConnell Y, Frager G, Levetown M. Decision-making in pediatric palliative care. In: Carter BS, Levetown M, editors. Palliative care for infants, children and adolescents: a practical handbook. Baltimore (MD): Johns Hopkins University Press; 2004. p. 69–111.

[81] Nitschke R, Humphrey GB, Sexauer CL, et al. Therapeutic choices made by patients with end-stage cancer. J Pediatr 1982;101:471–6.

[82] Kreicbergs U, Valdimarsdóttir U, Onelöv E, et al. Talking about death with children who have severe malignant disease. N Engl J Med 2004;351:1175–86.

[83] Mearns SJ. The impact of loss on adolescents: developing appropriate support. Int J Palliat Nurs 2000;6:12–7.

[84] Nolbris M, Hellstrom A-L. Siblings' needs and issues when a brother or sister dies of cancer. J Pediatr Oncol Nurs 2005;22:227–33.

[85] Davies AM. Death of adolescents: parental grief and coping strategies. Br J Nurs 2001;10: 1332–42.

[86] Giovanola J. Sibling involvement at end of life. J Pediatr Oncol Nurs 2005;22:222–6.

ELSEVIER
SAUNDERS

Child Adolesc Psychiatric Clin N Am
15 (2006) 717–737

CHILD AND
ADOLESCENT
PSYCHIATRIC CLINICS
OF NORTH AMERICA

Nursing Interventions in Pediatric Palliative Care

Kristen M. Powaski, RN, BSN, CPON

Department of Pediatric Hematology and Oncology, The Children's Hospital at The Cleveland Clinic, 9500 Euclid Avenue, Desk S20, Cleveland, OH 44195, USA

Parents and healthcare professionals face numerous challenges as they care for critically and chronically ill children and children who have a diagnosis associated with poor prognosis. Although most children meet their developmental milestones and make plans for their future, others undergo treatments, both experimental and routine, and deal with their side effects. The potential for cures for life-limiting illnesses has drastically improved, as has the treatment of chronic illnesses, and yet children suffer in spite of their treatments. Many experience pain and other distressing symptoms caused by the disease process. Whether treatment is aimed at curing the disease, controlling the symptoms, or extending life, children benefit when palliative care specialists are involved with the child and the family early in the diagnostic period. Palliative care teams facilitate medical decisions; offer support to the patient, family, and healthcare professionals; and offer expert advice on symptom management. The palliative care team may remain involved throughout the course of illness, regardless of the outcome.

Nurses have a unique role in the support of patients and family as they journey through the course of illness. The pursuit of a cure may lead families down avenues they would never anticipate. Nursing staff must be available to foster hope, recognize each family's unique challenges, and advocate for specialized palliative care services to support the patient and family. As the child's disease progresses, or as the quality of life becomes less than optimal, "roads less traveled" in pediatrics can be difficult for families to navigate alone. Pediatric palliative medicine teams help navigate the winding roads of the healthcare system and provide nurses and families with a holistic support structure.

E-mail address: powaskk1@ccf.org

doi:10.1016/j.chc.2006.03.001

childpsych.theclinics.com

Current technology focused on cure

The development of national, multi-center clinical trials and the technological advances in surgical and critical care medicine are creating new and promising treatment options every day. These technological advances are increasing the number of live premature births, prolonging the lives of those diagnosed with chronic and acquired diseases, and offering hope for curing others. Children now survive with chronic conditions that may offer a poor quality of life, and long-term morbidity. Efforts that focus on eliminating physiological dysfunction, life extension, and cure, often supersede the obligation to discuss palliative treatment options [1]. "Successful integration of palliative care perspectives following diagnosis means finding sensitive ways of providing parents—whatever their values and background—with timely and appropriate information about palliative care options and then encouraging their timely consideration of these options and goals of care" [2]. The gap between curative therapies and palliative treatments may be a difficult one to fill. Parents often equate palliative care with death, rather than with a service that can increase quality of life and help with medical decision-making, and so they find the discussion of palliative care intolerable until death is imminent or it becomes abundantly clear that life-prolonging treatments are ineffective [2].

Many seriously ill children experience multiple near-death events that are avoided because of the excellent advances in pediatric intensive care units. A child may have experienced multiple lifesaving interventions, such as intubations, and become well enough to be taken off the ventilator. This may create the expectation that every trip to the intensive care unit and course of intubation will result in restored health for the child. Parents may, however, neglect to consider the natural course of the disease process, or the sequelae from treatments or complications over time.

As healthcare professionals, it is important to recognize when death is a likely outcome. Intubation technology is not conducive to promote the final moments of closure for families during what may be the last moments of the child's life. When intubation is emergent and the child is unlikely to become stable enough to come off the ventilator, families may feel as if they haven't been able to say goodbye. Palliative care teams can facilitate discussions with the patient and family to clarify their wishes before times of crisis, which can prevent some guilt and regret that families experience if they have not had the chance to say goodbye. This is obviously difficult because the family may view these discussions as negative and a sign that their medical team has lost all hope for their child's recovery. Palliative care teams are able to frame discussions to foster simultaneous hope and preparation.

It is impossible to predict the future, but it is vital to inform the parents and child (whenever appropriate) of all possible outcomes. The challenge is to decide when it is appropriate to discuss the possibilities and to help prepare the family for a poor outcome. It can be difficult for the primary care team to discuss the possibility of death or severe morbidity, because they don't want to be seen as giving up hope. A palliative care team can work with the primary team to open these lines of communication; however, it can be difficult to introduce the palliative care team at the time of crisis, especially if they are viewed by the parents as less than hopeful.

Goals of care

Openness and honesty about prognosis, and realistic treatment goals, however difficult the discussion will be for both the parent and the primary care provider, will promote the development of a trusting relationship. For patients whose prognosis is likely to be poor, or for patients whose disease-related symptoms are temporarily or permanently debilitating, palliative care should be offered simultaneously with curative efforts to help prevent and ease suffering during treatment. This will also create ongoing relationships that can ease the transition of care goals if a cure is not possible.

When treatment fails and/or disease progresses, it is nearly impossible to transition the care goals from a solely curative intent to a strictly palliative intent. This is especially true if the family has not had a team focused on their child's comfort and the parents understanding of the situation. Healthcare providers can ease this transition by communicating early on that the treatment is aimed at curing the child, but if the disease is resistant to the treatment, the child will continue to receive care even if cure is no longer possible.

Families fear abandonment from their healthcare provider when they hear the words "nothing more can be done." However, there is never "nothing" left to do. When parents hear those words from physicians, many never believe them. In their hearts, parents believe there must be something else that can be done. No parent is willing to give up on their child, nor do physicians want to be viewed as giving up on their patients. Parents have a need to do something, anything, to contribute toward the care of their child. In today's computer literate world, parents often search the Internet for any information that might offer the slightest hope of a cure or at least life extension for their child. Families often use information gathering as a way to cope in response to disappointment or desperation when a treatment fails. They may search the Internet, shop for alternate institutions, or seek second, third, or fourth opinions. In an effort to prolong life, parents and healthcare providers might explore experimental treatment options that have high risk for side effects and low chance for cure. During the discussion of treatment options, treatments should be discussed in terms of whether they are "doing to" rather than "doing for" the child. It becomes the responsibility of healthcare providers to fully explore and discuss all treatment options, including the option to pursue no further treatment with curative intent, with both the parents and the child when possible.

When considering the goals of care, potential treatments, and likelihood of cure, it is critical to explore how the proposed treatments will affect the child and the family's quality of life. The definition of quality of life is unique to each child and family. To determine what quality of life means for a family, discussions should include the family's values, the likelihood and severity of potential side effects, time away from home or school at an outpatient clinic or in the hospital, and any financial strains that might be placed on the family. During these discussions, nurses can offer medical information in terms a family can understand, and give the parents time to process the information, and generate questions. It is important for the healthcare team not to monopolize the conversation. To formulate a treatment plan, several lengthy discussions will be necessary. Nurses can facilitate the decision-making process by being available to the family for questions as they arise.

As it becomes apparent that treatment is failing and disease is progressing, the options can become limited and more risky. It is important for the physician to offer—and for families to consider—the option to discontinue treatment for curative intent, and aim further treatment at palliation. Some examples of palliative treatment are anti-neoplastic drugs to slow cancer growth and spread, which relieves and sometimes prevents symptoms; radiation for pain relief and to restore function; or narcotics or other agents to relieve associated symptoms and promote comfort.

Families may elect to consider alternative or complimentary therapies such as nutritional supplements, herbal treatments, acupuncture, and therapeutic touch. When alternative therapies and herbal supplements are considered, there again should be a discussion of the risks and benefits. Points to consider include whether there are specific health risks associated with the supplement, and if the supplement will burden the child and caregiver with a large quantity of pills. A large number of pills may create unnecessary stress on the caregiver and child if the caregiver has to struggle to get the child to take them. Some children benefit from the herbal supplements because they feel like they are still being treated. Parents also benefit when they feel like they are doing something. It is crucial not to dismiss any option a parent believes will have a positive effect on their child, unless it has the potential to create more harm than good. Nurses can help the team to support alternative therapies and offer them in conjunction with other palliative options to promote the optimal quality of life.

The palliative medicine consult

Although 75%–85% of children who die do so in institutional settings [2], some families prefer to care for their child at home. A smooth transition from the hospital setting to the home setting can be facilitated through a pediatric hospice referral. Pediatric hospice programs are a specialty service that is not yet available in all areas of the country. In cases where pediatric hospice is not yet available, a close working relationship between the available home care agency and the palliative care team can facilitate this transition home.

Nursing care must always be delivered in a manner that reflects the personal, cultural, and religious values of the child and family. Patient-centered supportive interventions strive to meet the physical, psychological, social, and spiritual needs of the patient and family. It is difficult if not impossible for a busy bedside nurse to fulfill all of these needs. Palliative care teams aim to utilize the expertise and combined efforts of the interdisciplinary team including nurses, child life specialists, social workers, clergy, bereavement specialists, pharmacists, physicians, dieticians, music and art therapists, and counselors, to provide the holistic, comprehensive care that no one person or discipline can address alone.

Palliative care teams promote the opportunity for positive experiences even in the face of illness and suffering. Both children and their caregivers experience a wide variety of emotions as health declines and death approaches. The team can facilitate a more peaceful end of life by offering support to the family and helping them to address fears and unresolved issues, which can alleviate emotional suffering. The nurse must try to recognize the patient and family concerns, which are not always communicated in words. Presence, attentiveness, and a willingness to listen are paramount skills in this situation.

The palliative medicine team can serve as objective partners in the decision-making process. This multi-disciplinary team has the time and resources to devote to family-centered, holistic care. When consulted early, the palliative medicine team can develop a trusting relationship and discuss delicate issues over weeks and months as a disease progresses or regresses. These are not one-time discussions, because the goals of care change when the patient's condition declines or improves. Early involvement of a pediatric palliative medicine team can (1) prevent prolonged suffering for the patient; (2) for adolescents, promote a sense of ownership over their disease as they participate in discussions about their care; (3) promote closure at the end of life; and (4) give parents the opportunity to discuss medical issues and ask questions repeatedly. The primary medical team benefits because the palliative medicine team can take on the burden of some of these time-consuming, repetitive conversations.

The palliative medicine team can bridge the gap from acute hospital care to home hospice care. It is often the palliative medicine team that offers to place the consult to hospice services. Before hospice services are offered, the presenters need to educate themselves on what services the hospice has to offer. Many families are immediately turned off when they hear the word "hospice," but may be more accepting of the services when they hear what hospice has to offer. Hospice may be only associated with dying. If the potential to make the living better is presented, hospice may take on new meaning associated with hope for a better quality of life.

Nurses foster hope

No matter how close a child may be to his or her death, it is critical that they maintain hope. The dying process can challenge, temporarily diminish, or change the meaning of hope, but it does not inevitably bring despair. Maintaining a person's unique sense of hope throughout illness, even in the face of disease progression or impending death, can enhance quality of life and contribute to a process of dying that is meaningful to the child and family [3]. In most cases, parents remain hopeful for a miracle cure even until the time of death. And, families find new hopes.

Nurses foster hope without even thinking about it; they do it through everyday discussions in which they reminisce about past and present joys, share positive experiences, use lightheartedness and humor. The team should feel free to communicate hope to the family. Dialogue may offer hope for the patient's future, but also hope for the family's future. Hope for the future of the child [3] and for the preservation of the family structure can be communicated by discussing future events such as what the child wants to be when he/she grows up, the child's first or next day at school, or when he/she gets married or goes off to college. Other interventions to foster hope for parents or children may include encouraging religious rituals, suggesting keeping a journal, reading books or watching movies that are uplifting and highlight the joys in life. Children can be encouraged to illustrate their joys through art, and then decorate their home or hospital room with their drawings. Well siblings can create special artwork to brighten up their ill sibling's room. Nurses can take time to listen to music the child enjoys and explore if there is special meaning associated with it. This can facilitate a sense of openness between the nurse and the patient. This openness may encourage a dialogue about hopes for the future and also encourage verbalization of fears [3].

The discussion of hope does not eliminate the discussion of fear. Adults and children have different fears about illness and death. Children's fears focus on who will be with them if they die, who will take care of them, and whether or not their family will be able to function without them. It is important to keep in mind that it is common for children not to express their true emotions in an effort to protect their family from burden or additional worries, especially their parents [4,5]. The child may express their fears in artwork or writing. Parents also pretend they are not afraid because they don't want to worry their children [6].

Anticipating symptoms and needs

It is important to anticipate the child's needs and possible impending symptoms based on the course of the disease and to prepare the family for the management of potential upcoming events. Preparation should include comfort measures and a teaching plan for what to do and who to call in the middle of the night if concerns arise when the child is being cared for at home. (Defining this "go-to" team for off-hours care might be the door-opener for initiating a palliative care consult.) These discussions are likely to invoke many emotions. When the child is in pain or has other distressing symptoms, the caregiver will be under great stress. It will be difficult for them to recall such information from memory, therefore, the family should have "who to call" information written down and kept in an easily accessible location. Nurses can encourage the family to keep important phone numbers handy because the primary caregiver(s) may not always be available 24 hours a day, 7 days a week.

Early on in treatment, it is the nurse's responsibility to educate parents about the importance of early intervention in pain and symptom management. Children have the right to live out their last days free from pain and other distressing symptoms. The child should not be presumed comfortable if he/she does not complain of pain. Waiting to assess or medicate a child until he/she is crying in pain is too late. The nurse should explore with the parents how the child exhibits signs of pain. Parents will be able to provide subjective data. Asking children "Are you in pain?" or "Do you hurt?" may be ineffective. Ask the caregiver what word the child uses for pain. Use the child's language. Does the child have "ouchies," or "boo-boos"? It may also be ineffective to ask the parents of young patients, "Is your child in pain?" because for some, comfort may be a different concept than pain. Think of rephrasing such questions to ask, "Does your child appear comfortable?" Nurses should buy and read children's books to learn their language and their thought process.

Instruct the parents to view the child's behavior as an indicator of comfort. Respect their judgment when it comes to the child's behavior, as they know their child best. However, parents may not realize how gradually uncomfortable their child has become. Discuss with the parents that it is unacceptable if the child's only state of comfort is if he/she stays still on the couch. Explore the recent level of activity the child has been participating in. Has the child been actively playing games on the floor with his siblings, only to suddenly want to lie still and watch movies? Assess the child's mood: is he/she withdrawn and quiet, or unusually clingy to one or both parents? Assess the child's appetite because it may decline if the child is in pain. Review the child's sleep patterns, because a child in pain will often not sleep through the night. Examine the child's ability to maintain his/her activities of daily living. An astute nursing assessment and intervention can optimize how well the child can feel when they are properly treated for pain. A trial of pain medicines is often all it takes for the parent to recognize the difference proper interventions can make towards their child's quality of life.

Why do parents and nurses have to advocate so strongly for symptom control? Ninety-one percent of surveyed physicians rated themselves as "very competent" in their pain management skills [7], however, when 103 parents were surveyed, 82% of them reported their children suffered "a great deal" or "a lot" from pain at the end of life [8]. Of these patients, 76% were treated for pain; this treatment was seen as effective by parents in only 27% of patients. Poor pain control is unacceptable. In the hospital setting the nurse administers the prescribed medications, so it is the nurse's responsibility to routinely assess and reassess for pain or other distressing symptoms. Pain assessment scales must be age-appropriate, reliable, and valid. The nurse must assess both qualitative and quantitative aspects of the child's pain, because each patient may experience pain from many sources [9]. Objective data such as the child's appearance, vital signs, and response to touch or movement also must be considered. Assess the parents' level of understanding and educate them about other factors that may influence the child's pain including: the frequency of the pain, fatigue, anger, depression, fear, and anxiety [10].

An individualized, flexible plan of care that is based on the latest research must be established for the management of pain and other distressing symptoms. The plan must be consistently evaluated because the child's symptoms at the end of life can change rapidly and require prompt assessment and aggressive treatment. Parents must be kept informed as the plan of care changes. Interventions must be planned to promote the parents understanding of the care plan. Parents need to be educated about the medications being used and their potential for side effects. Nurses can address any fears or misconceptions the parents may have regarding opioids (eg, addiction and respiratory depression). When aggressive doses of opioid analgesics are administered, a common fear among health care providers is that respiratory depression will shorten life. However, the use of aggressive doses of opioid analgesics to control terminal pain is considered appropriate according to the principle of double effect [11]. The principle of double effect occurs when the intended action (pain control) is good and sincerely intended, but there is potential for an adverse secondary side effect (respiratory depression). In this case, the opioid is given to control pain and suffering, and therefore is acceptable. Narcotics should not be withheld or limited by traditional milligram-per-kilogram dosing when a child is in pain at the end of life. Doses of opioids may be rapidly titrated until intolerable side effects are present or until there is no increase in analgesia [9].

Constipation and urinary retention are two symptoms that can be caused by the disease process itself, or by side effects related to the treatment of symptoms. A nurse can assess a child's ability to void and defecate independently as he/she normally did. Incontinence can be embarrassing to a school-age child or adolescent. Regardless of cause, these symptoms require aggressive management.

Interventions for pain management may be both pharmacological and non-pharmacological and work best when implemented together. It can be particularly helpful to include the multidisciplinary team members when implementing the non-pharmacological measures. Some measures that may be implemented and taught to parents include guided imagery, distraction techniques, deep breathing exercises, a warm bath or shower, hot or cold packs, prayer or meditation, gentle massage, art, music, play or pet therapies, all of which can be easily accomplished whether the child is at home or in the hospital setting. Nurses may teach these techniques to parents. A sense of usefulness and partnership with the care team is fostered in a situation where the parent often feels helpless against the disease.

Support from the bedside nurse

Because it is the bedside nurse who spends more time with the child and family than any other member of the health care team, the nurse has a unique and very special role. As the nurse consistently meets the family's needs, a special bond is created. The nurse's "presence may be in fact be our greatest gift to these patients and their families" [12]. Being present with dying children and their families allows the nurse to enter into the world of the patient and respond with compassion [13]. Parents often trust their nurse with intimate thoughts and questions they may not feel comfortable asking others. They often realize there are no answers to the questions they pose. Nurses should not fill the gaps of silence with false hope. Answers are sometimes nonexistent and nurses need not fill the air with words, nor try to "fix" things as some things cannot be fixed [14,15]. Important concepts include

- We cannot change the inevitability of death.
- We cannot erase the anguish felt when someone we love dies.
- We all must face the fact that we too will die.
- No matter how hard we try, perfect words or gestures to completely relieve child and family distress rarely, if ever, exist.
- It is sometimes enough to just be with the child and parents.
- There is always an opportunity to heal, even when cure is not possible.

Support from the bedside nurse is crucial as he/she is the hands-on care provider and the one most readily available to the family as questions arise and conditions change. It is imperative that the nurse convey the same sense of concern and caring during times when the patient's condition changes; even when a decision has been made to designate the patient "Do Not Resuscitate." In the course of patient care there may once have been an urgency to escalate ventilator support or increase pressor; now there may be a shift to an urgency to promote comfort. Some comfort measures may be pharmacological, but their effectiveness may be enhanced when used in conjunction with nursing measures such as suction, massage, positioning, and even a warm or cool blanket. Altering the environment to make it quiet, warmer or cooler, darker or lighter, or by playing soft music may also facilitate patient and caregiver comfort.

The nurse must not neglect the basic needs of the child such as mouth care, clean linens, feeding, or bathing. Neglecting these basic needs can convey a sense that because this child is dying, he/she is less important than other children who will recover from their illness. If a nurse is nonchalant about providing care for basic needs and providing comfort measures, the family will immediately detect a sense of abandonment and all trust will be lost.

Some family members may wish to take care of the child's basic needs because it strengthens the bonding experience and facilitates the need the parents have to be doing something for the child. The nurse can offer to assist where the family feels unskilled. When it comes to comfort measures, family members should not be neglected. The nurse must be creative when promoting the bonding experience between parent and child. It is often the nurse who offers to organize intravenous lines, monitors, and multiple tubes so a baby in the neonatal or pediatric intensive care unit may be held. Parents may be so intimidated in these settings that they don't even know they can ask for this assistance. When this happens, parents feel like the nurse has given them a real gift.

Nurses are often the first to see the mental, physical, and emotional exhaustion in caregivers. Nurses must encourage caregivers to take care of themselves as well as their child. Offering to stay with the child while the parents take care of their own basic needs, such as going to the cafeteria to get a meal, using the restroom, or taking a shower, are often things a parent will recall about a nurse or nursing assistant.

The nurse can promote parent–child bonding by providing quiet, uninterrupted family time. They can encourage family time for rituals the family practiced before the illness took over. Visits from friends or extended family can be encouraged. The child may benefit from time alone for reflection, but alone time should be balanced with family time to prevent isolation.

Planning a care conference

It may be a nurse who recognizes the need for a care conference. Staff may recognize the need for a care conference if they believe that the care goals are discongruent with the care being provided. Another excellent reason for a conference is to address the needs of the family if they are unclear about the direction their child's care is headed. The nurse who organizes the conference should inform other members of the multidisciplinary team involved in the child's care and make sure they know what the impending issues are, so all come prepared. It is best to plan the conference at a time when those staff intimately involved with the family have blocked time, and will not have to rush out. Abrupt endings can communicate a sense of trivializing the meeting and leave parents with a sense of abandonment.

The nurse should plan to reserve a quiet, private room that will not have interruptions. The registered nurse should sit with the family, in order to convey that time is available for them. Staff should place pagers on vibrate so they will not distract from the meeting. Tissues should be available for the family, as should paper, in the event they want to take notes. The nurse may help the family to organize their thoughts and formulate questions ahead of time. Parents should be encouraged to bring their written questions with them.

When planning a care conference, allow the family the opportunity to identify those staff they would like to have present. Although it is important to facilitate a multidisciplinary approach, too many staff can easily overwhelm the family. This may be a time to ask those not intimately involved with the family to excuse themselves. The introduction of the palliative care team is best facilitated before the patient is actively dying, so that a trusting relationship can be established over time. A meeting that includes the primary care and pediatric palliative medicine teams will communicate cohesiveness to the family, and show that the staff is working together to provide the best care for the child. It is also a chance to demonstrate to the reluctant physician staff that this team does not "take over" the care of the patient (unless directly asked to do so).

A nurse from the primary care team, who regularly cares for the child, should be included at family meetings to offer the family support from a familiar face they trust. The nurse must assess and advocate for the patient's needs. The bedside nurse may be the one to highlight what it takes to care for the child and what needs can be anticipated for transitioning care home. Recognizing strengths and weaknesses can identify education deficits. The nurse can participate in care planning to support the family's strengths, and intervene to address their weaknesses. When planning interventions to address education deficits, the nurse must be sure to evaluate the caregivers' educational level, and the learning style in which they learn most effectively.

Discuss with the family whether the child is to be present, and how much information the family wants shared with the child. If the child is to be present, allow the child to ask questions and let them guide the discussion. A Child Life professional can make a great partner to the nurse in these efforts. It is important to offer an adolescent a confidential meeting without the presence of the parents.

If the parents wish to have medical decision-making discussions without the child, a nurse can determine with the family what information is to be shared with the child, and who will communicate it. A nurse can also offer to present the information to the child, be with the family for support if the parents wish to share the medical information themselves, and offer the child opportunities to ask questions.

The conference should be planned for a time when the family has no other distractions (eg, attending to other children at home, attending to their own basic needs, going to work). If the child will not be attending the care conference, the nurse should ask the parents to have another family member or friend sit with the child during that time. This will alleviate the fear that their child's needs are not being met in their absence.

To avoid miscommunication, and to ensure both parties are given the opportunity to speak or ask questions, the conference should occur when both parents are available to participate in the medical decision-making process. Determine the primary support system. Caregivers need as much support as possible, and in some cases, the parents may also request outside parties such as grandparents or close friends be present for support.

Determine who the head of the family is and who is likely to be the speaker for the family. Consider that the head of the family may be different from what your culture is accustomed to. Offer an interpreter from the hospital staff if English is not the primary language. Consider religious or cultural factors that may inhibit family members from being present or may affect the outcome of the discussion. Offer to contact a member from the family's religious affiliation to be present for support.

Discussions to determine the goals of care and make treatment decisions can go from several minutes to an hour or more. As the family provides verbal and non-verbal cues, meeting participants should evaluate how much the child and family want to know, keeping in mind that too much information in one sitting can be overwhelming. Although silence may feel uncomfortable for some, allow for it, as this will allow the family time to gather their thoughts and generate questions. There may be times the family asks questions the nurse doesn't have the answers to. Assure the family where there are answers to be found, they will be sought out. It is acceptable to verbalize that modern medicine doesn't have all the answers. This will convey openness and honesty, and solidify trust.

At the end of the care conference it needs to be communicated to the parents that all involved medical staff will be informed of the goals of care, and that treatment will be based on them. It is the responsibility of whoever is deemed in charge of the conference to ensure clear communication to those who could not attend, including documenting these discussions in the medical record. One or two people should be appointed for the family to go to, to be a consistent source of information. As the family goes forth, they will undoubtedly reflect on the discussion that took place. The family should be encouraged to write down questions as they arise. At the conclusion of the care conference, the nurse can offer future opportunities for meetings, as the family would like. Communicate to the family that their decision(s) are supported and their opinions are valued. Identify their strengths in their coping mechanisms and reinforce them. An excellent strategy is to have one person stay behind to take questions that may be easier asked one-on-one, and when the doctors have left.

Discussions that require complex medical decision-making may need to be repeated, either as a formal care conference, or as general conversation ensues. It is not uncommon to repeat the same discussion just days or weeks apart. The family may come to different decisions after each discussion. This can be exhausting, confusing, and frustrating for staff. What the family needs to hear is that no matter what decision they make for their child, they know what is best for the child, and that all involved care providers will support the family's wishes even if it means changing the plan of care.

Determining quality of life

When discussing quality of life with the child and or family, it is important to consider the child and family as the unit of care. The family itself defines the concepts of healing and quality of life. Attention must be paid to ascertain what healing is to the family as it is multidimensional in influencing one's quality of life [16]. Children learn from their caregivers; thus, their definitions of quality of life often mirrors that of their caregivers, but do not assume this.

When assessing quality of life, nurses should consider the physical, emotional, psychological, social, and spiritual well-being of both child and family. Neglecting the psychological and spiritual needs of children and families coping with life-limiting illnesses may intensify suffering [17]. The nurse must assess and include both positive and negative aspects of all facets. For example, focusing only on negative attributes such as fears doesn't give the child the opportunity to discuss hopes, and vice versa.

Assessment of physical well-being includes the child's functional ability for developmental level. Is the child able to accomplish the same tasks he/she was doing a few months or even days ago? Is he/she learning new skills and taking on new tasks? Is she/he able to keep up with siblings, or frustrated with fatigue?

Nurses may encourage the family to eat together, because meals are a social time in our culture. Is the child able to keep food down without having nausea and emesis? Nurses may encourage pre-medicating meals with anti-emetic drugs, or even anti-anxiolytics as ordered by physicians. Facilitate a calm environment that is pleasant for mealtimes. Unpleasant procedures should be avoided close to meal times. Eliminate foul smells that may nauseate the child to the point of food aversion. As the disease process progresses, the child may eat only a few bites and become full. Early satiety is distressing to parents because feeding their child is something ingrained from the moment of birth and is a significant part of our culture and rituals. During times where health is declining, the nurse can try to reassure the caregivers by gently explaining that the body needs fewer calories and will try to conserve energy as the body's natural processes slow down.

Getting on the scale at the doctor's office can be a source of significant stress for both the child and parents. Weight loss and/or extreme weight gain may be a focus of intervention during active or palliative treatment. Cases of extreme weight gain, such as a child on steroids, can be an opportunity for nurses to promote health by educating families on healthy eating choices. This can be challenging because during times of already heightened stress, it is difficult if not impossible to change longstanding habits.

An assessment of the child's coping ability is imperative to his/her mental, emotional and spiritual health. Does the child exhibit symptoms of anxiety such as sleeplessness, clinging to one or both of the parents, or constant crying? Is the child withdrawn and refusing to play with siblings? Does the child exhibit fear in his/her behavior, play, or artwork? Has the child regressed and now wants to sleep with the parent? Nightmares can be a sign of significant stress in the child. Does the child/adolescent exhibit emotional outbursts? The pediatric palliative medicine team can utilize its members from multiple disciplines to address these concerns.

Does the child show joy when participating in activities? Assess the quality of schoolwork being completed, and the motivation to complete it. The child's attention span may also be greatly effected by significant stress. Even young children can become depressed and should be assessed by a psychiatrist, psychologist, or other professional trained in pediatrics. It will be helpful if such a professional has established a prior relationship, because establishing new relationships can be challenging during a time of crisis. In any case, the earlier the treatment can begin the better.

A change in body image can be devastating to adolescents. Is outward change effecting the child's self-esteem and thus quality of life? Has the adolescent isolated himself, or just stopped going out with friends? Does the adolescent refuse friends' phone calls? Have the adolescent's friends isolated him/her and stopped calling or stopping by? Have boyfriend/girlfriend relationships stopped? Loss of peer support is devastating for the adolescent.

The course of the illness and hospital stays may put financial strain on the family. Families may drain life savings when caring for terminally ill children in order to pay for medical and non-medical needs not covered by insurance [16]. Caregiver burden can put strain on the family structure and marriage; the child will sense this strain and has the potential to feel like a burden.

Is the role of the "big brother" or "big sister" threatened? Well siblings now have to help care for their ill sibling, where he or she previously could care for her/himself. The well sibling may have the responsibility of caring for another child because the parent is too busy with the sick child. Are there more chores at home for the well siblings since the ill sibling isn't able to contribute to the household? The additional responsibilities can create animosity in the household. The nurse may facilitate discussions with the siblings to encourage verbalization of these frustrations.

Does the child/adolescent continue to express hopes and dreams? Do they speak of growing up and short or long-term goals they want to accomplish? Do they make plans for next week, next month, or their next birthday? Do they talk of plans for the prom, getting their driver's license, or attending college? Even in the light of suffering, do their spirits remain hopeful for cure? Do they express a faith that someday "everything will be okay"? This is not denial. This is hoping for the best, and nurses will still find evidence of the child/adolscent preparing, in their way.

Although parents almost always maintain hope until their child takes their last breath, the anticipatory grief work begins. Parents struggle with the milestones their child will not get to achieve such as the first day of school, getting a drivers license, or graduating high school. Parents and family experience unique sorrows surrounding a child's death: loss of future, loss of dreams attached to the child, loss of a part of self, failure to protect the child, survivor's guilt, reversal of the natural order of death, and changes in family roles and functioning [18]. Grandparents may have difficulty coping because they struggle with sorrow for themselves because their role of grandparent may be threatened, but at the same time feel saddened for the loss their child will endure.

After the death of an only child, parents struggle with the thought that "I'm not even a parent anymore," especially during holidays like Mother's Day, Father's Day, or Christmas. No Mother's or Father's Day cards will be opened, and waking up Christmas morning will never be the same. Other parents struggle when strangers ask them how many children they have. The question becomes: "Do I include my deceased child in the number?" Some parents find it easier to avoid explaining the circumstances to a stranger, and exclude the deceased child, but then can feel guilt later. The bereavement staff on the palliative medicine team can help in the weeks and months that follow a child's death.

Both the family and child suffer

In the face of life-limiting or life-threatening illness, suffering is almost universally experienced, but the degree of suffering can vary greatly. Suffering is the state of severe distress associated with events that threaten the intactness of the person [19]. The intactness of the whole person includes the physical, psychological, social, and spiritual self. Suffering can arise when any aspect of the person is threatened [20]. The degree to which one experiences suffering depends on the significance or personal meaning of the actual loss sustained. It is impossible to assume the presence or absence of suffering in another [19,21]. The components of suffering are variable and may include but are not limited to the physical aspects. The suffering of patients and their parents is widely experienced and recognized by nurses.

Parental suffering may be recognized at any or all phases of a child's treatment. It may be recognized the most as the disease progresses. The parent may experience emotional suffering and believe they are being punished by God, and have caused their child's illness. Physical signs of illness impact the suffering of parents. For example, alopecia may be equally as or more distressing for the parent because now their child "looks the part" of a cancer patient. Both patients and parents must deal with what the hair loss represents. Parents are also affected by direct physical evidence such as surgical scars that are a constant reminder of a traumatic time in the child's recent or distant past. Parents also suffer from the loss of the intactness of the family as a whole, from the loss of professional and social roles and relationships, and from financial burdens that may affect the family's lifestyle.

Emotional suffering for the adolescent may center on the loss of self-concept and physical changes such as hair loss, acne, a dramatic surgical scar, and weight loss or gain. Adolescents suffer as social changes in their peer group emerge. The adolescent who once was a leader may now be isolated from or by their peers. Adolescents miss out on the meaningful experiences their peers may take for granted. They may begin to resent their friends as they become jealous of their "normal life" [22]. Research supports that chronically ill adolescents want healthcare professionals to "treat me like a person, try to understand, don't treat me differently, give me encouragement, don't force me, give me options, have a sense of humor, and know what you're doing" [23].

Although it is impossible for one person to assume the presence or absence of suffering in another, it is possible as a healthcare provider to explore what suffering may occur in any given family [19,21]. Lengthy hospital stays and the involvement of multiple specialties and multiple staff for each specialty can make it challenging to establish and maintain good continuity of care. Fragmented care is a common problem in complex medical illness. Families find it difficult to know who is the "go to" person directing the care. The potential for fragmented nursing care exists as they rotate in 4-, 8-, or 12-hour shifts. Without good continuity of care, exploring personal issues such as suffering may be limited because most people would rather ignore it or keep it to themselves. Festering issues like emotional suffering are extremely draining, but can be addressed to lighten the family's burden with a good rapport on an intimate level. The bedside nurse may be the one constant who is able to predictably come and go, but also address such issues.

Although palliative care aims to prevent and relieve suffering, not all suffering can be avoided. All dimensions of suffering should be assessed on an ongoing basis, and the plan of care should be modified accordingly. For some, suffering leads to finding meaning in the experience of the illness, and of life. For others including children, and especially adolescents, an opportunity exists to overcome the physical, emotional, and spiritual distresses that occur at the end of life in the midst of struggles.

Facilitating a good death

Of the 53,000 deaths annually in the United States, 75%–85% take place in the hospital [2]. There has, however, been a recent shift to home hospice care which assists those who choose to live out their last moments at home. There is no right way or right place to die. If possible, the nurse should help the family to plan ahead of time where the death will take place, whether in the hospital or home, ideally with specialists trained in pediatric hospice support. There are families who don't know home is an acceptable option for their child's final days, or how to get the support they need to be able to care for their child at home.

When death is inevitable, no matter what the setting, nurses can facilitate a "good death." They can determine with the family what will make any aspect of the dying process easier, offer a presence, but also allot the family time alone and provide a quiet environment with as few interruptions as possible. Families should be encouraged to make the hospital environment as home-like as possible, by bringing in pictures, blankets, and any items that offer the comforts of home. Exceptions can be made in the case of visiting restrictions.

When a child dies

After the death of a child, knowing the right thing to do or say in every situation is nearly impossible. Some tips from those who have journeyed through this experience may be helpful. Any sentence that starts "At least..." is usually something to avoid, whether it's "...they didn't suffer" or "...you can have more children," explains Wayne Loder, public awareness coordinator for The Compassionate Friends, a not-for-profit self-help bereavement organization [24].

Nurses should avoid comparing life and death; do not make comments such as "You're lucky your child died because another who lived had it so much worse." Instead, acknowledge "it must be the worst thing you can experience, and all I can say is I'm sorry," says Loder, who lost two children in an automobile accident. No matter how uncomfortable the moment, it is important not to withdraw from grieving families. Remember, sometimes it is just a presence that is important [24].

Nurses are often the first and last health care contact for grieving families after the child's death. Physicians move on, leaving nurses to escort the family out of the hospital and perform post-mortem care. After death, it is crucial to give families the opportunity to grieve. They need privacy and time. They need to tell their story over and over. Reliving the child's experiences, both good and bad, will offer comfort and help the family to make sense of the tragedy that has just occurred. However difficult and time consuming it may be, nurses need to listen, and listen again. Palliative nursing is not only "doing for," but also sometimes just "being with," caring not only for patients, but offering holistic care to the family.

All health care providers intimately involved with a child's death must be aware of their own grief. It is important to not over-empathize. "If we over-identify, we grieve with parents too much instead of letting them grieve,' cautions a nurse who lost her 17-year-old son in an auto accident. Stay compassionate as professionals, but seek comfort from peers, not parents [24].

Making positive memories is something nurses can facilitate throughout the course of illness, and at the time of death. Encourage parents to scrapbook and take plenty of pictures, to document the journey the family has lived. From the parent of an infant who died shortly after birth: "One stunning shot was taken by a nursing assistant moments after he was born. He is under warming lights in a bassinet, bathed in a golden glow. Visible are the gloved hands of a neonatologist, listening with a stethoscope to Gabriel's heart. Gabriel is crying and so clearly alive. Whoever that nursing assistant was, thank you" [25]. Encourage the child, parents, and siblings to create art projects together. Plan the activity around having fun and celebrating life, not as creating memorials. Preserving the projects in a scrapbook can facilitate bonding between the siblings and create positive memories for all involved. Many families choose to bring these scrapbooks to the memorial service to share. Doing so, may help other family members who may not have been present during the course of illness, to recognize the journey the family has been through from wellness, through treatment, and death.

Whenever possible, parents should discuss ahead of time where they want the siblings to be at the time when death is impending. Ask parents if they want close family members present when death is near. Parents may also want to consider how and when other family members such as grandparents wish to say goodbye, whether that is to be before or after death or both.

If children are to be present at the time of death, or shortly thereafter, they must be prepared for what they may see, hear, and feel. Nurses and other multidisciplinary team members can give parents the words to prepare their children, or actually take place in the discussion of what to expect. The developmental level of the child must be considered when trying to prepare them for the impending death of their brother or sister. Some will respond to play, puppets, books, or music. A pediatric nurse who is experienced and comfortable with the discussion of death should facilitate this. A nurse can initiate the discussion of what the body will look and feel like. It is the bedside nurse who is present with the family at the time of death and for the care of the child after he/she has died. Encouraging siblings and parents to view or touch the body can help the survivors' transition from denial to awareness and promotes closure. The nurse might ask if the family would like to have a lock of hair, or a hand or footprint. The nurse should always ask permission for such activities, and consider the culture of the family, as some cultures would find this offensive. Some families wish to take photographs. This is especially important for parents of infants as they have a need to solidify their memories, the relationship, and the death.

When a child dies in the hospital, the family leaves behind what may be their strongest support system. Families often refer to staff as their "hospital family." Often it is the hospital staff who has spent the most intimate moments with the family. Parents may feel as if the extended family just doesn't understand the journey the family has traveled.

When the child dies, the abrupt loss of the hospital support system may feel like abandonment and increase the sense of loss for the family. Pediatric palliative care programs and hospice agencies offer formalized bereavement support services that extend beyond the funeral services. Ongoing bereavement support is crucial to support the healthy grieving process. What long-term, follow-up support hospitals may not be able to provide, hospice services are equipped to handle. This is one major benefit to having a hospice service or pediatric palliative medicine team involved.

Nurses cope

Caring for the child at the end of life may be the most life-altering experience of one's career. "The consistent question to those who care for dying children is 'How do you do it.' The answer is life. Life in it's fullest form, because no one makes you appreciate each ordinary, laughing, fighting, and crying moment of life better than a child" [26]. The moment of death is but the briefest of moments, but how the child and family arrive at that final moment can make all the difference in the end [26]. Nurses have a great impact on creating positive experiences and more peaceful memories. Other than the moment of their birth, the parent will remember no other moment more clearly than the moment of death. Parents will relive over and over in their minds who was present and what they did at the moment of death. It isn't only the parents who will have these most vivid memories. There are those patients who died in our care that we, too, as nurses remember as if it were yesterday.

Opportunity exists for profound change in our own lives based on experiences working with dying children and families. In 1959, Victor Frankl, a psychotherapist and concentration camp survivor wrote: "We must never forget that we may also find meaning in life even when confronted with a hopeless situation, when facing a fate that cannot be changed....When we are no longer able to change a situation, ...we are challenged to change ourselves" [27]. Nurses must face the inevitability of their own mortality. It can force them to look more deeply at their own priorities in life, along with their own beliefs and values and instill some positive change. There probably isn't a nurse in practice who hasn't been changed positively by a patient in some way.

Summary

Caring for chronically ill children whose health is declining and those children who are critically ill is stressful and can be overwhelming to both healthcare professionals and parents. Palliative care teams aim to provide the multidisciplinary and holistic support staff and families need. Families, nurses, and primary medical teams value the involvement of a pediatric palliative medicine team to improve the quality of living. The bedside nurse is a vital part of the support system and is ready and available to be present with the palliative care team to support families no matter what the circumstances. Advocating for the patient; creating a culture of flexibility; anticipating, identifying, and responding to the patient and family needs; fostering hope; and providing the support needed for the parents to make informed decisions, are keys to providing quality patient care. Nurses are in the position to positively influence each of these areas of patient care in a positive manner.

References

[1] Scanlon C. Defining standards for end-of-life care. American Journal of Nursing 1997; 97(11):58–60.
[2] Field MJ, Behrman RE. When children die: improving palliative and end-of-life care for children and their families. Report of the Institute of Medicine Task Force. Washington, DC: National Academy Press; 2003.
[3] Ersek M. The meaning of hope in the dying. In: Ferrell BR, Coyle N, editors. Textbook of palliative nursing. New York: Oxford University Press; 2001. p. 339–51.
[4] Shapiro B. The suffering of children and their families. In: Ferrell BR, editor. Suffering. Sudbury (MA): Jones and Bartlett; 1996. p. 67–93.
[5] Sumner L. Pediatric care: The hospice perspective. In: Ferrell BR, Coyle N, editors. The textbook of palliative nursing. New York: Oxford University Press; 2001. p. 556–69.
[6] Goldman A. Care of the dying child. Oxford (UK): Oxford University Press; 1994.
[7] Hilden JM, Emanuel EJ, Fairclough DL, et al. Attitudes and practices among pediatric oncologists regarding end-of-life care: results of the 1998 American Society of Clinical Oncology Survey. J Clin Oncol 2001;(19):205–12.
[8] Wolf J, Holcombe EG, Klar N, et al. Symptoms and suffering at the end of life in children with cancer. N Engl J Med 2000;342(5):326–33.
[9] Hockenberry-Eaton M, Barrera P, Brown M, et al. Pain management in children with cancer. Austin (TX): Texas Cancer Council; 1999.
[10] Association of Pediatric Oncology Nurses/American Nurses Association. Scope and standards of pediatric oncology nursing practice. Washington (DC): APON/ANA; 2000.
[11] Siever BA. Pain management and potentially life-shortening analgesia in the terminally ill child: the ethical implications for pediatric nurses. J Pediatr Nurs 1994;9(5):307–12.
[12] Borneman T, Brown-Saltzman K. Meaning in illness. In: Ferrell BR, Coyle N, editors. Textbook of palliative nursing. New York: Oxford University Press; 2001. p. 415–24.
[13] O'Conner P. Clinical paradigm for exploring spiritual concerns. In: Doka K, Morgan J, editors. Death and spirituality. New York: Baywood Publishing Company; 1993.
[14] Rando TA. Grief, dying and death: clinical interventions for caregivers. Champaign (IL): Research Press Company; 1984.
[15] Yates P, Stetz KM. Families' awareness of and response to dying. Oncol Nurs Forum 1999; 26(1):113–20.
[16] Byock I. Dying well: the prospects for growth at the end of life. New York: Riverhead Books; 1997.
[17] Ferrell BR. Humanizing the experience of pain and illness. In: Ferrell BR, editor. Suffering. Sudbury (MA): Jones and Bartlett Publishers; 1996. p. 3–27.
[18] Lattanzi-Licht M, Mahoney JJ, Miller GW. The hospice choice: in pursuit of a peaceful death. New York: Fireside Publishers; 1998.
[19] Cassel E. The nature of suffering and the goals of medicine. N Engl J Med 1982;306(11): 639–45.
[20] Spross JA. Coaching and suffering. In: Ferrell BR, editor. Suffering. Sudbury (MA): Jones and Bartlett Publishers; 1996. p. 3–27.

[21] Kahn DL, Steeves RH. An understanding of suffering grounded in clinical practice and research. In: Ferrell BR, editor. Suffering. Sudbury (MA): Jones and Bartlett Publishers; 1996. p. 3–27.

[22] Attig T. Beyond pain: the existential suffering of children. J Palliative Care 1996;12(3):20–3.

[23] Woodgate R. Healthcare professionals caring for chronically ill adolescents: adolescent's perspectives. J Society of Pediatr Nurs 1998;3(2):57–67.

[24] Bonifazi W. When a child dies. Nursing Spectrum 2004;5(8):17–8.

[25] Kuebelbeck A. Waiting with Gabriel. Chicago: Loyola Press; 2003. 118.

[26] Sumner L, Hurula J. Making the most of each moment. Nursing 1993;93(August):50–5.

[27] Frankl VE. Man's search for meaning. New York: Washington Square Press; 1984. 135.

ELSEVIER
SAUNDERS

Child Adolesc Psychiatric Clin N Am
15 (2006) 739–758

CHILD AND
ADOLESCENT
PSYCHIATRIC CLINICS
OF NORTH AMERICA

Program Interventions for Children at the End of Life and Their Siblings

Janet Duncan, MSN, CPNP[a],*,
Marsha Joselow, LICSW[a], Joanne M. Hilden, MD[b]

[a]Pediatric Advanced Care Team, Children's Hospital Boston and Dana-Farber Cancer Institute, 44 Binney Street, Dana 3, Boston, MA 02115, USA
[b]Pediatric Oncology, The Children's Hospital at The Cleveland Clinic, 9500 Euclid Avenue, Cleveland, OH 44195, USA

"How can I tell my child she is dying?" "What should I tell him?" "I'm afraid she'll give up if we tell her the truth." "I don't want to destroy his hope." "He's too young to understand."

"I don't want her sister and brother to see her this way." "I don't want this to be the last image they have of him." "What should I tell her brothers and sisters?"

"I still pray for a miracle."

As children, teenagers, and parents ask questions, the health care providers struggle to find answers that will make sense in an apparently senseless situation. For both the child who has a life-threatening illness and the sibling left behind, there are common themes that suggest possible interventions. Appropriate and helpful interventions will be based on a family's style, values, spirituality, and culture. Interventions are also selected based on the child's style, values, spirituality, culture, and ways of relating to and interfacing with others in his or her world.

The goal of the interventions is to maximize the child's quality of life. The goals of interventions for the siblings are to provide a supportive structure to maximize the relationship with the dying sister or brother and to lay a pathway for processing grief after the death. Clearly, sibling bereavement lasts throughout life [1], and as for parents, certain events may trigger renewed grief. The bereaved sibling, needs to know that this is normal.

Common themes need to be considered, such as the importance of communication. It is clear from recent research that parents highly value

* Corresponding author.
E-mail address: janet.duncan@childrens.harvard.edu (J. Duncan).

1056-4993/06/$ - see front matter © 2006 Elsevier Inc. All rights reserved.
doi:10.1016/j.chc.2006.02.002

childpsych.theclinics.com

communication with their health care team. Specifically, ratings of high satisfaction with physician care were directly correlated with receiving clear communication around end-of-life issues, delivered with sensitivity and caring; such communication included speaking directly to the child when appropriate [2]. Another theme is that of protection [3]. The ill child wants to protect his or her parents or siblings; similarly, the parents want to protect the ill child and the siblings. It is a two-way street. Hence communication is complicated. We need to honor the family's communication style while offering new options. We must never lie to a child, or we risk losing trust. However we may need to reframe a question or offer an answer with the parents present [4].

Developmental aspects of the child and siblings need to be carefully considered [5]. How old is the child? What life experiences has he or she had? Has the sibling been included in frank discussion about the ill child's condition? How long has the child been sick? How often has he or she been hospitalized? Has the child seen others die? What is the "role" of the ill child in the family—oldest, peacemaker, clown, star athlete, troublemaker, the "good child"? What is the child's experience of death in the family? Have grandparents died? What is the parents' experience? How does that influence the family's belief system and the fears its members might have surrounding death?

Another theme is "keeping hope." Hoping for that miracle is real and can and does coexist for parents with an ability to face the more likely reality of death. Listening to children and families speak about the future even as they face the reality of disease or illness may help them keep the focus on living even while dying. Helping them plan big events or little events that reaffirm relationships and focus on the child's life may allow events to become meaningful experiences that build memories to cherish.

The team can ask several questions that help it to focus on and plan interventions. For instance, does the family have a strong religious faith [6]? Does it influence how they think about life and death? Are there supports within their faith community? Do their beliefs or their culture incorporate particular rituals or traditions that may help them to "get through" the crisis of death and the subsequent recovery?

What is the psychologic health of the family? Are the parents married or divorced? Does the family have support of extended family and their community? Is the family very private, or is it able to accept help and support? Does anyone suffer from pre-existing conditions, such as anxiety disorder or depression?

Finally, there is the possibility for growth of the children and parents through this painful experience [7–9]. Parents often shift priorities to caring for the ill child or keeping home a safe and predictable place for the siblings. Siblings may not want to speak about the ill brother or sister, but they may choose to write about their experience. Often when a child is near the end of life, parents recount how the brother or sister helps out by offering the ill child food, playing games, or even helping with physical care, such as turning or ambulating. As experts avow [1], when children are included in the process and are prepared for what lies ahead, their experiences are validated, often yielding a positive outcome.

Common barriers to interventions for children also exist, such as myths about how children do or do not grieve [10] and geographic distance of the child or siblings from hospital supports, community-offered groups, or extended family. Family stressors, such as a single parent or divorced parents, may limit or complicate the availability of interaction. Escalating illness and loss of function may alter the ways in which the ill child is able to interact, for instance, if he or she loses the ability to speak. Finally, individual and family coping styles may affect the interventions that are seen as acceptable, such as a provider speaking to the child alone, bringing up the subject of limited days to live, or talking with siblings about ways to "say goodbye."

Lessons must be continually learned from children and families and continually taught to medical and community providers. Each child is unique, as is each family and each circumstance. The challenge then is to respond out of our humanity and our caring [11].

Program intervention for the seriously ill infant and bereaved infant

Interventions for the seriously ill infant and bereaved infant are dependent on interventions with parents. Common to both are finding ways to "normalize" daily activities. For example, when an infant is in an intensive care unit, finding ways to let the parents hold, bathe, or feed the infant is important. It may be possible to allow the parents and baby to take a walk in a garden or visit a nearby museum. Doing these kinds of activities together will help create memories and a family legacy, and staff should encourage and offer resources for the taking of photographs during these times.

Ensuring consistent caregivers and routines for the seriously ill infant or bereaved infant will promote trust and decrease anxiety or irritability. In the hospital setting, providing consistent medical caregivers can create a safe holding space for parents, allowing them to focus on "being mom and dad" and not on the medical technology surrounding their infant. Anticipating parental anxiety and stress and finding interventions to decrease them is important. Depending on the physical and emotional availability of the parent, especially in the home, it may be helpful to enlist a surrogate caregiver to maintain daily routines and provide respite for the parent.

Parents are often grateful when they are offered memory-making ideas, such as making footprints and handprints, cutting a lock of hair, or putting special mementos in a memory box [12]. Also, promoting documentation through photography, video, scrapbooking, or creating a baby journal provides tangible things that may help not only the parents but also bereaved siblings remember, especially when a life is brief.

Furthermore, for the bereaved infant, creating future opportunities as he or she develops and matures to remember, reprocess, and celebrate the life of the deceased sibling will facilitate open communication about this life-changing family experience.

Program intervention for the seriously ill toddler and bereaved toddler

As with the infant, it is important to maintain routines for the seriously ill toddler. Having some structure to the day and maintaining family rules and values allows the toddler to feel safe. Keeping consistent expectations for behavior and limit setting, when appropriate, will increase the coping of the ill child. This practice will also remind the sibling that there are uniform family expectations for all the children.

In explaining things to toddlers or allowing for expression, several interventions using symbolic representation may be helpful. Bibliotherapy or play therapy with puppets, toy figures, paint, or storytelling may allow toddlers to ask questions, express what they know or have heard, release feelings, and cope with the situation. The siblings may be invited to draw a picture or help decorate the room of the ill child.

In the authors' clinical experience, parents are often astounded by how even very young children assimilate and express family cultural or spiritual values. Prayer, belief in a higher being, and acknowledgment of what may happen to a brother or sister may be explained in a matter of fact way, such as when Charlotte, the 3-year-old sister of a dying infant, explained to her mother that her baby sister was going to grow wings and be an angel in heaven. Another 3-year-old, who was imminently dying, awoke and said to her mother that she wanted to "go up there," pointing to the ceiling of her hospital room. "There's food up there," she added (she had not been able to eat for days). Finally she patted her crying mother's hand and reassured her, "It'll be all right, Mommy."

To allow for these unexpected proclamations, questions, and feelings, parents must be vulnerable and open to hearing and responding. Providers should therefore help them to anticipate these potential questions. In the acute phase of grieving after the loss, the parents may need to rely on other friends and family members to be present in this way to their surviving children. It may be too overwhelming and painful to be helpful to the other children. Many parents express feelings of guilt that they cannot "be there" to help the sibling on the grief journey, because they are so consumed by their own. As the sibling grows and matures, questions and feelings most likely will arise, so creating opportunities to remember and celebrate the life of the deceased sibling is important [1]. Furthermore, acknowledging the true nature of the brother or sister, the positive attributes and the not-so-positive ones, may allow the bereaved sibling not to feel diminished or threatened by an older "perfect" sibling, now dead.

Aaron's story is a poignant example of the importance of interventions by a neonatal intensive care unit (NICU) staff and palliative care consult service.

Aaron's mother's pregnancy was unremarkable until the week of his birth. Because Aaron had a typically developing 3-year-old sibling, Aaron's birth was anticipated with much joy and little worry. Aaron's mother presented in labor to a local hospital and, because of a previous history of Group B streptococcus–positive pregnancy, was treated with penicillin. Unexpectedly, she had an anaphylactic reaction to the penicillin that resulted in severe perinatal depression for Aaron. He suffered significant hypoxic ischemic encephalopathy, resulting in severe breathing difficulties and requiring ventilatory support. From a neurologic standpoint, Aaron was without movement or respiratory effort, had large, nonreactive pupils, and was without reflexes. His medical team believed there was no chance of any meaningful recovery for Aaron, together with his family decided to withdraw ventilatory support. Aaron died at day 2 of life.

The palliative care referral came from the NICU within hours of discussions about redirection of care. In addition to supporting the family in the hours immediately after Aaron's birth, the referral was intended to assist the parents in discussing Aaron's imminent death with their 3-year-old daughter Amelia. Aaron's parents reported many concerns that her brother's death would traumatize or psychologically scar Aaron's sister. The mother was also certain that Amelia would be unable to understand what had happened to Aaron or to understand the concept of death. Their worries included questions about Amelia's participation in the funeral and the impact of her seeing Aaron's body at a wake. These are common worries among parents of young children.

The palliative care team met with Aaron and his parents in the NICU family room. Amelia was with extended family in another room. In reviewing what Amelia had been told to that point, it was learned that her parents had explained to her that Aaron had a "booboo" on his head and that he would not be coming home. Instead, he would stay at the hospital with his nurses and doctors. Her parents' choice of language came from their deep hopes of protecting Amelia from pain and fear at the same time that they let her know that Aaron would not be coming to their home, which had been prepared for the new baby's arrival.

The team took the opportunity to discuss some general developmental themes of preschool-aged children and suggested some ways in which their earlier presentation to Amelia might be expanded to incorporate strategies that have been helpful to other young bereaved children.

Aaron's parents and the team discussed ways to expand their earlier description to prevent future fears Amelia might have about her own minor injuries, which are referred to in this family as "booboos." Concerns that she might extrapolate from this story that she too would need to stay in the hospital with a "booboo" and never return home were discussed. In addition, discussion about the initial story that Aaron would remain at the hospital was needed to help Amelia understand the wake and funeral that were to follow and the grief and sadness that would surround her.

Considerable time was spent with the family to help them find their "own" language that would enable them to feel comfortable and to reproduce the message over time. The explanation needed to incorporate the word "dead" and the idea of permanence and the lack of bodily function associated with death in simple and clear terms. As an intervention, this one is crucial, because each individual and family has a unique communication style reflecting personal values, culture, and religious or spiritual beliefs. It is particularly important for the young child that the adult be able to present a consistent and simple retelling of events. The young child often requires multiple recountings of the facts, particularly in a situation such as this, where some corrective work was indicated.

Aaron's parents chose language that was comfortable for them and incorporated earlier words shared with Amelia. They told her that Aaron had a "booboo" on his brain that, no matter how hard they tried, the doctors were unable to fix. The "booboo" was so bad that Aaron died. Conversation included reassuring Amelia that she and her parents were healthy and safe. Reassurances that others are safe and will be there for him or her are important, particularly for the very young child. Safety was an important concept for this family because of the mother's severe medical reaction to the antibiotic and the earlier concern for her survival around this event. Both parents were open to this intervention and used role play to "practice" this message for Amelia. Other members of the extended family joined in, so that consistent language and messages would be provided by those caring for her at a time when her parents might be less available.

Amelia's parents decided that she would be allowed to be present at the wake in their home. This way her parents could "protect" Amelia from parts of the experience while allowing her to participate with extended family in the way most comfortable to them. They chose not to have her attend funeral services. Amelia's parents were also given several developmentally appropriate picture and workbooks to use at that time and in the future as questions about Aaron's death might arise. In a follow-up phone call to the family, the team learned that Amelia was doing well and was asking many questions about Aaron and his death. At the time of the telephone call, Amelia and her father were in the backyard planting a "memorial garden" in Aaron's memory with the plants that were sent to the family at the time of Aaron's death and funeral. This idea of the family's was a beautiful way to involve Amelia indirectly with the funeral, to create a special place within the family to remember Aaron, and to offer the chance for informal conversation and questioning between Amelia and her father as they planted their garden (Box 1).

Program intervention for the seriously ill school-aged child and bereaved school-aged child

Case study: Nikki is 6 years old and has been living with her cancer for 3 years. It appears that no further chemotherapy will arrest the growth of

---

Box 1. Preparing children and families: a palliative care approach

- Maximize the function and coping of each parent so that he or she in turn may be open and available to the seriously ill child and the siblings [7].
- Identify and harness extended family and friends to provide support and care for the sibling if the parents' emotional, physical, or spiritual resources are "unavailable."
- Make available the hospital multidisciplinary team—social work, psychology, chaplain, child life, psychiatry, interpreters, parent-to-parent program, volunteers, and medical staff.
- Mobilize community, hospice, school, and spiritual resources for the family.
- Encourage and provide resources for meaning-making experiences, such as journaling, scrapbooking, and special family events.
- Suggest "normal" activities, such as eating together 1 night a week and celebrating birthdays and holidays.
- Involve siblings as much as possible.
- Prepare the parents for what may happen as the disease/condition progresses, thus optimizing the timeliness of interventions [2].

---

tumors. She has several new growths along her jaw and most recently one on the back of her head. Nikki has always been concerned about her appearance, and when her G-tube was inserted she was worried about what the other children would say. Nonetheless, she wanted to go to school in the fall. She wanted to be with friends, do schoolwork, and be a part of that community. Nikki's parents were not sure that they wanted to send her. They wanted to be with her for whatever time they might have. They finally decided to let Nikki make her own decision, and she started school in September.

Finding ways for children to continue their "work" of school can be meaningful. This may mean simply allowing them to attend school when possible and adjusting the assignments to individual need and ability. It means working with the teacher and classmates to understand and have compassion and acceptance [12]. The ill child may be able to go for special events or even half days, depending on the situation. If the child is unable to attend school, often the classroom may be extended into the hospital room or home with videos, cards, tape recordings, or pictures [3]. Schools have used video phones and computer technology to bring the classroom to the child and the child into the classroom.

One particularly resourceful family turned its "sunroom playroom" into a classroom each day so that the ill child could go out the back door, around the yard, and into the "classroom" for a few hours each day with his tutor. Another family showed pictures of how the whole elementary school, in costumes for Halloween formed a parade and walked to the house of a homebound child. Needless to say, both for this young boy, his classmates and his parents, it was a special holiday.

Many parents ask how honest they should be in giving information to their seriously ill child. They ask how they can possibly tell the child that he or she is dying. Given that most seriously ill children are perceptive and intuitive, particularly in regard to what is going on in their own bodies [13,14], parents should be encouraged to find words and explanations with which they themselves feel comfortable. This may not be "telling" but rather finding ways to acknowledge together what the child knows already but may not be able to express in words. Children as young as 3 years may "tell" us, through play, of their fears and hopes about and understanding of their dying [14]. One mother related how she had told her 7-year-old that the medicines were no longer working to fight his tumors; she asked whether he knew what that meant. He responded that it meant he would be going to heaven to be with his grandpa. Significantly, in a recent study in Sweden [15], researchers found that none of the parents who talked with their child about death regretted it.

Asking about and listening to the child's priorities and providing choices, when possible, may allow the child to participate in life-enhancing experiences even at the close of life. This may mean a cherished trip to Disneyworld or simply making cards from photographs for special family members. Children often want to leave a legacy [6]. They want to be remembered.

Children at this age in particular may be interested in family traditions, rituals, and spiritual beliefs. Incorporating and observing these despite illness may help keep the focus on living each moment and day fully. Often aunts and uncles or other extended family members may be able to continue or create special relationships with the ill child that are enriching and give respite to parents. One aunt, who worked close to the hospital, made a daily trip to spend her lunch hour with her ill niece. This practice allowed the mother a brief respite and created a unique bond between the child and her aunt.

The following family situation illustrates frank and open communication, particularly between a son and mother, as well as the importance of legacy and family traditions. Bobby was 11 years old when he was diagnosed with metastatic bone cancer. He was an avid athlete, loving soccer and school. His mother, Molly, described knowing from the outset that "he wouldn't make it." She consented to conventional treatment as a way to treat the painful side effects of his widely spread cancer. Her approach to Bobby from the beginning was to tell him that "We're not in charge of everything" (referring to her belief in a Higher Being) and that her job was to be "a babysitter who would feed him, take care of him, and enjoy him." She told him that his job was to "be a kid, play, take your medication, and pretend you're not sick." They settled into a routine of frequent hospital stays alternating with time at home, when Bobby always insisted on going to school.

Several months before his death, Bobby and Molly traveled to another treatment center in hopes of enrolling him in an experimental protocol. There Molly described Bobby's overhearing a comment by the consulting physician, who was explaining that Bobby wasn't going to make it. He asked his mother, "Mom, you heard I'll never get better?" Molly said that she initially dismissed this by saying that the doctor must have been tired and certainly didn't know what he was talking about, but she knew Bobby didn't really believe her.

Not long after, a close hospital friend died, Bobby asked, "Why do kids die?" Molly explained this by saying that sometimes, when you get sick, your body gets tired and God says it's time to come home...and play. Bobby asked, "Am I going to die, too?" Molly again offered the reply, "Would I come here for no reason? I come because I hope some people will get better." She reassured Bobby that "I'll let you know when you won't get better and then I'll stop treatment." He appeared content with this explanation for a time, but one day "from nowhere" he asked, "What if I don't make it?" Molly responded, "I'll be devastated. I'll be missing you, but you'll be enjoying yourself in heaven—riding a bicycle, playing soccer...you'll be okay." Subsequently they talked about the (hospital) children who had died and spoke about them as angels, along with his Grandma Angel and Grandpa Angel.

The hard times would come in the middle of the night, when Molly would find Bobby not sleeping and ask what he was thinking about. "What do you think...my life!" Molly believed that often Bobby struggled alone, trying to deal with this by himself.

Molly recalled one night when Bobby woke her and asked her, "What am I good at?" She began thinking and responded, "Well, you're a good listener, a good partner." Bobby quickly said, "I don't want that mushy stuff." She continued, "Good at soccer, the champion of Game Boy."

Bobby also participated in his legacy by dictating painfully honest letters to his teachers shortly before his death. He made Molly promise to deliver these after his death. He thanked the principal for giving him the "angel pin" and accepting him; he thanked his kindergarten teacher for being the best teacher ever. He wanted to tell another teacher that he knew the teacher didn't like him but was nice because he had cancer; finally, he wanted to tell another teacher to "stop being mean to the kids."

Molly was able to ask Bobby about his funeral arrangements. She recalled saying, "I need to ask you something sad. You know when you die you have a special bed; what color do you want for your special bed? Sometimes they put something special inside with you, like a cross or flowers; what do you want? What color do you want us to wear at your celebration? What do you want to wear?" In answer to these questions, Bobby was able to say that he wanted Sponge Bob stickers, that he wanted to wear a favorite sweatshirt and have the angel pin from the principal, and that his family should wear red, blue, and black.

This topic led to a more serious discussion between them one night as they were driving home and were nearly involved in a car accident. Molly expressed her feeling that "I wish I could die for you, you're just a kid." Bobby replied, "No, you have my sisters and so many kids to take care of. You have to let me die. I'm okay."

Bereaved siblings often want to know what is happening to their brother or sister. They need information about the disease and the treatment. Their imagination about what is happening in the hospital may be worse than the day-to-day reality. Information regarding what to expect as their sibling gets sicker and what to expect at the time of death may be helpful. They also need to know that they are not responsible for what is happening [9]. The medical team can include them by learning their names, encouraging their participation, and giving them the opportunity to express their feelings.

Program intervention for the seriously ill adolescent and bereaved adolescent

Working with the adolescent involves particular challenges. Instead of becoming independent and separating from parents, the adolescent with a life-threatening illness is thrown into a dependent and more connected situation. The adolescent may feel out of control, not old enough to make decisions legally but old enough to understand the risks and benefits of treatments offered. The teenager may understand the prognosis but deny it on another level so as to live fully.

For the adolescent it is particularly important to balance optimal care while supporting the age-appropriate developmental striving toward autonomy and self-definition. The goal of many of the strategies is to find opportunities to support and respect the teenager's need for autonomy within the context of a family system that has by virtue of the illness taken over many aspects of the adolescent's physical care. Because the seriously ill teenager often requires extensive physical care, the capability of the adolescent to create emotional distance and space is extremely compromised.

The health care team is ethically bound to involve these adolescents in decision making even when exposing the adolescent to these decisions may appear to impose an overwhelming burden. It is important to let families know that open communication may alleviate some of the stress and anxiety for everyone and allow for individual growth and understanding.

Peers remain supremely important to the adolescent and may be a blessing or a disappointment. Many adolescents want to be supported and hear about the "normal" happenings of their friends, even as they find that this knowledge brings an increased sadness about what they are missing and unable to participate in. Nonetheless, this situation is preferable to that of abandonment, when peers may be too frightened or uncomfortable to know how to continue a relationship with a friend who is dying. Creating opportunities to support the peer group can enhance the experience for peers and the seriously ill teen. One mother decided to invite her son's friends to their home and give them suggestions about things that would be helpful to her 15-year-old son, who was very close to death. Other times, caregivers may visit a school and have discussions with the peer group so that peers may talk about their fears, learn ways to cope, and stay in the relationship. Hospital-based outreach programs to schools can be effective in assisting parents and children in meeting these goals.

Of utmost importance for this age group is the connection of the ill adolescent to the normal activities of his or her peers. Depending on the child's medical status, this may take the form of a modified return to school. This choice often requires a flexible approach, with room to adapt to the teenager's changing needs. Engaging the special education system in the school may be necessary to address evolving educational and learning needs as illness progresses.

Inducing adolescents to communicate their feelings, fears, or hopes may be a challenge. Many teenagers may not want to speak to hospital providers or family and friends. They may not have available art supplies, music, or a camera to use for their expression. Sometimes it is only after the death that it is learned that a teenager wrote extensive poetry related to this living and dying process or had conversations with a sibling that were not shared with parents at the time.

To illustrate how these interventions may flow into a patient's and family's life, the authors offer this case example with the permission of Valerie and her family:

Valerie was a 20-year-old woman who was diagnosed with neurofibromatosis type I at 5 years of age. The early stage of her illness was marked by some facial disfigurement and increasing physical disability. She had a progressive form of the disease leading to multiple surgeries throughout her life. One year before her death, she underwent a final surgery to remove tumors along her spinal cord that left her with spastic quadriparesis marked by further deterioration in mobility, increased difficulty in breathing and handling her secretions, intractable pain, and overall loss of function. Toward the end of her life, Valerie lost her ability to speak as a result of pain, weakness, and increasing pressure from neurofibromas in the cervical-spinal region.

Despite her illness, Valerie remained cognitively intact. She was an intelligent and motivated young woman. She was deeply connected to her Catholic religion and found great comfort in prayer. She was committed to her education and was able to complete 1 year of college. Her goal was to become a defense lawyer and eventually a judge. She also hoped to marry and have children of her own. She enjoyed writing poetry and had several of her works published in school and community publications.

Valerie was remarkable in her strength of character and compassion for others. She was the conduit through which love in her family passed. Pain was a symbol of weakness and increasing illness for her and her family. She often expressed concern about others and did not want to "bother" or worry them with her illness. This characteristic of Valerie's created challenges for the medical team trying to treat her pain. When her mother was in the room, she would say that she felt fine and rated her pain at two to three (where zero is no pain and 10 is the worst pain imaginable). When her family was out of earshot, she would tell the team how much pain she was in and rate it an eight or nine.

As Valerie's illness progressed, so did her level of disability. Among her greatest losses from her disease was her inability to go back to college. Her ability to communicate both verbally and through the computer was also compromised and, toward the end of her life, completely lost. For a young woman who used both spoken and written language for emotional and intellectual expression and connection, this was a loss of great magnitude for her and her family. Another complication for Valerie was that of finding ways to experience the normal developmental challenges of separation from parents and movement toward her independence as a young adult, while remaining deeply dependent on her parents for every aspect of her life.

Valerie had a remarkable and close-knit family. Her nuclear family included her mother, father, and three siblings: Eric, aged 17, Amy, aged 14, and Katie, aged 10. Her close extended family included her maternal aunts and, most significantly, her maternal grandmother, who was very close to Valerie and stayed with the family for long periods to provide support to her while keeping the basic family routines intact.

Valerie completed public high school and, before her last surgery, was able to attend one semester of college. When return to college was not possible, her family worked toward providing her with opportunities to continue her studies with an online college computer course. Because of her increased motor impairment and changes in her voice due to weakness, even voice activation of the computer was inconsistent and frustrating.

Because the family still wanted to support Valerie's intellectual and emotional sides, a writing tutor was found to come to her home and assist her with her poetry, but unfortunately Valerie never returned home.

When these obstacles were too great, her family and psychosocial team worked on other opportunities to allow Valerie to "keep her voice" and independence and give meaning to her life. For her, sharing her ideas and feelings was paramount. Her hospital social worker met with Valerie on a regular basis to become her "scribe" and vehicle for writing and distributing the poetry she wrote to others. As one example, she wrote a stunning thank-you poem for those attending a community fundraiser.

Valerie and her family had a strong need to continue fighting her illness and "not give up." Until several days before her death, Valerie continued to write, although her voice was barely audible. This type of writing offered

Valerie and her family symbolic ways to "say goodbye" and share their love without needing actively to concede victory to her illness. At the same time, wonderful expressive memories were created.

Before her last hospitalization, Valerie's palliative care social worker made regular home visits for home-based psychotherapy. Most of these sessions revolved around the frustration Valerie felt at being so dependent on her mother as well as lacking the ability to do things on her own schedule. For example, when her mother had time, then she was bathed and needed to get out of bed and dressed, often earlier and with greater speed than she would have done when she had more independent adaptive skills.

For Valerie, as for other teenagers with life-threatening illness, maintaining her physical appearance and interacting in normal teenage activities (shopping at the mall, wearing makeup, having that first drink at the bar at age 21) were important and meaningful. She had created a design encompassing the initials of her parents that she hoped to have tattooed on her chest on her birthday. Efforts were made to coordinate and facilitate this last wish for her while an inpatient. She wore her tatoo proudly at her hospital-based 20th birthday party 3 days before she died.

For the bereaved adolescent sibling, some of the same challenges exist. Even as parents struggle with what to tell them, siblings most often want to be a part of what is happening and to be informed. Parents may not fully appreciate the bond that exists and the need for healing or for having lasting, meaningful experiences [16]. At the same time, siblings desperately want to be "normal," so acknowledging the life-changing event of the brother or sister, who may die, often complicates the feelings they have and the activities they choose. Parents therefore may not appreciate the sibling's turmoil or realize just how affected he or she is (Box 2).

Following her death, the palliative care team has had the opportunity to follow Valerie's entire family for the past year, including her three siblings, Eric, aged 17, Amy, aged 14, and Katie, aged 10.

Katie, who has similar facial features to Valerie, has assumed the role that Valerie had in the family. She is protective of her mother and loving toward her. She writes beautiful, always optimistic poems to everyone and in her journal draws pictures of butterflies and angels. She speaks of Valerie as her guardian angel and, although she is sad that she has died, she is happy that Valerie is always in her heart (Fig. 1).

Eric says that, although he misses and grieves for Valerie, he has a need to "be a normal teenager." He points to the back of his head and says, "I keep Valerie here. She's always with me, but I still need to go to school, be with my friends, and play sports...keep moving forward."

Amy, who is a young teenager, describes a more multilayered grieving process. In her own words: "Losing a sibling is the worst loss. You do everything with a brother or sister. You eat together, you play together, you have holidays together. It's not like losing a grandmother. I love my grandmother and I'm close to her, but this is different."

Box 2. Common themes and experiences of bereaved siblings [8]

- The siblings must come to terms with the knowledge that their parents have changed following the loss and that along with that change comes a sense of loss of safety and routine. An additional shift is that the bereaved sibling sometimes believes that with the child's death, his or her relationship with the parent will be restored.
- Loss often brings an increase in maturity for the bereaved sibling accompanied by complex feelings that may lead to isolation from his or her former peer group.
- The deceased sibling frequently takes on an idealized role in the family or that of guardian angel.
- Often the loss is accompanied by feelings of shock and disbelief.
- It is common to question faith and God's role in suffering.
- Friends and peers can provide substitute care, support, and connection when family life is disrupted by sibling loss.
- Death of a sibling can promote growth and change.

Like other bereaved siblings, they must often come to terms with the parallel loss of their parents' emotional or physical availability. Older children often take on a parental role to "keep the family going." In Amy's words, "My mom falls apart every time she sees or thinks about Valerie. And she's telling me to be strong? My dad just smokes and smokes. He usually gets sad, nervous, or scared, so he goes and sits outside smoking two or three cigarettes. He's smoking way too much. I'm scared for him. I wish he would stop. Sometimes I don't like going to school because I don't want to leave my family."

For Amy, the loss of her sister has been accompanied by an increase in maturity, leading at times to feelings of isolation from her peers. She says, "It gets me mad when people say they hate their mom or dad or brother or sister. I mean, okay, you might be mad at them for that moment, but 'hate'? It gets me even more mad when they hope a certain someone in their family dies. I don't think they mean it or even understand what they are saying. They won't and don't understand what they are saying until, God forbid, it happens. I try to get that point across to people, but they don't understand the true meaning or feelings they would go through."

Often a feeling of shock or disbelief accompanies the loss. Amy says that "I am still in shock of her death. I hate accepting it. I don't want to. Nothing or no one can make me feel better. I wish I could see, hear, or feel her once more."

Amy joins her parents in being strongly connected to their Catholic faith. Despite this, she questions her faith and God's role in suffering. "I'm so angry

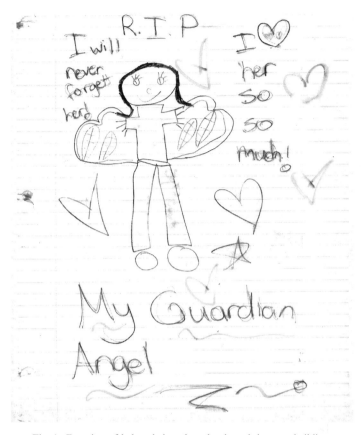

Fig. 1. Drawing of beloved sister by school-aged, bereaved sibling.

that I can't see or feel her. She did not deserve to be taken away from us. She was better off here...How could God have the power to cause a person so much pain?"

As in the cases of other bereaved siblings, the life of her sister with her medical illness and subsequent death has had an enormous impact on Amy's values and may shape her life and career goals. Amy speaks about writing a book for teenagers dealing with loss. She believes that her experiences were growth inducing and that she has a powerful story to share with other siblings. She also speaks about career goals of becoming a physician to discover a cure for Valerie's disease. She says that, as a physician, she will sit down and talk with sisters and brothers of sick children and tell them that she had a sister who died. She believes this will allow them to trust her. She says she will spend a lot of time explaining to them what is happening to their brother or sister. One goal she would have is never to remove their hope or scare them.

Neither Amy nor Katie found that counseling offered at school was helpful to them. They both speak of the importance of not having to retell their stories about Valerie. The best support for them came from those who had been part of Valerie's life, including the treating hospital clinicians. Amy says that her best friend has been the most reliable source of support for her. She describes this best friend as someone who knew Valerie almost as a sister but who could talk to Amy and know what it meant "to lose Valerie without really losing her."

They also speak of the support from their church youth group. The common theme is that these peers knew Valerie and the entire family. Amy says that, although they are all praying for different things, there is enormous "strength in group prayer."

When asked what helped them most toward the end of Valerie's life, both Amy and Katie describe an afternoon spent in Valerie's hospital room with the child life specialist. Their mother went home for the day, and the girls spent the entire afternoon decorating Valerie's hospital room. They describe how this "normal" activity together was very helpful.

Amy also describes how she often felt left out of discussions among the medical team around Valerie. She says it would have been valuable for the medical team to discuss the seriousness of Valerie's illness directly with her. Almost a year after Valerie's death, when asked, she says she has unanswered questions that continue to haunt her. These include concerns that the family "gave up too soon" and that they should have found ways to bring Valerie home to die.

Strategies for supporting children at the end of life and their bereaved siblings

- Preparation is essential and makes a difference.
- Ongoing conversation with families to know their goals, coping styles, and natural and community support systems makes possible an individualized approach to end-of-life care and sets the stage for bereavement care.
- One may incorporate the skills of child life, social work, chaplaincy, psychology, psychiatry, and other specialists will provide comprehensive care for children and their siblings.
- It is important to identify and respond to specific sibling needs and concerns, including direct information from medical care providers.
- Enlist community support, including the school system, hospice resources, pediatricians, and others in the community. It is important to provide the community with educational opportunities and resources to help provide this assistance.
- Provide concrete supports, including counseling (both individual and group), books, Internet sites, camp opportunities, bereavement mailings.
- Provide medical center–based memorial services to allow families to participate with other bereaved families and to feel their child is remembered.
- Acknowledge the importance of continuity of care during the child's life and following the family into bereavement.

Box 3. Books that may be helpful for families before the death:

Drescher J. The Moon Balloon: a journey of hope and discovery for children and families. Waltham (MA): Arvest Press; 2005.

Heegaard M. When someone has a serious illness: children can learn to cope with loss and change. Minneapolis (MN): Woodland Press; 1991.

Mellonie B, Ingpen R. Lifetimes: a beautiful way to explain death to children. New York: Bantam Books; 1983.

Miller JE. When you know you're dying. Fort Wayne (IN): Willowgreen Publishing; 1997.

Stickney D. Waterbugs and dragonflies. Cleveland (OH): The Pilgrim Press; 1982.

Zolotow C. When the wind stops. New York: Harper Collins; 1969, 1995.

Books that may be helpful for families after the death:

Dodge N. Thumpy's story: a story of love and grief shared by Thumpy, the Bunny. Charles (MO): Prairie Lark Press; 1984 [Available in Spanish.].

Grollman E. Straight talk about death for teenagers. Boston: Beacon Press; 1993.

Heegaard M. When someone very special dies: children can learn to cope with grief. Minneapolis (MN): Woodland Press; 1988.

Munoz-Kiehne M. Since my brother died: desde que murto mi hermano. Omaha (NE): Centering Corp.; 2000.

Romain T. What on earth do you do when someone dies? Minneapolis (MN): Spirit Publishing; 1999.

Schwiebert P, DeKlyen C. Tear soup. Portland (OR): Grief Watch; 2003.

Scrivani M. When death walks in: for teenagers facing grief. Omaha (NE): Centering Corp.; 1991.

Sims AM. Am I still a sister? Louisville (KY): Carrario's Art-Print & Pub.Co.; 1998.

Box 4. A sampling of internet resources that may be helpful:

www.centering.com. A catalogue of grief resources and books
from a regional office for bereaved children and parents.

www.compassionatefriends.org. National self-help organization
that offers friendship, understanding, and hope to bereaved
parents, grandparents, and siblings.

www.hopingskillscompany.com. Started by a bereaved mother
and child life specialist. Offers resources for family members,
a newsletter, keepsake gifts, and links.

www.geocities.com/ethanshouse provides this small site for
bereaved parents who have suffered the loss of children or
infants. Includes a Dad's Network area.

www.griefnet.org. Large site for adults and children. Specializes
in "e-mail support groups" where peers provide support while
being monitored by trained therapists and a licensed
psychiatrist. Site for children (www.kidsaid.com) includes
support for typical childhood/adolescent issues (eg, peer
pressure, dating, family relationships).

www.grievingchild.org. Web site for the Dougy Center,
a nationally renowned center for work with grieving children
and teenagers. Information also provided to assist with the
grief experienced when someone at the child's school dies.

www.juliesplace.com. Created by a teenager who lost her sister,
this site is designed to help other kids and teens who have lost
a sibling. There is a section for children 6–12 and one for
teenagers 13–18.

Intervention models

To look more specifically at intervention models for the child facing the
end of life and the bereaved sibling, we must consider where the child is living. For the ill child, the hospital needs to provide support, as do the school,
religious community, neighborhood, and home care agency. The same is
true for the bereaved sibling. It also makes sense to think about the natural
communication style between children and other family members. Providers
may take this opportunity to introduce new strategies to encourage open
and honest communication.

Promotion of self-expression, both for the ill child before death and the
sibling before and after the death [17], may only be limited by the degree
of willingness of others to engage in this activity. Communication may
take many more forms than talking, although talking is not to be minimized
[4]. It is a gift to be able to tolerate speaking about a child's hopes or fears

and questions about what happens at death or after. Other possible avenues of expression are music, journaling, dance, video/photography, play with puppets [18], dolls, or stuffed animals, poetry, letter writing, a workbook, scrapbooking, pictures, or another kind of project [19].

Support after death for siblings may be provided by trained individuals, such as a social worker, child life specialist, psychiatrist, psychologist, pediatrician [3], or chaplain. It may also be offered by significant others in a child's life, such as a teacher, special friend, or relative [20].

Bibliotherapy may allow children, adolescents, and adults to read about things that are difficult to discuss and thereby open the door to difficult feelings and topics [4]. Some suggested books and online resources to use before death are listed in Boxes 3 and 4.

Finally, groups may be formed and utilized in various ways. For the ill child, there may be groups or camps that are illness specific, such as those for children who have cancer or cystic fibrosis or those for any child who has a life-threatening illness. Some examples are the Hole in the Wall Gang Camp (www.holeinthewallgang.org), the Imus Ranch, The Canyon Ranch Camp, and Dream Street (www.dreamstreetfoundation.org).

For bereaved siblings, depending on geographic location, there may be minimal resources or there may be a variety of programs, bringing together age-based groups for a specified number of sessions to explore, process, and express grief after the death of a loved one. Because parents continue to play a pivotal role in the life of the bereaved sibling, it is often recommended that any intervention be geared toward the family unit [20]. Community-based organizations that support bereaved siblings, family members, and classmates may be found through local hospitals, religious organizations, and hospice groups. Some groups meet separately, with points of integration for siblings and parents. Some meet for just 1 day or a weekend [21–23]. Because the death of a child is relatively rare, sibling groups often mix those who have lost a brother or sister from any disease or condition with those who have lost a parent.

An analogy may be drawn between readying a family for the birth of a child and readying a family for the death of a child. Both experiences bring about an intense fusion of the emotional, physical, and spiritual realms for those bearing witness. Preparation, communication, and collaboration are essential to provide optimal support for the children at the end of life, the parents, and the brothers and sisters.

References

[1] Davies B. The grief of siblings. In: Webb NB, editor. Helping bereaved children: a handbook for practitioners. 2nd edition. New York: Guilford Press; 2002. p. 94–127.

[2] Mack JW, Hilden JM, Watterson J, et al. Parent and physician perspectives on quality of care at the end of life in children with cancer. J Clin Oncol 2005;23:9155–61.

[3] Lewis L, Brecher M, Reaman G, et al. How you can help meet the needs of dying children. Contemp Pediatr 2002;19(4):147–59.

[4] Wolfe J, Grier HE. Care of the dying child. In: Pizzo P, Poplack D, editors. Principles and practice of pediatric oncology. 4th edition. Philadelphia: Lippincott Williams & Wilkins; 2002. p. 1477–93.

[5] Hurwitz C, Duncan J, Wolfe J. Caring for the child with cancer at the close of life. JAMA 2004;292(17):2141–9.

[6] Thayer P. Spiritual care of children and parents. In: Armstrong-Dailey A, Zarbock S, editors. Hospice care for children. 2nd edition. New York: Oxford Press; 2001. p. 172–89.

[7] Davies B. After a child dies: helping the siblings. In: Armstrong-Dailey A, Zarbock S, editors. Hospice care for children. 2nd edition. New York: Oxford Press; 2001. p. 157–71.

[8] Silverman P. Never too young to know: death in children's lives. New York: Oxford University Press; 2000.

[9] Walker CL. Sibling bereavement and grief responses. J Pediatr Nurs 1993;8(5):325–34.

[10] Himelstein BP, Hilden JM, Boldt AM, et al. Pediatric palliative care. N Engl J Med 2004; 350(17):1752–62.

[11] Browning D. To show our humanness—relational and communicative competence in pediatric palliative care. Bioethics Forum 2002;18(3–4):23–8.

[12] Field MJ, Behrman RE, Institute of Medicine (US). Committee on Palliative and End-of-Life Care for Children and Their Families. When children die: improving palliative and end-of-life care for children and their families. Washington, DC: National Academy Press; 2003.

[13] Bluebond-Langner M. The private worlds of dying children. Princeton (NJ); Princeton University Press; 1978.

[14] Sourkes BM. The broken heart: anticipatory grief in the child facing death. J Palliat Care 1996;12(3):56–9.

[15] Kreicbergs U, Valdimarsdottir U, Onelov E, et al. Talking about death with children who have severe malignant disease. N Engl J Med 2004;351(12):1175–86.

[16] Evans M. Teenagers and loss. Int J Palliat Nurs 1996;2(3):124–30.

[17] Davies B, Worden W, Orloff S, et al. Bereavement. In: Carter B, Levetown M, editors. Palliative care for infants, children, and adolescents: a practical handbook. Baltimore (MD): The John Hopkins University Press; 2004. p. 196–219.

[18] Harris A, Curnick S. Group work with bereaved children. In: Smith SC, Pennells M, editors. Interventions with bereaved children. Philadelphia: Jessica Kingsley Publishers; 1995. p.193–203.

[19] Fry V. Part of me died, too: stories of creative survival among bereaved children and teenagers. New York: Dutton Children's Books; 1995.

[20] Stokes J, Pennington J, Monroe B, et al. Developing services for bereaved children: a discussion of the theoretical and practical issues involved. Mortality 1999;4(3):291–307.

[21] Creed J, Ruffin JE, Ward M. A weekend camp for bereaved siblings. Cancer Pract 2001;9(4): 176–82.

[22] Kramer R. A weekend retreat for parents and siblings of children who have died. Interview by Samantha Libby Sodickson. J Palliat Med 2002;5(3):455–64.

[23] Potts S, Farrell M, O'Toole J. Treasure Weekend: supporting bereaved siblings. Palliat Med 1999;13(1):51–6.

ELSEVIER
SAUNDERS

Child Adolesc Psychiatric Clin N Am
15 (2006) 759–777

CHILD AND
ADOLESCENT
PSYCHIATRIC CLINICS
OF NORTH AMERICA

Palliative Medicine in Neonatal and Pediatric Intensive Care

Brian S. Carter, MD[a], Chris Hubble, MD[b], Kathryn L. Weise, MD[c],*

[a]Pediatric Advance Comfort Team, Department of Pediatrics, Vanderbilt Children's
Hospital (Neonatology), 11111 Doctor's Office Tower, Nashville, TN 37232-9544, USA
[b]Pediatric Advanced Comfort Care Team (PACCT), Children's Mercy Hospital and Clinics,
2401 Gillham Road, Kansas City, MO 64108, USA
[c]Pediatric Critical Care Medicine and Bioethics, Pediatric Palliative Medicine,
The Cleveland Clinic Foundation, 9500 Euclid Avenue, Cleveland, OH 44195, USA

Most childhood deaths within the hospital, whether anticipated or unexpected, occur in areas primarily designed for providing acute, life-saving care—the emergency department, the neonatal ICU (NICU), or the pediatric ICU (PICU). Although palliative care services for children are becoming an accepted element of comprehensive, family-centered care, the current nature of ICU settings presents special challenges to providers and families in need of these services. Potential barriers include implicit expectations of families and providers for curative medicine; the belief that these expectations exclude palliative medicine team consultation; commonplace use of highly technical equipment and often painful procedures; and providers self-selected and trained for provision of aggressive, often invasive, life-extending care. Because of the common misconception that palliative care is synonymous with giving up, the palliative care provider is often unwelcome in the ICU. Despite these challenges, palliative care can and should be provided concurrently with aggressive, curative care for all patients, especially patients at highest risk of dying. This article addresses the unique challenges of providing palliative care in the ICU and offers examples of how several current programs have integrated this type of care in the PICU.

* Corresponding author.
E-mail address: weisek@ccf.org (K.L. Weise).

1056-4993/06/$ - see front matter © 2006 Elsevier Inc. All rights reserved.
doi:10.1016/j.chc.2006.02.008

childpsych.theclinics.com

Defining pediatric palliative care

In the Institute of Medicine report, *When Children Die: Improving Palliative and End-of-Life Care for Children and Their Families,* palliative care is broadly defined as seeking to:

> ...[P]revent or relieve the physical and emotional distress produced by a life-threatening medical condition or its treatment, to help patients with such conditions and their families live as normally as possible, and to provide them with timely and accurate information and support in decision making. Such care and assistance is not limited to people thought to be dying and can be provided concurrently with curative or life-prolonging treatments. End-of-life care focuses on preparing for an anticipated death (e.g., discussing in advance the use of life-support technologies in case of cardiac arrest or other crises or arranging a last family trip) and managing the end stage of a fatal medical condition (e.g., removing a breathing tube or adjusting symptom management to reflect changing physiology as death approaches) [1].

Many aspects of this definition apply equally well in home, hospice, and ICU settings.

Major domains of palliative care have been described by Ferrell [2] (Box 1).

These domains are consistent with the World Health Organization definition of palliative care because they are active, are comprehensive, and focus on improving the quality of life of patients in whom a life-limiting or life-threatening condition is expected to lead to premature death. They have been explored further in the development of holistic, emotionally supportive, and compassionate pediatric palliative care services in the NICU and PICU [3,4]. The successful application of these palliative care principles benefits at least three parties, or stakeholders, in the ICU: the patient, the family, and the staff working in the ICU.

Rationale for offering palliative care in the ICU

The rationale for offering palliative care in the ICU is summarized in Box 2.

Epidemiologic studies attest to the heavy burden of childhood death seen in NICU and PICU patient populations. More than half of all annual child deaths in the United States occur before the first birthday, and more than half of these are related to conditions of the perinatal period. Although infants may be discharged from the NICU after lengthy stays for management of prematurity, congenital anomalies, or infection, many return in the first year of life to be hospitalized in the PICU for complications of heart or lung disease, infection, or surgical correction of anomalies. The Institute of Medicine [1] report noted that "more children die in the first year of life than in all other years of childhood combined," and that the preponderance

```
┌─────────────────────────────────────────────────────────────┐
│ Box 1. Domains of palliative care                           │
│                                                             │
│  • Structure and process of care                            │
│  • Physical aspects of care                                 │
│  • Psychological and psychiatric aspects of care            │
│  • Social aspects of care                                   │
│  • Spiritual, religious, and existential aspects of care    │
│  • Cultural aspects of care                                 │
│  • Ethical and legal aspects of care                        │
│  • Care of the imminently dying patient                     │
└─────────────────────────────────────────────────────────────┘
```

of these deaths occur in the neonatal period. Thirty-four percent of all childhood deaths occur in the neonatal period, defined as the first 28 days of postnatal life, and more than a quarter of all childhood deaths occur as a result of shortened gestation, complications of pregnancy, conditions of the placental cord or membranes, congenital heart disease, respiratory distress, or congenital anomalies [1]. Other studies reporting on the location of or circumstances around pediatric death identify the NICU and PICU as the site of 85% or more of inpatient deaths. Death after accidents and trauma typically occurs before hospitalization, in the emergency department, or in the PICU [5–10]. A disproportionate number of PICU admissions for severe, acute illness occur among children with chronic health conditions [11], a population well served by the kind of anticipatory care that a palliative medicine consultant can provide when a life-threatening event occurs. This facet of palliative care is particularly important in providing continuity of care through the many phases of chronic illness that face these children and families.

In the NICU or PICU, many children have an uncertain long-term prognosis, and aggressive curative care is initiated with the knowledge that at least some of these children will die. When delivered appropriately,

```
┌─────────────────────────────────────────────────────────────┐
│ Box 2. Rationale for providing palliative care in the ICU   │
│                                                             │
│  • Heavy burden of complex illness and childhood death in ICU│
│  • Frequent uncertain long-term prognosis                   │
│  • High potential for painful or fearful interventions      │
│  • Need for facilitation of complex care planning           │
│  • Need for continuity of care through successive phases    │
│    of diagnosis and illness                                 │
│  • Shared goals of optimizing quality of life between ICU   │
│    and palliative care teams                                │
│  • Facilitation of end-of-life planning, when appropriate   │
└─────────────────────────────────────────────────────────────┘
```

palliative care supports the hope for cure that parents and caregivers should maintain and complements the technology-based, curative therapy of modern medicine. Not only is this humane, complete (holistic) medicine, but it also sets the foundation of trust needed between ICU health care providers and families for making difficult decisions in the event that curative treatment fails [12]. Early involvement of palliative care personnel also establishes relationships that continue long after the child is discharged from the ICU, providing much needed continuity for the child's health care journey.

Integrating interdisciplinary and comprehensive palliative care principles in the NICU is not a new concept. Incorporating hospice approaches in the management of certain newborns was described in 1982 in the United States [13]. In this setting, it is well acknowledged that although care must revolve around the newborn patient, it must be equally supportive of families. In recent years, family support systems have become increasingly present in the NICU. In some institutions, however, integral parts of a comprehensive interdisciplinary palliative care service (eg, social work, pastoral care, child life specialists, behavioral health services, staff support programs, clinical ethics) may be lacking, difficult to access, or inconsistently or poorly coordinated in accomplishing patient-focused, family-centered care. It is easy—given the history of success in neonatology and the technologic environment of the NICU in which the physicians feel comfortable—for physicians to retain a cure-oriented, life-extending interventional approach to care that demands attention to what is currently "urgent." In so doing, clinicians may push aside any consideration or preparation for plausible, or even probable, anticipated mortality. What results is a lack of time for team and family preparedness, coordinated support services, and anticipatory grief work. Also, when called on late in the child's course, the palliative care team members are strangers to the parents, when instead they could have begun the hardest conversations in the context of an established relationship.

Developing similar supportive services in the PICU differs from the NICU in large part as a result of differences in patient diagnosis, medical history, and disease course. Many patients are postsurgical, having brief PICU stays with rapid recovery and prompt transfer out of the PICU. Similarly, most children admitted to the PICU with nonsurgical problems improve rapidly or die soon after arrival. Both groups of patients differ greatly from premature infants who may spend weeks to months in the NICU before discharge home or death. In total, less than 5% of PICU patients stay longer than 12 days, although these patients often account for a higher proportion of PICU patient days [14–16]. In addition, many PICU patients already have established medical providers before the PICU admission. It is not surprising that few PICUs have established extensive programs focused on the long-term, family-centered, patient care teams similar to those in many NICUs. Differences in patient populations between PICUs and NICUs and the presence or absence of preexisting family-centered teams would affect the integration of palliative care services into the ICU.

Despite the differences between NICUs and PICUs, both ICUs have a great deal in common that necessitates palliative care support services, as follows: (1) Many patients have a significant risk of dying during the hospitalization, (2) patient care often involves highly invasive, painful technology, (3) patient and family routines are disrupted to a greater degree than during a ward admission, and (4) many patients who survive do so with significant morbidity and the likelihood of returning to the ICU or dying in the future.

During the patient's ICU stay, the neonatologist, surgeon, or pediatric intensivist usually assumes the role of primary medical manager. For a patient in the NICU, this is often the beginning of an intense, extended health care relationship. Previously healthy children who have an acute onset of illness experience a similar introduction in the PICU. Chronically ill children who are admitted to the PICU often have well-established relationships within a health care system, however, and the PICU team's medical management is often viewed as a disruption to continuity of care. The complex medical patient who survives an ICU stay subsequently has their medical management transitioned back to their original provider or, in the case of a new diagnosis, to a completely new health care provider. Palliative care teams often can smooth these transitions between different health care teams, providing continued support throughout the patient's medical journey and a consistent voice representing the patient and parents as new care providers are encountered.

Palliative care medicine does not preclude the appropriate application of life-sustaining therapies, especially when a life-limiting or life-threatening condition has not yet been confirmed, and it addresses the necessary management of physical symptoms. Palliative care goals remain focused on the child's best interests and on attaining an acceptable quality of life, while contributing a continuity role in helping parents with medical decision making over time. Even in the case of sudden, unexpected trauma or illness, the umbrella of palliative care facilitates addressing the psychosocial, spiritual, cultural, and ethical aspects of care for the patient and family, who now are facing difficult days and decisions [2]. Some studies attest to the length of stay of NICU and PICU patients exceeding days to weeks—even after acute illness or trauma—before ultimately dying [5,6]. Such lengthy time frames necessitate the introduction and coordination of palliative care services while the patient is in the ICU. After even the most sudden death, supportive care services that are culturally sensitive and congruent with families' faith communities also can prove beneficial. Palliative services may be the bridge to such care in some institutions.

ICU patients identified as benefiting from palliative care include patients with lethal anomalies, complex anomalies with a poor prognosis, anticipated severe chronic disease or anticipated complex care regardless of prognosis, and conditions requiring intensive treatment to prolong an acceptable quality of life [17,18]. Such patients represent a large number of the patients admitted to pediatric and NICUs. Few data are available to assess the impact of palliative care consultation in the ICU [4]. A discussion of ethics and palliative care consultation in the adult ICU describes their potential benefits, however, characterizing them as existing on a continuum from a "facilitation" to a "care provider model" [19]. Parallels can be drawn to pediatric and NICUs, but further studies of effectiveness are lacking at this time.

Aspects of intensive care pertinent to palliative care

Aspects of the ICU that are pertinent to palliative care are presented in Box 3.

Circumstances of admission to neonatal or pediatric intensive care

Patients are admitted to an ICU under a variety of circumstances. Although there is an increasing societal awareness of the tragedy of chronic pediatric illness, and there will always be the acute and sometimes unavoidable presentation of children to the critical care setting, society does not routinely accept the death of a child as natural. For some parents, the news of a potentially life-threatening illness for their child may come as a complete surprise. Whether facing a newborn with a previously undiagnosed, life-threatening congenital heart lesion or a previously healthy 5-year-old with

---

Box 3. Pertinent aspects of ICU care

- Frequently unexpected or sudden presentation of declining health
- ICU staff may meet family for the first time during a crisis
- Issues surrounding first exposure of family and patient to ICU
- Discontinuity of care: changes in medical team composition and control
- Communication: potential for differences of opinion and conflicting information
- Training issues and care paradigms: ICU staff trained for rapid, aggressive interventions; palliative care staff may be less familiar with critical illness physiology and potential for recovery
- Intensivists and palliative care staff may function in both roles: confusing for colleagues and families
- Difficulties in initiating end-of-life discussions in critical care setting

severe traumatic brain injury after a motor vehicle accident, parents experience an immediate, significant loss of their previous hopes or expectations for a healthy child. Historically, critical care teams have not been structured or trained to dedicate significant attention to helping families process this immediate loss, but rather have focused on the curative, lifesaving efforts of the critical care environment. With an increased presence of support staff, such as chaplains, child life specialists, and social workers, and the increased awareness of palliative care practice by nurses and physicians, critical care settings may become better equipped to acknowledge and address the immediate loss experienced by the patient and parents.

In the NICU, prenatal diagnosis increasingly helps families prepare for the potential illness their child will face and the potential questions they might face as surrogate decision makers. Although pediatric physicians and genetic counselors meet with parents to discuss the implications of a prenatal diagnosis, few centers have integrated the palliative care team at this early stage of care, arguably when parents have the most questions and most need the support of the health care team. In the case of older children with a life-limiting condition, the potential for advance planning occurs when families, physicians, and health care support personnel are honest about the possibility for treatment failure. Starting at the time of diagnosis and readdressing them when critical events arise during medical treatment, such discussions maintain a balance between hope for medical cure and the reality that medical treatments may not work, resulting in the death of the child. The tone and balance of these conversations must change to accommodate alterations, good and bad, in the patient's medical condition. Although some physicians believe that any discussion of treatment failure with the family or patient implies weakness or a lack of conviction in the curative efforts, these are often the same physicians who effectively abandon their patients when there is no curative care to offer or continue to provide futile care that is potentially painful or limiting to quality-of-life goals of the family.

Inclusion of palliative care in the ICU can occur in two ways—as continuation of a service already involved before a particular patient's ICU admission or as a new concept to a family dealing with a decline in their child's health. A family already involved with a palliative care team might expect or hope that their child's care still would be managed by the palliative care team in the ICU, but would find that in most neonatal and PICUs, care instead is managed by the ICU team or by a collaboration between surgical and intensivist teams. The palliative care team most often assumes a consulting role and may be advising groups who are neither familiar with nor accepting of a palliative care approach. In this case, continued involvement of the palliative care team is especially important to the family and child as they work with a new group of physicians and nurses who may not be accepting of a team often associated with giving up hope. The mere situation of being in a unit in which success may be defined in different terms—long-term survival, a successful operation, or distinct physiologic improvement—may be disconcerting if the concepts of palliative care are not promoted by the entire staff.

Neonatal and pediatric critical care workers share the challenge of first meeting patients and families during a time of crisis. Parents with a worrisome prenatal diagnosis occasionally have the benefit of meeting the staff and seeing the NICU before the infant is born. For the most part, such previews are rare. Unless the parents and child have had prior experiences with a critical care environment, they typically are exposed to things for which they have no frame of reference. The parent–NICU relationship is formed around the shared experience of the critically ill neonate and typically starts when the newborn is gravely ill. The subsequent medical course of the newborn affects the relationship between the parents and the staff. Bonds form between staff, child, and family, especially when the hospitalization is for a prolonged period, as is often the case for premature infants. As in the NICU, a large proportion of PICU patients have never been exposed to a critical care setting. The critical care setting is a new and, in many ways, fearful environment because of the technology and accompanying risk of side effects; different and, in some cases, more restrictive visitation policies; different noises; and often increased level of activity. Before arriving in the ICU, parents may not acknowledge that children die in critical care settings, but after becoming aware of the death of other children, they may question their own child's chance for survival.

Although families experience loss from the point of prenatal diagnosis, premature or complicated delivery, or the acute medical deterioration of a chronically ill patient, the ultimate message of a limited life span or impending loss of an infant or child's life brings discomfort for families and staff alike. In the NICU and PICU, stress around these matters has been well studied and measured. Little has been presented in the way of beneficial interventions, however, using psychological consultation or other behavioral health means of interventions to assist these parties [20–24]. There is a role for the palliative medicine team in assisting with these stressors.

Communication issues

Families are at risk for receiving mixed messages from the myriad ICU staff members involved in the care of critically ill children [25]. A study of staff perceptions of end-of-life care in the PICU revealed that nurses and physicians encounter conflict arising from multiple sources, many relating to communication difficulties [26]. Because families often seek updates and opinions from multiple caregivers, communicated differences in views on prognosis and goals may worsen the uncertainty faced by the parents of critically ill infants and children [27]. Recognition of these phenomena by the palliative care team can provide a valuable opportunity to work with families, patients, and staff toward a rich understanding and more consistent presentation of expectations and hopes.

Effective education, identification of preferences, and advance planning before admission to the ICU facilitates decision making by focusing on patient quality-of-life values. This process better prepares parents and guardians for new questions they will face during crisis situations. The pros and cons of invasive therapies can be discussed before use, allowing more realistic expectations and a better knowledge of the implications of using such technology. Data from a PICU imply that a perception of their child's quality of life is the family's primary factor in end-of-life decision making [28]. Including older children and adolescents in these discussions validates the importance of patient preferences and choices, making the older child or adolescent a more active participant in the medical decision-making process. At least some bioethical experts have advocated for increasing the role of minors in their own health care decision making [29–33].

Staff and environmental issues that affect palliative care in the ICU

ICU staff are trained to act decisively. Decisions may need to be made in a rapidly analytical manner, relying on physiologic data, laboratory and imaging studies, and surgical or procedural techniques. In the usual paradigm, the intent is first to stabilize altered physiology and to save the child's life. Only after such action can attention be diverted to ascertaining just "who" this child is—his or her place in the family, typical daily activities or baseline limitations of function, life goals, close kinship to a special sister or aunt—and what values are driving decisions to continue life support, restore function, or begin the long road of rehabilitative treatment.

Resources brought to bear in the ICU are vast and complex and almost always bring with them a high level of activity or perceived commotion. Invasive procedures (endotracheal tubes, intravenous catheters, chest tubes, surgical drains, and urethral catheters) and extensive monitoring are second nature to workers in the ICU, but are often new, painful, and anxiety-provoking for the patient and family. Nurse-to-patient ratios often exceed those on general wards, and immediate physician presence is often more noticeable to families. Coupled with the higher level of monitoring, the patient is under almost constant observation. This observation often includes more and different noises, less privacy, disruption of sleep-wake cycles, and physical and emotional discomfort for the patient and often the family. Many ICUs have restrictive visitation policies. High-technology resource measures are often used, such as renal dialysis or extracorporeal membrane oxygenation. At times, it may seem to families that there is no limit to what resources may be used, and this may imply that there is no limit to what critical care medicine has to offer. It is often only after an initial stabilization that the need for values assessment relative to a specific patient is recognized. In this situation, it may seem to a family or staff that a seemingly abrupt shift in the goals and direction of care is occurring.

Difficulty initiating end-of-life discussions in the ICU

For many clinicians, introducing end-of-life or palliative care issues for a critically ill newborn or child who is not actively dying might seem untimely—acknowledging that the moment, content, and delivery of such conversations with families would affect their understanding and acceptance of the communication. Providing a clear prognosis to parents may be especially difficult for many ICU patients. In the NICU, where survival rates of extremely low-birth-weight infants have improved dramatically over the last several decades, morbidity for survivors remains quite high and is not always easily predicted [8,34–39]. Even when reasonable mortality data are known, patients and their families often are not effectively informed of the prognosis, or they are informed but are unable to understand the information within the same timeframe as members of the medical care team [40].

An example would be a bone marrow transplant patient who develops complications requiring transfer to the PICU. Such a patient has undergone a high-risk procedure, often overcoming significant challenges in the medical journey, with much investment of time, energy, and hope for cure. When the patient subsequently develops a complication requiring admission to the PICU, the child, parents, and oncology specialist all experience loss and may interpret the change as only a "step backward," rather than acknowledging the life-threatening nature of the event. Although these patients have a poor survival rate when intubated (2-year survival rate of approximately 10–20% and worse in the case of multiorgan system involvement), the families and clinicians often find it difficult to limit curative care [41–45]. The parents of these children may not grasp their child's high risk of death or the quality-of-life implications of aggressive ICU care until after it has been initiated. Even when the probability of a poor outcome is known for a given circumstance or patient population, families may not have the opportunity to process this information in advance and seldom have an opportunity to process it until their child's acute deterioration forces the issue. In addition, many families understandably resist the prediction of a poor outcome and may believe that a poor prognosis is the result of working with the wrong physician or wrong hospital. This dynamic makes conversations about palliative approaches even more difficult for caregivers who already are uncomfortable with the subject.

Acknowledging the complementary nature of critical care and palliative care

Integrating a palliative care approach in the NICU or PICU requires mutual understanding of each discipline's goals and processes across a range of clinical situations. Both teams must recognize the wide range of outcomes of critically ill infants and children and the uncertain prognosis of many patients. Both teams must recognize that neither discipline hopes for death, but for improving the quality of life, whether long or short. The palliative care team must recognize which critically ill patients have a reasonable expectation of survival with an acceptable quality of life to be accepted as colleagues and to communicate effectively with the ICU team and the family. Conversely, the ICU team should recognize that the laudable goal of providing lifesaving treatment does not confer an absolute prerogative to preserve life without consideration of the perspectives of the moral communities to which the child and family belong [36]. A palliative care consultation can facilitate information transmission and decision making over a long hospitalization that ends in cure and in so doing make a real contribution to the family's experience. A clear elucidation of the goals of care must be approached in the context of time, resources, and values assessment with continued re-evaluation as the patient's condition evolves.

A challenge to families and staff relates to confusion of perceived roles of the providers. Especially when the palliative care specialist is also an intensivist, colleagues may assume that the goals of that provider are in conflict when caring for a critically ill patient. Picture a postoperative patient with complex congenital heart disease who has developed multiple complications and now faces a prolonged course with less than a 10% chance of survival. The hopeful family, surgeon, and critical care team may believe that continued aggressive measures remain appropriate as long as any chance of recovery exists. Providing intensive lifesaving therapies simultaneously with palliative measures that include attention to long-term goals, assistance with decision making, psychological care of the patient and family, ethical issues, cultural differences, and intensive comfort measures may be appropriate as long as medical team goals and family goals are concordant. If the primary team in the ICU believes that palliative care goals are in conflict with, rather than concordant with, ongoing critical care, team interactions may be compromised. Because optimal care in the ICU includes communication and cooperation, it is incumbent on the intensivist/palliative care specialist to work with colleagues toward a better understanding of how palliative care can complement intensive care, rather than undermine its potential curative goals.

Family and patient support, communication, and continuity

Palliative care teams often serve as the communication hub or coordinators of information for the family and the health care team, to represent the family and to ensure that the family and patient's voices are heard by the entire health care team, especially as the primary team experiences changes in who is in charge over time. The palliative care team focuses on the patient and family response to the disease course and supports their care needs beyond strictly medical needs. This support often requires the incorporation and coordination of social workers, child life specialists, behavior medicine specialists, and chaplains in the care of the child and family [25].

Patient-focused documentation tools help identify and organize the numerous patient preferences, medical indications, quality-of-life issues, contextual or social circumstances, and objectives of care and may set target dates for completion, when appropriate [46]. The process of compiling the information often helps families and patients prioritize the many challenges they encounter—both immediate and potential future crises. With appropriate updates, such tools also help family members and new providers communicate more efficiently and ease transitions to new providers inside or outside of their current center. Examples of ICU patients who might benefit from such a tool include a former premature neonate who is going home and will be followed by a special care clinic and a PICU patient who is recovering from a life-threatening illness but will require extensive medical care on the ward, who remains at risk of dying, and who still may face challenging decisions regarding care in the future.

Examples of palliative care systems

Four models of palliative care services with extension into the PICU and NICU are presented. All models involve multiple caregivers that interface with other care providers when in the ICU.

Children's Mercy Hospitals and Clinics

The Pediatric Advanced Comfort Care Team (PACCT) at Children's Mercy Hospitals and Clinics formed in 2000 and has been providing palliative care for patients since 2003. Although initial efforts focused on education, the team is now established as a clinical consultation service, serving more than 14 different medical and surgical sections throughout the hospital, consulting on almost 100 new patients in 2005, and carrying an average census of 80 to 85 patients. The team currently is composed of one full-time and two part-time nurses who serve as PACCT clinicians, a chaplain who is the education coordinator, an intensive care physician who serves as the medical director, and an operations manager who develops organizational structure, including a computer program for patient tracking and interface with the electronic medical record. Since 2000, PACCT has benefited greatly from countless hours of work from hospital staff who have volunteered on a task force committee. A dedicated administration has secured start-up funding and provided personnel support.

Currently, the PACCT team does not include dedicated support staff, such as a social worker, chaplain, or child life specialist. Instead, the PACCT clinicians integrate into individual medical and surgical sections, identifying and collaborating with each patient's primary physician, nurses, and support staff who already are dedicated to that particular medical section and patient. This integration ensures continuity for the patient and family and is intended to encourage earlier consultations, ideally at the time of diagnosis, while curative therapy is still ongoing. This strategy helps share the workload among support staff for the PACCT patients and has increased the interactions between PACCT clinicians and the general health care staff throughout the hospital. Integrating the PACCT clinician role into the primary care team in this manner (1) builds trust with the patient, family, and health care team; (2) provides a more complete understanding of the patient's medical journey for the palliative care clinician; and (3) helps prevent PACCT from being viewed only as an "end-of-life" or inpatient "hospice" service. When patients switch primary physician or nurse providers, they maintain the same support staff of social worker, chaplain, child life worker, and PACCT clinician. To date, PACCT has not assumed the primary care role for patients, and the medical director is not involved in direct patient care.

Integration of PACCT within the NICU and PICU began in early 2005. Initial discussions were held between the physicians of both sections to outline the spectrum of PACCT services and to identify appropriate patients for potential referral. Although there remain issues of acceptance and overcoming the viewpoint by some that PACCT is an end-of-life service, health care workers are increasingly accepting the role of the PACCT clinician as part of the health care team in the ICU. Currently, PACCT is not consulted in either the NICU or the PICU when the child is not expected to live more than a few days. When the child shows a chance for survival of at least a few weeks to a month, PACCT is consulted to assist with the decision making and long-term planning for the child with a limited life expectancy or significant morbidity. PACCT participation has increased continuity for patients because NICU and PICU attending staff rotate at relatively frequent intervals (1–2 weeks). When involved in patient care, PACCT also helps ensure that quality-of-life issues are addressed adequately. PACCT has been particularly helpful in the care of medically complex, critically ill children when they are discharged from the ICU to (1) the general wards, where the supervision of care is switched to different physician providers; (2) home with follow-up by different physicians inside or outside of hospital system; or (3) home with the local hospice team (Carousel–Kansas City Hospice). For 2005, PACCT has been consulted on more than 25 patients in the NICU and more than 35 patients in the PICU.

Cleveland Clinic

The Helping Hands Pediatric Palliative Care team at the Cleveland Clinic Foundation comprises physicians, a palliative care nurse, a care coordinator with social work training, child life specialists, and a pediatric psychologist. The physicians involved with the team include intensivists, pediatric oncologists, a pediatric anesthesiologist, and a pediatric psychiatrist, two of whom are certified by the American Board of Hospice and Palliative Care Medicine. Although this array of providers insures clinical expertise in oncology, pain management, critical illness, and psychological support, the nonphysician members of the team provide the primary support and continuity of care with patients and families.

When an established palliative care patient is transferred from the ward to an ICU, the care coordinator and palliative care nurse round daily or as needed with the ICU team and are available at all times to work with the family or to attend family meetings. They play a large role in helping the family to process new information and communicate their understanding of these issues back to the ICU team. In addition, members of the palliative care group attend PICU rounds several times a week and are participants in weekly multidisciplinary rounds in which all PICU patients are discussed.

New patients appropriate for advanced illness care planning and palliative care are identified by physicians, nurses, or other staff members, and families have access to information about these services through brochures available on most hospital wards. It is common for families to request input from the service for its role in interpreting complex medical information from multiple caregivers. The goal is to provide continuity of care to complex patients before death is seen as likely.

Despite an active presence of the palliative care team in the NICU and PICU, barriers to its acceptance remain. Some ICU and surgical attending physicians have expressed frustration when palliative care team members did not understand critical care physiology as it related to condition and prognosis, fearing that mixed messages would be sent to families and other staff. This situation has improved as the palliative care team has gained familiarity with practices and outcomes in these units, and as the ICU teams have gained an understanding of the role of the palliative care team members. In addition, there remain specialty services that believe that their role is to provide only aggressive lifesaving measures, and that their approach to death, when it is inevitable, is excellent. The palliative care team continues to work to offer services beyond what services with more limited time can provide, including family support, sibling support, follow-up after discharge, or bereavement care. Numerous services have become more accepting of the palliative care service after members of the team have provided interventions not classically seen as end-of-life care, but within the purview of the team, such as coordinating transport back to a home institution. Occasionally, the team has agreed to assume primary attending status of ICU patients when a surgical team did not think it had expertise in providing comfort care after families decided not to pursue further surgical intervention. Numerous approaches to increasing acceptance of the palliative care team in the ICU have been effective, including continued availability and visibility in the ICU, encouragement of all teams to understand what the others have to offer, demonstration of family and physician satisfaction with care measures provided, and willingness to assume important aspects of care that others are uncomfortable providing.

Vanderbilt Children's Hospital

In the neonatal and PICUs, consultative services through the Pediatric Advanced Comfort Team (PACT) are available when requested by any clinical staff member or family member. On receipt of a consult, the nurse clinical coordinator for PACT contacts the attending physician to notify him or her and proceeds to meet with the staff and family. An intake form is used to document information about the patient and family, medical condition, current understanding of the goals of care, patient/family values and preferences, and options for providing comprehensive, interdisciplinary, compassionate care in a setting or environment most conducive to meeting patient/family goals. At times, coordination of spiritual, social, and psychological support predominates. At other times, symptom management is a key area of concern. Social workers, chaplains, community clergy, child life specialists, case managers, and specialty physicians (pain and anesthesiology, oncology, palliative medicine) all work in a coordinated manner with unit nursing staff to effect comprehensive care. Parents are engaged in decision-making processes. Choices for the location of care may include the ICU, a ward room, home with home health or hospice services, or inpatient hospice (coordinated through Alive Hospice in Nashville).

More recent experiences include the adjustment of analgesia and sedation; managing withdrawal from life-sustaining measures such as assisted ventilation or dialysis; helping families with decisions concerning palliative surgical interventions, home care needs, and sibling support; grief and bereavement counseling, and staff support in the ICUs and on the wards after the death of children following a prolonged hospitalization. Numerous cases have involved oncology diagnoses, terminal pulmonary hypertension in infants and children with congenital heart disease or diaphragmatic hernia, and a variety of congenital anomalies with no curative interventions. In some instances, neonatal-perinatal loss has been supported.

It has been noted that having key personnel from the PACT on staff in each unit enhances the receptivity to palliative care and incorporating it concurrently with critical care. Acceptance has been enhanced by regularly attending care conferences and reviewing with other ICU team members cases that prove most challenging by virtue of length of stay in the ICU, complex diseases, multiple caregivers (including multiple consulting physicians or services), and recognized family coping issues. The concordant use of ethics consultation also has helped in some cases.

Palliative care services at Vanderbilt Children's Hospital have proved helpful in furthering research in this area. Projects conducted in 2002–2003 involved establishing baseline data regarding palliative care of children hospitalized at Vanderbilt Children's Hospital. The first study described the circumstances surrounding the deaths of hospitalized terminally ill children, especially as they pertain to pain and symptom management by the multidisciplinary pediatric care team. A second study involved interviews with consenting parents of these children by telephone to assess their satisfaction with end-of-life care. The survey included a 14-item, Likert-type scale and 2 open-ended questions. A third study involved a survey of interdisciplinary staff in the NICU, the PICU, and cardiology and oncology units to determine their knowledge, understanding, and concerns about end-of-life care for infants and children. In 2003–2004, the use of monthly Morbidity and Mortality Conferences to enhance end-of-life education and improve care provision and its documentation was studied. Presently, research is addressing communication and coping mechanisms within families after a child is diagnosed with a life-limiting condition.

Two additional services of a palliative care effort in the ICU may include care for the caregiver support services and critical incident debriefing. Caregiver support programs are often at the nursing or unit level, but may be directed toward entire staff, focused on housestaff, or adapted as needed [47]. These programs may include wellness themes or activities or may be more focused on team or unit needs, such as dealing with loss or stress, recognizing compassion fatigue, avoiding burnout, anger/stress management classes, ethics discussions, breakout groups on professionalism, mentoring, or peer support. Critical incident debriefing may be coordinated after a significant event or after a cumulative number of losses [48–50].

Children's Hospital of Wisconsin

The Palliative Care Program at the Children's Hospital of Wisconsin dates back to the early 1980s, largely as a home-based nursing service. In 1994, the inpatient consultation service started, and an outpatient clinic was added in 2001. A monthly joint clinic with physical medicine and rehabilitation was added in 2004. Current staffing consists of two nurse clinicians, an advanced practice nurse, a medical director, a masters-prepared program coordinator, and research staff. Funding for these positions comes from a complex combination of billings/charges, philanthropy, grants, contracts, the pediatrics department, and the hospital.

The core consultation team typically consists of a physician and a nurse, often with students, residents, or fellows joining. Social work, chaplaincy, child life, case management, and other essential ancillary services are not part of the core palliative care team; rather, they are drawn from unit-specific or service-specific personnel. Typically, 100 to 120 new patients/y are seen, and 75 to 80 children are followed at any given time. The average length of stay is approximately 3 months. Major diagnostic categories include neurologic conditions or neurologic complications of other disorders, genetic and chromosomal problems, problems associated with low birth weight or short gestation, and cancer.

The service is available "24/7/365," with first coverage provided by a combination of nurses and the medical director. Attending backup coverage is provided by the medical director and two physicians from the chronic pain team. The team also offers services in pain and symptom management and assistance with decision making and advance care planning, prognostication, home care and hospice service coordination, care coordination, and staff support and education.

In addition to traditional consultation and home-based practice, the palliative care program has established several liaison practices, in which palliative care personnel join with other clinical team staff to provide support and expertise in palliative care. Services currently seen in this fashion include oncology/stem cell transplant, neurology, physical medicine and rehabilitation, tracheostomy/ventilator program, and the children with special health care needs program. The team rounds weekly in the NICU, alternating between the two attending services, and currently is working closely within a task force to try to create a palliative care extension team in the PICU.

Through a contractual arrangement, the palliative care program director is also the pediatric medical director for the Visiting Nurse Association of Milwaukee Hospice, with a typical pediatric census of 15 to 20 children at a time. The program provides education to M2, M3, and M4 students, the latter through a combined adult/pediatric selective. The program has a combined pediatric/adult palliative medicine fellowship, and a resident rotation is available.

Summary

Patients and families in NICU and PICU settings can be well served by fundamental palliative care approaches during curative and end-of-life care. A wide variety of patients are suitable for these services. Although barriers exist to implementing these teams within the ICU, the concepts remain sound, and models for successful integration of practices in these settings exist.

References

[1] Institute of Medicine, Field MJ, Behrman RE, editors. When children die: improving palliative and end-of-life care for children and their families. Washington, DC: National Academic Press; 2003.
[2] Ferrell BR. Overview of the domains of variables relevant to end-of-life care. NIH State-of-the Science Conference on Improving End-of-Life Care, December 6–8, 2004; Program and Abstracts. pp. 29–31.
[3] Gilmer MJ. Pediatric palliative care: a family-centered model for critical care. Crit Care Nurs Clin North Am 2002;14:207–14.
[4] Pierucci RL, Kirby RS, Leuthner SR. End-of-life care for neonates and infants: the experience and effects of a palliative care consultation service. Pediatrics 2001;108:653–60.
[5] Carter BS, Howenstein M, Gilmer MJ, et al. Circumstances surrounding the deaths of hospitalized children: opportunities for pediatric palliative care. Pediatrics 2004;114(3):e361–6. Available at: http://www.pediatrics.org/cgi/content/full/114/3/e361.

[6] Feudtner C, DiGiuseppe DL, Neff JM. Hospital care for children and young adults in the last year of life: a population-based study. BMC Med 2003;1:3. Available at: http://www.biomedcentral.com/1741–7015/1/3.

[7] Garros D, Rosychuk RJ, Cox PN. Circumstances surrounding end of life in a pediatric intensive care unit. Pediatrics 2003;112:e371–9. Available at: http://www.pediatrics.org/cgi/content/full/112/5/e371.

[8] Burns JP, Mitchell C, Outwater KM, et al. End-of-life care in the pediatric intensive care unit after the forgoing of life-sustaining treatment. Crit Care Med 2000;28:3060–6.

[9] van der Wal ME, Renfurm LN, van Vught AJ, et al. Circumstances of dying in hospitalized children. Eur J Pediatr 1999;158:560–5.

[10] Feudtner C, Christakis DA, Zimmerman FJ, et al. Characteristics of deaths occurring in children's hospitals: implications for supportive care services. Pediatrics 2002;109:887–93.

[11] Dosa NP, Boeing M, Kanter RK. Excess risk of severe acute illness in children with chronic health conditions. Pediatrics 2001;107:499–504.

[12] Meert KL, Thurston CS, Sarnaik AP. End-of-life decision-making and satisfaction with care: parental perspectives. Pediatr Crit Care Med 2000;1:179–85.

[13] Whitfield JM, Siegel RE, Glicken AD, et al. The application of hospice concepts to neonatal care. Am J Dis Child 1982;136:421–4.

[14] Marcin JP, Slonim AD, Pollack MM, et al. Long-stay patients in the pediatric intensive care unit. Crit Care Med 2001;29:652–7.

[15] Goh AY, Mok Q. Identifying futility in a paediatric critical care setting: a perspective observational study. Arch Dis Child 2001;84:265–8.

[16] Sachdeva RC, Jefferson LS, Coss-Bu J, et al. Resource consumption and the extent of futile care among patients in a pediatric intensive care unit setting. J Pediatr 1996;128:742–77.

[17] Himelstein BP, Hilden JM, Boldt AM, et al. Pediatric palliative care. N Engl J Med 2004;530:1752–62.

[18] Levetown M, Liben S, Audet M. Palliative care in the pediatric intensive care unit. In: Carter BS, Levetown M, editors. Palliative care for infants, children, and adolescents. Baltimore: Johns Hopkins University Press; 2004. p. 273–91.

[19] Aulisio MP, Chaitlin E, Arnold RM. Ethics and palliative care consultation in the intensive care unit. Crit Care Clin 2004;20:505–33.

[20] Franck LS, Cox S, Allen A, et al. Measuring neonatal intensive care unit-related parental stress. J Adv Nurs 2005;49:608–15.

[21] Mitchell ML, Courtney M. Reducing family members' anxiety and uncertainty in illness around transfer from intensive care: an intervention study. Intensive Crit Care Nurs 2004;20:223–31.

[22] Spear ML, Leef K, Epps S, et al. Family reactions during infants' hospitalization in the neonatal intensive care unit. Am J Perinatol 2002;19:205–14.

[23] Balluffi A, Kassam-Adams N, Kazak A, et al. Traumatic stress in parents of children admitted to the pediatric intensive care unit. Pediatr Crit Care Med 2004;5:547–53.

[24] Cook P, White DK, Ross-Russell RI. Bereavement support following sudden and unexpected death: guidelines for care. Arch Dis Child 2002;87:36–8.

[25] Contro NA, Larson A, Scofield S, et al. Hospital staffs and family perspectives regarding quality of pediatric palliative care. Pediatrics 2004;114:1248–52.

[26] Burns JP, Mitchell C, Griffith JL, et al. End-of-life care in the pediatric intensive care unit: attitudes and practices of pediatric critical care physicians and nurses. Crit Care Med 2001;29:658–64.

[27] Weise KL. Finding our way. Hastings Cent Rep 2004;34:8–9.

[28] Meyer EC, Burns JP, Griffith JL, et al. Parental perspectives on end-of-life care in the pediatric intensive care unit. Crit Care Med 2004;30:226–31.

[29] Bartholome WG. Hearing children's voices. Bioethics Forum 1995;11:3–6.

[30] Midwest Bioethics Center, Task Force on Health Care Rights for Minors. Health care treatment decision-making guidelines for minors. Bioethics Forum 1995;11:A1–16.

[31] Committee on Bioethics of the American Academy of Pediatrics. Informed consent, parental permission, and assent in pediatric practice. Pediatrics 1995;95:314–7.

[32] Bartholome WG. Informed consent, parental permission, and assent in pediatric practice. Pediatrics 1995;96:981–2.

[33] Hinds PS, Drew D, Oakes LL, et al. End-of-life care preferences of pediatric patients with cancer. J Clin Oncol 2005;23:9146–54.

[34] Piecuch RE, Leonard CH, Cooper BA. Infants with birth weight 1,000–1,499 grams born in three time periods: has outcome changed over time? Clin Pediatr 1998;37:537–45.

[35] Wilson-Costello D, Friedman H, Minich N, et al. Improved survival rates with increased neurodevelopmental disability for extremely low birth weight infants in the 1990s. Pediatrics 2005;115:997–1003.

[36] Sharman M, Meert KL, Sarnaik AP. What influences parents' decisions to limit or withdraw life support? Pediatr Crit Care Med 2005;6:513–8.

[37] Frader JE. Global paternalism in pediatric intensive care unit end-of-life decisions? Pediatr Crit Care Med 2003;4:257–8.

[38] Roig CG. Art of communication. Pediatr Crit Care Med 2003;4:259.

[39] Brahm G, Merkens M. End-of-life in the pediatric intensive care unit: seeking the family's decision of when and how, not if. Crit Care Med 2000;28:3122–3.

[40] Wolfe J, Klar N, Grier HE, et al. Understanding of prognosis among parents of children who died of cancer: impact on treatment goals and integration of palliative care. JAMA 2000;284: 2469–75.

[41] Jacobe SJ, Hassan A, Veys P, et al. Outcome of children requiring admission to an intensive care unit after bone marrow transplantation. Crit Care Med 2003;31:1299–305.

[42] Hagen SA, Craig DM, Martin PL, et al. Mechanically ventilated pediatric stem cell transplant recipients: effect of cord blood transplant and organ dysfunction on outcome. Pediatr Crit Care Med 2003;4:206–13.

[43] Keenan HT, Bratton SL, Martin LD, et al. Outcome of children who require mechanical ventilatory support after bone marrow transplantation. Crit Care Med 2000;28:830–5.

[44] Rossi R, Shemie SD, Calderwood S. Prognosis of pediatric bone marrow transplant recipients requiring mechanical ventilation. Crit Care Med 1999;27:1181–6.

[45] Todd K, Wiley F, Landaw E, et al. Survival outcome among 54 intubated pediatric bone marrow transplant patients. Crit Care Med 1994;22:171–6.

[46] Hays RM, Haynes G, Geyer R, et al. Communication at the end of life. In: Carter BS, Levetown M, editors. Palliative care for infants, children, and adolescents. Baltimore: Johns Hopkins University Press; 2004. p. 131–8.

[47] Ewing AC, Carter BS. Once again, Vanderbilt NICU in Nashville leads the way in nurses' emotional support. Pediatr Nurs 2004;30:471–2.

[48] Reddick BH, Catlin E, Jellinek M. Crisis within crisis: recommendations for defining, preventing, and coping with stressors in the NICU. J Clin Ethics 2001;12(3):254–65.

[49] Caine RM, Ter-Bagdasarian L. Early identification and management of critical incident stress. Crit Care Nurse 2003;23(1):59–65.

[50] Rushton C. The other side of caring: caregiver suffering. In: Carter BS, Levetown M, editors. Palliative care for infants, children, and adolescents. Baltimore: Johns Hopkins University Press; 2004. p. 220–46.

ELSEVIER
SAUNDERS

Child Adolesc Psychiatric Clin N Am
15 (2006) 779–794

CHILD AND
ADOLESCENT
PSYCHIATRIC CLINICS
OF NORTH AMERICA

Children Facing the Death of a Parent: The Experiences of a Parent Guidance Program at the Massachusetts General Hospital Cancer Center

Susan D. Swick, MD, MPH[a], Paula K. Rauch, MD[b],*

[a]Department of Psychiatry, Harvard Medical School,
Massachusetts General Hospital, Boston, MA 02114, USA
[b]Child Psychiatry Consultation Service and MGH Cancer Center Parenting Program,
Massachusetts General Hospital, WACC 725,
15 Parkman Street, Boston, MA 02114-2696, USA

Apart from the loss of a child, few issues raise the kind of overwhelming sadness and anxiety for a family that the loss of a parent can elicit. Parents of young children may die suddenly and unexpectedly or may die after a long illness, with its associated ups and downs and eventual deterioration in health and functioning. This extended timeline offers the opportunity to address the needs of the children with the intent of supporting the children's coping during the end of the parent's life and beyond. What can be expected from the short-term and long-term development of a child who loses a parent? How might the child's chances of developing along the best possible trajectory be optimized? Given the answers to those two questions, how can parents be helped to anticipate and manage their children's needs under these challenging circumstances?

Parenting At a Challenging Time: PACT

PACT (Parenting At a Challenging Time) is a parent guidance program at the Massachusetts General Hospital Cancer Center that was created to address these issues for patients in the Cancer Center who were the parents of young children (≤ 18 years old) [1]. PACT is a consultation service staffed by three child psychiatrists and two child psychologists (Susan Swick, MD,

---

* Corresponding author.
  E-mail address: prauch@partners.org (P.K. Rauch).

1056-4993/06/$ - see front matter © 2006 Elsevier Inc. All rights reserved.
doi:10.1016/j.chc.2006.02.007

Paula Rauch, MD, Stephen Durant, EdD, Cynthia Moore, PhD, and Anna Muriel, MD). To make the program accessible to patients regardless of their insurance coverage, institutional and philanthropic funding supports PACT. It is available free to all patients at the cancer center. It remains available to families after the cancer-related death of the parent. Staff members see inpatient and outpatient consultations, with referrals coming from oncologists, palliative care physicians, nurses, and social workers. Regular in-service educational programs are offered to providers of different disciplines. In addition to work with individual families, weekly drop-in groups that patients and spouses can make use of as needed are ongoing.

PACT uses a parent guidance model of treatment. PACT does not offer conventional psychotherapy for families, couples, or individual parents or children. The goal is to support parents' existing skills at this critical time, when their distress and their children's needs are especially great. Parents are recognized as the experts on their own children. They want to be the ones to help them, and they are best equipped to do so. Children's questions are most likely to arise at home, and their parents will have been mediating their understanding of illness or death in this setting. With guidance, parents can field these questions better and organize the most supportive home environment possible under the circumstances. Most children do not need a psychiatric intervention, and for the children who do, their parents can best provide effective screening for clinically significant distress or impairment.

The posture at PACT is supportive; the aim is to contain parents' strong emotions, rather than draw them out. Doing so is often necessary to persuade parents that although their circumstances feel extraordinary, their parenting skills remain intact. Individualized education is provided for parents about their children's development and likely understanding of and reactions to death. Parents are reassured about what to expect, and strategies are devised to improve communication and emotional support within the family. The clinicians at PACT want to help the parents identify their greatest concerns, then devise an approach for handling them. Clinicians review other challenges the parents have faced and managed as a family and identify and engage their existing supports. When it is needed, clinicians provide a referral for ongoing psychiatric treatment or useful resources within the family's community [2].

Guiding principles

Based on clinical experiences with families, four general principles have proved especially useful in helping children to cope with the illness or loss of a parent. Interventions at PACT are guided by these principles, which are shared with parents to help organize their efforts with their children.

Communication

The first and most important principle is to support open, honest, clear, child-centered communication within the family. A parent's illness or death can precipitate intense anxiety and uncertainty for everyone in a family. Open and appropriate communication is essential to manage this anxiety and uncertainty. This statement is straightforward enough, but parents often want to protect their children from painful facts. The parents often are surprised to discover the degree to which their children are already aware that something troubling is going on in their family. The children are likely to experience their parents' "protection" as exclusion. Although they may believe that a parent's health status is threatened (based on what they see or the emotional climate at home), the parents' silence provides no access to family support. The absence of open communication delivers the unintentional message that the parent's illness is too terrible to be discussed, or that the child is not valued enough to be addressed directly. Parents may prefer to use euphemisms when they wish to protect children from painful facts such as a diagnosis of a brain tumor. Euphemisms, such as boo-boo or lump, typically raise anxiety (eg, about a child's own boo-boos) and create confusion.

The worst way for a child to hear bad news is to overhear it. In a home with an ill parent, conversations about the illness or prognosis are common. Children, who are always paying attention to adults' conversations, are likely to overhear frightening information. Parents can provide their children with the best protection from uncertainty and anxiety by fostering open, warm, age-appropriate communication, offering information and reinforcing family cohesion and integrity at a time when it feels threatened.

The crucial feature of communication that relieves anxiety is that it be child-centered. The substance and style should be appropriate to the child's age, and the communication should be facilitated, not forced. Parents should welcome questions. They should check in with their children at times and places where they usually like to talk, but not force them to talk. When children do have questions, parents first should figure out what the child is really asking and not make assumptions. Clarifying with questions such as, "What are you wondering about?" or "Where did you hear that?" sometimes reveals a different (and possibly easily answered) question. Parents should remember that questions do not require immediate answers. Merely stating, "That's a great question. I'm not sure of the answer, but let me talk to dad," for example, provides reassurance and support. The key to facilitating communication is that children are included and supported; they are not left to worry alone.

Minimize disruption

The second principle is to minimize the disruption of a child's life and routine. Although some disruption is unavoidable, there are often straightforward ways that it can be minimized. Even under normal circumstances, children depend on predictability and routine for a sense of security. Preserving regular routines during a parent's serious illness is even more important. Ideally, school can be maintained as an oasis of normalcy, and children are supported so that they can continue with favorite extracurricular activities, hobbies, or just time with friends. Minimizing disruption is often the result of the combined efforts of parents, relatives, and family friends. It may include a parent making a comprehensive list of their children's likes, dislikes, and rituals so that another caregiver can step in and manage them if needed. Designated familiar adults may help keep track of school assignments or activities for a child, to ensure they do not fall between the cracks. It often feels especially upsetting to a child whose parent is dying to find at school that he or she does not have the appropriate materials for a school project. It is helpful to designate a point-person at school, chosen in conjunction with the child, whom the parent can keep informed about developments within the family. This is the person the child can go to if he or she feels overwhelmed or needs to talk while at school. This teacher, school nurse, or other member of the school staff can keep the parent informed about how the child is coping while at school.

Another way to decrease disruptions in a child's routine is to designate a "Minister of Information" and a "Captain of Kindnesses". Phone calls from well-wishers can occupy considerable amounts of a parent's time typically during key family time after school and in the evenings. A Minister of Information is the one person who gets updates from the parents and who can keep others informed about how the ill parent is faring without precious family time being spent reporting and re-reporting the same illness information to each caller. Likewise, the parents may designate a Captain of Kindnesses, who keeps a list of the family's specific needs and to whom all offers of assistance can simply be referred. Often this individual organizes the meals delivered to the family and can offer to put a cooler by the family's front door so that the meal delivery does not cause unwelcome social interactions during family time.

Maximize family time

The corollary of minimizing disruption is to maximize and optimize the meaningful time that the family can spend together. Having a Minister of Information or Captain of Kindnesses can facilitate this. Simply turning off the phone ringer can help to preserve an uninterrupted mealtime where families can catch up on details about school, sports, and other topics. Serious illness in a parent often causes financial hardship and can place great demands on the well parent's time and energy. Although many of these new responsibilities cannot be deferred, continuing with important family rituals, holiday plans, and even vacations, within the bounds of what is realistic, can be reassuring for children and meaningful for the entire family.

Legacy leaving

The final principle is to facilitate thoughtful planning for the family's emotional adjustment and financial well-being. Often parents and children need to identify things they want to be sure to have said to one another. Parents want to identify the adults who will help the child lovingly remember the deceased parent. They may want to anticipate special events, write letters, or organize photos into albums with dates and descriptions. They also must address financial and legal planning, with an eye toward minimizing the children's disruptions and maximizing their supports. Moves or school changes are always difficult and best avoided in the aftermath of losing a parent. Providing the surviving parent with supports can be especially helpful. Any custody plans that do not involve a biologic parent must be addressed with an attorney and discussed openly with the children and affected adults to alleviate uncertainty and avoid conflict.

Background

Rather than being primarily research-driven, these principles have grown out of clinical experiences working with families facing life-threatening illnesses. Research on parental illness and loss provides some information about what might be expected for the children, and it suggests what kinds of interventions may offer them the greatest protection from untoward outcomes. Most of the research on children who lose a parent has had small numbers and has been limited by groups and variables that are mixed (uncontrolled). Five percent to eight percent of children lose a parent before age 18, and approximately 75% of these deaths are anticipated [3]. Psychological outcomes of bereaved children vary. There is a modestly increased risk of major mental illness; a significantly increased risk of potentially serious psychiatric symptoms; and frequent milder difficulties of social, emotional, and educational adjustment. Parental death is a tremendously difficult event that requires significant adjustment and is re-experienced with new meanings throughout the life of the child.

A common expectation is that bereaved children develop depression, and symptoms of sadness and anxiety are common in these children. Weller et al [4] assessed bereaved children within 3 months of their parent's death and found that 60% were dysphoric, and 37% were severely depressed. Several studies have shown that parents underreport the symptoms of bereaved children. Weller et al [4] found that 26% of 38 bereaved children met criteria for major depressive disorder compared with only 8% by their surviving parent's report. Although bereaved children may not fit the criteria for major depression neatly, studies have shown that parents and children report high rates of distress (manifested as irritability, somatic complaints, and sadness) and behavioral disturbances, such as separation anxiety, regression, excessive dependency, nighttime fears, and bedwetting. Within 1 year of the parent's death, 20% to 30% of bereaved children develop symptoms that require psychiatric referral [3]. In the Harvard Children's Bereavement Study, Silverman and Worden [5] showed that 1 year after the death of a parent, 20% of children still had problems sleeping and frequent headaches, and 15% had frequent or constant difficulty concentrating. Additionally, the rates of aggressive, intensely withdrawn or somatically preoccupied behaviors were two to six times higher than in nonbereaved children 1 year after their parent's death. Such symptoms pose challenges for the surviving parent and can cause impairment in emotional, social, and academic development.

The research also addresses risk and protective factors for bereaved children. In her meta-analysis of the literature on the psychiatric sequelae of parental loss, Dowdney [3] identified several factors that increase a child's risk of poor adjustment, including the presence of a preexisting psychiatric condition or learning disability, poor socioeconomic status, limited social supports, and mental illness in or poor adjustment of the surviving parent. Dowdney [3] also described several studies that showed that children who had emotional difficulties that preceded the illness and loss of their parent faced a particularly high risk of serious psychiatric problems immediately after their parent's death and continuing into adulthood. Beyond their own innate cognitive and psychological resources, a child's ability to cope with the loss of a parent is shaped by the well-being of the surviving parent; the harmony among and availability of family members and other caretakers; and the stability and supportiveness of their living circumstances, school environment, and peer relationships. The centrality of the surviving parent to this adjustment cannot be overstated. Children at the highest risk of disturbance are those from families with a prior history of parental conflict, separations, and divorce [6,7]. The surviving parent faces tremendous challenges; widowed parents have higher rates of serious problems than married parents, including depression, alcohol abuse, deteriorating physical health, and risk of suicide [8]. Support of the surviving parent can be crucial to maintaining the integrity of a child's environment and fostering the child's healthy adjustment to the loss of a parent.

The cancer literature addresses children facing a serious or terminal illness of a parent. Parents may report less distress than their children do, and children and adolescents report significant distress after their parent's diagnosis [9,10]. Higher continuing levels of anxiety are reported by children who describe an inability to discuss their parent's illness or decreased time in age-appropriate activities [11]. Children who have been given specific information about their parent's illness describe lower rates of anxiety [12]. Children whose parents are terminally ill with cancer seem to be more vulnerable to depression, anxiety, low self-esteem, fears, misconceptions, and behavior changes [13–15]. Finally, a relatively large, prospective study of parental loss at the University of Michigan found that children who experience the anticipated loss of a parent are more likely to have behavioral problems and psychiatric symptoms than children who experience the unanticipated loss of a parent [16]. This finding runs counter to the conventional wisdom that children who have had the chance to prepare for their parent's death have better outcomes. The study suggests, however, that it is not the anticipation itself that predicts a poor outcome, but rather the nature of a protracted parental illness in which the healthy parent has been too busy or distressed to be fully available to the children, whose other resources (financial, social, and emotional) also may have been depleted by the parent's long illness.

Child-centered interventions: developmental stages

Significantly, the research suggests that children facing the loss of a parent experience distress that may be ameliorated with information and support. Bereaved children experience anguish, and mild-to-moderate depressive symptoms are frequent and may persist for 1 year or longer. Most commonly, bereaved children present with a wide variety of emotional and behavioral symptoms that do not meet formal psychiatric criteria for a mood or anxiety disorder, but that nonetheless interfere with their daily lives. Of bereaved children, 20% to 30% experience symptoms that are serious enough to merit a psychiatric referral. Although some risk factors for serious symptoms cannot be modified (eg, preexisting psychiatric illness or learning disability in the child or surviving parent), the stability, supportiveness, and harmony of their social network can be prioritized and cultivated in the effort to improve children's adjustment to this enormously difficult loss. It is worth underscoring the converse: If 20% to 30% of children have symptoms warranting psychiatric referral, 70% to 80% of children adapt to this significant life event without requiring this intervention.

To provide useful guidance to parents, it has been essential to organize an approach not only by certain principles, but also around children's distinct developmental stages. A child's particular developmental tasks, abilities, and requirements determine their understanding of and responses to a parent's death. Helping parents to understand or anticipate their children's responses and particular needs is reassuring for the parent and protective for their children. The clinician's work is primarily educational, framing a child's questions or behaviors within a developmental context. The clinician specifies the likely understanding of and responses to death by developmental stage to support and organize the parents' nurturing and appropriate approach to their children.

Infants and toddlers

Because the central social and emotional task of children through toddlerhood is attachment, their crucial need is for the predictable responsiveness of their caregivers and consistency in their routines. Infants and toddlers have no meaningful understanding of death, but they notice the absence of a familiar caregiver and sense distress in a present caregiver. They are most sensitive to disruptions in their routines. Such disruptions can trigger fussiness or eating and sleeping problems in infants. Toddlers may be more prone to tearfulness and tantrums, particularly around transitions or separations, such as day care dropoffs or bedtime. Toddlers also may have a harder time trying new things, from foods to skills. Toddlers usually regress behaviorally when faced with the practical and emotional upheavals of parental loss. When the authors work with the parents of infants and toddlers, the recommendations are similar to the recommendations offered parents of children this age without an illness in the family. The authors recommend that parents focus on maintaining the routines and caregivers within their child's microenvironment. One practical suggestion is that parents create detailed lists of preferred foods, bedtime rituals, favorite games and books, and household rules and consequences so that other caregivers can step in as seamlessly as possible if it becomes necessary. If the parent is hospitalized but awake and interactive, toddlers typically do well with regular, brief visits. Toddlers should be told with age-appropriate language what to expect from a visit to the hospital. If they resist or get distressed, the visit should not be forced. Hospital visits should include an adult the child knows and trusts who is available to go on a walk with the child should he or she want to leave while the other parent or siblings stay.

Legacy leaving is often the primary concern for the parents of infants and toddlers because their picture of the deceased parent will have to be constructed by others. Some parents write letters for important future events in the lives of their children, create photo albums rich with details, or film videos. Helping families to identify the important adults who will be available to the children to answer questions and lovingly teach them about who their parent was is an important and meaningful part of this planning.

Preschoolers

Preschoolers strive to develop independence, manage frustration, and learn about social relationships. Although they typically have impressive verbal skills, their thinking remains concrete, limited by associative logic and relentless egocentrism. Preschoolers need interested, patient adults who provide calm, consistent limit setting, listening, and clarification and lots of cheerleading. They may be able to parrot an understanding of death, but have no meaningful appreciation of death's finality. Preschoolers usually require repeated explanations. They often offer "solutions" to the problem of death, have magical expectations ("Can we call heaven?"), and create self-centered explanations for a death or a survivor's reactions to it. Missing their parent distresses preschoolers, as does the distress evident in other adults and the disruptions in their routines. Their moods can shift quickly so that sadness easily gives way to delight and back again. Imaginary play often involves themes of death and loss because preschoolers gain mastery of most subjects (especially scary ones) through play. They often regress to earlier coping behaviors: using their words may revert to using hands or teeth, sharing is harder, and bedwetting may return. Preschoolers are especially prone to distress and behavioral problems around separations from the surviving parent, becoming clingy at preschool or refusing to sleep in their own bed.

When working with the parents of preschoolers, the authors remind them how important it is for them to explore their preschoolers' understanding of the situation, offering reassurance and warmly correcting misconceptions. Parents need to be patient and prepared for disarming and often painful questions. They should not be surprised or worried when they have to answer the same questions over and over. As their preschoolers start to master this new information, they may be pleased with themselves. This can create a surprising discrepancy between what the parent is saying ("Dad isn't coming back") and the child's affect that looks happy or proud. Consistency of routines and limits are still crucial at this stage, and detailed lists can be helpful. This is not a time to suspend household rules or smother children with gifts because that might contribute to a child's sense of being unmoored from the predictable routine. If a parent is in the hospital, preschoolers should be offered regular, brief visits. It is important to prepare young children for what to expect, provide them with the option of leaving at any time, and provide them with alternative means of staying connected (eg, phone calls, listening to tape-recorded stories or messages).

Latency-age children

When children are old enough to attend school, their focus becomes mastery—of facts, rules, and skills in the social, physical, and academic realms. These children are developing the initiative, diligence, and patience necessary to master an undertaking. They must have some initiative and frustration tolerance to begin this process and must experience some successes to have it reinforced to believe that their hard work will pay off. School-age children have developed cause-and-effect logic, but they can be rigid in their thinking about causes and effects. They are very focused on fairness and predictability and are disturbed by events that do not follow the rules or seem fair. Coping with unfair events is especially hard because their emotional maturity tends to lag behind their cognitive and physical skills. Latency-age children need adults who facilitate their attempts at mastery, providing encouragement and comfort when things are unfair. They especially need friends, hobbies, and a stimulating and safe school environment in which they feel they fit in and can practice their new skills.

By latency, children have a mature understanding of time and appreciate that death is final and irreversible, but they do not have the emotional maturity or abstract reasoning to grapple with strong feelings and existential implications. They are especially vulnerable to sadness and anxiety that can feel overwhelming, as though it may never end, around the illness or death of a loved one. These children may be curious about religious explanations, but often struggle to develop anything beyond a concrete grasp of them. As they master new situations, particularly anxiety-provoking ones, by gathering information, they may ask very specific, detailed, and disconcerting questions. ("What happens in cremation? What exactly caused the death?") They may be especially preoccupied and angry about the unfairness of the loss. ("Dad didn't smoke. How come he got cancer?") Their drive to master other skills does not evaporate with the death of a parent. Periods of intense distress alternate with intense (and often happy) engagement in school, sports, or social events. They often feel confused or guilty about enjoying themselves, and adults can be bewildered by how seamlessly they seem to get on with their lives. Their understanding of death is such that they also can become worried about their vulnerability and particularly worried about their surviving parent's health. Their anxieties often manifest themselves as somatic complaints or problems at bedtime. The sadness they feel likewise is expressed indirectly as irritability, trouble concentrating, or withdrawal from friends or activities. Special accomplishments or milestones may become especially painful events, as these children miss showing off for their lost parent.

Parents of these children are encouraged to be prepared for many, sometimes disturbing questions. These children benefit from parents listening to questions, clarifying their underlying worries, and providing clear, accurate, and detailed explanations. Parents should emphasize the here and now, however, when their latency-age child has questions about existential implications ("Are we all going to die?") because it would be hard for children this age to bear the associated anxiety. Parents should expect them to cope by doing (eg, chores, practicing piano) and to want to be involved in practical matters, such as hospital visits and funeral planning, and they should facilitate this means of coping. Their timetable for coping should be respected; children should be reassured that continuing on with their activities is healthy and not a betrayal of the deceased parent. They should not be pushed to talk, but should be informed about things they may overhear and reminded to "never worry alone." These children especially depend on school as an oasis of normalcy, and it is crucial to them that they not be different from their peers. It is particularly important that parents help their children pick a point-person at the school who can be available at the child's request. The school should avoid announcements or well-meaning questions from teachers, instead being aware of what's going on and available to their student as needed.

Adolescents

Adolescents face the tasks of developing independence, establishing a nuanced identity and greater intimacy in their relationships, and managing their sometimes unruly impulses. They face these developmental tasks with fully mature cognitive skills: reasoning abstractly, analyzing situations within the framework of prioritized values, and managing uncertainty. There is often a mismatch, however, between their mature level of comprehension and their immature behavior, particularly under stress. They need parents who can balance their trials at independence with ongoing connection and appropriate limits, all while bearing the adolescent's apparent moodiness and frustrations. In addition, adolescents need friends and nonparental adults as confidantes and sounding boards as they build intimacy and their own identities.

Adolescents typically have a complete understanding of death—its finality, irreversibility, and universality. They have and express a full array of intense, adult emotions about loss. They may struggle with questions about faith, suffering, justice, and the meaning of life. Their relative (and developmentally appropriate) preoccupation with themselves may cause adolescents to focus on the personal consequences of a loss in ways that can feel selfish to surviving adults. These egocentric concerns can be reasonable and sophisticated, however. ("Will I be able to afford college?" "Am I vulnerable to the same illness?") As is the case when discord is present in adult relationships, the conflict that is typical between adolescents and their parents can complicate their grief. They may feel anger that the "wrong" parent died, guilt for actions taken or not taken, or regret for things said or left unsaid. Because they are so attentive to matters of individual style, they are often critical of how others respond to their parent's death. They may be sensitive as to how a loss sets them apart from their peers, but exploring and establishing their own identity (and how a loss may figure into it) is more important than sameness. Still, they typically experience a heightened need for the company and support of their friends and other important adults.

When working with the parents of adolescents, the authors remind them to respect their teen's established style of coping; this is not the time to expect that they suddenly become talkers or highly organized. Respecting their adolescent's coping style does not mean, however, ignoring dangerous behaviors or behaviors that suggest deeper problems (eg, alcohol abuse or profound withdrawal). When there has been a lot of conflict with the ill or deceased parent, it is vital that parents acknowledge the love that does exist, protecting the adolescent from guilt or being vilified by other family members. Adolescents may need to hear that it is not a betrayal of their parents if they turn to other, nonparental adults for support. It is crucial that parents not assume that their adolescents are essentially adult and best left alone. Adolescents need their growing independence, but it still must be balanced with support and reasonable limits.

Common questions

Although every family is unique, several questions occur, in one form or another, with some regularity, and these provide useful illustrations of the approach of PACT. The clinicians at PACT try to bring other important adults into discussions with parents—both parents, if they are able, and friends or relatives that are trusted and play an active role in the lives of their children, particularly if they are the adults that the children would turn to in the absence of their parents. If a parent is terminally ill, the clinician should gather specific information about the parent's understanding of prognosis and likely course of the illness, with particular emphasis on what the children are likely to see. The clinician should discuss the family's religious or other framework for understanding death and any prior experience of loss. The clinician should ask for details about the children, particularly about their temperament, strengths, and vulnerabilities. Gathering stories about the relationships within the family, including supportive and conflicted relationships, can be very helpful. Finally, the clinician should ask about what the parent has told the children and how it went. The clinician should pay particular attention to the language the parent uses and try to use the same language in helping the parent think about how to talk about these difficult topics.

Should I tell them?

The wish to protect children from such painful news as a parent's diagnosis with a terminal illness is natural, and this is a common question. Parents have described feeling like they will be injuring their children if they force this news on them. The clinician typically should start by finding out what responses the parents are most afraid of and to anticipate likely responses. The clinician should explore how much the child already may know, pointing out that the worst way for children to hear news like this is to overhear it. It is much more reassuring and supportive for children to be included in the circle of information and to have their sense of what is going on validated. The youngest toddlers need to have their misconceptions cleared up and to not be alone with their worries and fears. The oldest adolescents need enough information to make informed decisions about their future plans and to address unfinished business. The clinician typically should suggest to parents that they tell all children together so that there is no risk of overhearing or resenting that a sibling was told first.

How do I tell them I'm going to die?

The clinician typically should start by determining what the children already know. Is this going to be a shock, or has there been a long struggle with a serious illness already? Has uncertainty about the parent's future health been part of the ongoing discussion with the children? The clinician should discuss the family's previous losses and religious beliefs to help parents think about their own context for understanding death, anticipating likely questions and possible responses. Helping parents find language they are comfortable with that also would be developmentally appropriate is practical and organizing. Often parents find language that emphasizes the concrete and faultless nature of what they are facing: "The doctors say that we have done everything we could to fight this illness, but the illness is simply too strong and my body can't fight anymore." Parents typically can then follow their children's lead, with specific questions or the simple need for their parents' company and comfort. The clinician should try to help parents anticipate their children's specific questions, such as timeframe, type of death, or custody questions, so they have some chance to think about their responses.

Should I be at home or inpatient (hospice)?

This is an important question, and one where a little guidance can make a great difference in the quality of this time for the family. One should start with the likely course of the illness. What might the children see? Could the parent become delirious or agitated? What might the cause of death be? Anticipating events in the likely course of the parent's illness that could be traumatic for children to see can help guide this decision. It is important to consider how disruptive it would be for the parent to be in the home. Can the parent be in a room in the house that preserves private and play space for the children? Or would the parent be in a large bed in the living room in the wintertime? Would there be enough help at home to enable the other parent private time with the children, or would most of his or her time need to be devoted to the sick parent? What wishes has each member of the family expressed about this issue? A child is unlikely to say that he or she does not want the sick parent at home, but it is important to balance the wish to be together with the likelihood that the togetherness will be meaningful in a positive way. If there is a possibility that this situation could be traumatic or extremely disruptive for the children, the parents should consider carefully whether inpatient hospice would be more comfortable for the parent and manageable for the children. It also is important for the surviving parent to make time to spend with the children at home and to consider which other caring adults can be available for the children during this time.

My children won't talk about it. Should I be worried?

The short answer to this question is no. Not initiating conversations about emotionally charged topics is usually normal in childhood, and there is no correct style for coping or timeframe for talking or asking questions. Reassuring parents that this situation is normal is often helpful, as is reminding them to listen carefully to their children, who may be talking indirectly about their distress. Parents can consider the times and places where their children have been most likely to talk (eg, bedtime or in the car) and check in with them then: "I know there is a lot going on, and I wanted to see how you're feeling." Inviting children to talk, without pressuring them, and following their lead, while reminding them that they should "never worry alone," fosters child-centered communication and support. The age and previous coping and temperamental style of the child also are important factors. Parents may have developmentally inappropriate expectations about how their child should be managing a loss. They may need information about what a preschooler may actually understand, how a latency-age child may "cope by doing," or how adolescents typically seek out friends or nonparental adults. Placing their child's behavior in a developmental context can be heartening for parents and can help them to be available without being coercive.

Should they go to the funeral?

Children of all ages should be told in clear, developmentally appropriate language what to expect at the funeral and then given the choice about whether or not they want to go. This principle applies to toddlers and adolescents alike, who may grapple with a legacy of anger, deprivation, or guilt if they are not given a free choice in the matter. This means that parents must be supportive and understanding if the children wish not to go to the funeral. Some children may want to speak at the funeral. Supporting them, while providing them with the option of changing their mind (even at the last minute), is crucial. With younger children, it is wise to designate a loving, trusted adult who can be available for each child. That way, if they change their mind and want to leave, they can do so without making their siblings or parent leave also. The emphasis is on giving children a modicum of control, keeping them included in decision making, and providing them with support as they try to find the way of managing this loss that feels right to them.

Pitfalls and red flags

In some situations, it becomes complicated to help parents to help their children through the loss of the other parent. When there is conflict between caregivers (both parents or one parent and their in-laws), the adults sometimes do not act in reasoned or mature ways. This situation can exacerbate greatly the disruptions caused by the illness or loss of a parent. Sometimes, helping the adults involved to turn their attentions to the children's needs can remind them of what is important and facilitate resolution of the conflict, or at least a truce. Families with secrets pose a variety of challenges. If their style is to keep secrets, it may be difficult for them to start fostering openness at such a stressful time. If their secrets are more serious or criminal, they would be highly suspicious of any support or assistance that is offered.

In some families, particularly families with estranged parents, one parent may have been vilified, with or without good cause. This estrangement between a child and the dying or deceased parent can complicate grief greatly. It is especially important to help a child carefully consider the things they may want to ask of or say to this parent. It likewise would be important to identify other adults who could help the child lovingly remember the parent when deceased.

Families in which the parents seem to lack the expected level of distress about their children also pose difficulties. Other people providing care to such parents often feel intensely concerned for these children, and a parent guidance intervention for them may feel more like a confrontation. Although it may be possible to complicate their thinking about how best to protect their children, it is important not to expect to alter their parenting style drastically at a time of such great stress. Instead, providing some support and reassurance for the staff about the varieties of parenting styles and the value of parenting consistency around such a challenge as the loss of one parent can be most helpful for the staff and dying parent and perhaps indirectly for the children.

In addition to the times when the parent guidance model may seem inadequate, there are times when a psychiatric referral is recommended. Although grief typically mirrors depression (but is managed differently), there are times when grieving parents and children should undergo a psychiatric evaluation. If a parent is experiencing deteriorating function in several areas over the year after a spouse's death, if the parent is suicidal or expresses the belief that the children would be better off without him or her, or if the parent is unable to attend to the children's needs, a psychiatric referral is recommended. Likewise, some children ask to see a therapist, but more often individuals around a child suggest a psychiatric referral. Childhood grief typically is characterized by waxing and waning symptoms over many months. When the child's course is one of constant distress or symptoms are continuing to worsen after the first 4 to 6 months, psychiatric referral should be recommended. A child who is experiencing persistent (>6 months) difficulties in two out of three general areas of functioning (home, school, or social relationships) should be assessed, and any child who exhibits dangerous behaviors or expresses the wish to be dead should be referred for psychiatric evaluation. Lastly, when the surviving parent is unable to attend to a child's particular emotional needs (but is not abusive or neglectful), the child may be well served by an evaluation and psychotherapy. Whether it is because of a child's extraordinary needs, a parent's deficits, or a situation in which the surviving parent cannot help the child grieve because of his or her own feelings about the deceased, a trusting, meaningful connection to a therapist can make a crucial difference in the adjustment of these children.

Summary

Children facing the death of a parent are facing a major upheaval, a loss that will bring them emotional pain and will resonate in different ways at important points throughout their lives. Given the proper supports, most children can expect to adjust well to this enormous change and live happy, productive, and meaningful lives. Although some risk factors for poor adjustment are fixed, the parents themselves often can address others effectively. Clinicians can help the parents of these children facilitate their children's best possible adjustment by emphasizing the principles of facilitating communication, minimizing disruption, preserving family time, and attending to their legacy. Clinicians place their children's behaviors within the context of their developmental stage and help the parents find language and an approach that feels comfortable to them. The goal is to help parents relocate their bearings and realize they can use the parenting skills they already have. Guided by the goal of protecting their children, these parents can find purpose and strength. Reframing their circumstances as a painful and unavoidable challenge, but one that they can actively face, is organizing and fortifying for these families buffeted by loss.

References

[1] Rauch PK, Muriel AC, Cassem NH. Parents with cancer: who's looking after the children? J Clin Oncology 2003;21:117s–21s.

[2] Rauch PK, Muriel AC. Raising an emotionally healthy child when a parent is sick. Chicago: McGraw-Hill; 2005.

[3] Dowdney L. Childhood bereavement following parental death. J Child Psychol Psychiatry 2000;41:819–30.

[4] Weller RA, Weller EB, Fristad MA, Bowes JM. Depression in recently bereaved prepubertal children. Am J Psychiatry 1991;148:1536–40.

[5] Silverman PR, Worden JW. Children's reactions to the death of a parent. In: Stroebe MS, Stroebe W, Hansson RO, editors. Handbook of bereavement: theory, research and intervention. New York: Cambridge University Press; 1993. p. 300–16.

[6] Kranzler EM, Shaffer D, Wasserman G, Davies M. Early childhood bereavement. J Am Acad Child Adolesc Psychiatry 1990;29:513–20.

[7] Elizur E, Kaffman M. Factors influencing the severity of childhood bereavement reactions. Am J Orthopsychiatry 1983;53:668–76.

[8] Gersten JC, Beals J, Kallgren CA. Epidemiology and preventive interventions: parental death in childhood as a case example. Am J Community Psychol 1991;19:481–500.

[9] Compas BE, Worsham NL, Epping-Jordan JE, et al. When mom or dad has cancer: markers of psychological distress in cancer patients, spouses, and children. Health Psychol 1994;13:507–15.

[10] Compas BE, Worsham NL, Ey S, Howell DC. When mom or dad has cancer: II. coping, cognitive appraisals, and psychological distress in children of cancer patients. Health Psychol 1996;15:167–75.

[11] Nelson E, Sloper P, Charlton A, While D. Children who have a parent with cancer: a pilot study. J Cancer Educ 1994;9:30–6.

[12] Rosenhiem E, Reicher R. Informing children about a parent's terminal illness. J Child Psychol Psychiatry 1985;26:995–8.

[13] Siegel K, Mesagno FP, Karus D, et al. Psychosocial adjustment of children with a terminally ill parent. J Am Acad Child Adolesc Psychiatry 1992;31:327–33.

[14] Christ GH, Siegel K, Freund B, et al. Impact of parental terminal cancer on latency age children. Am J Orthopsychiatry 1993;63:417–25.

[15] Christ GH, Siegel K, Sperber D. Impact of parental terminal cancer on adolescents. Am J Orthopsychiatry 1994;664 604–3.

[16] Saldinger A, Cain A, Kalter N, Lohner K. Anticipating parental death in families with young children. Am J Orthopsychiatry 1999;69:39–48.

ELSEVIER
SAUNDERS

Child Adolesc Psychiatric Clin N Am
15 (2006) 795–815

CHILD AND
ADOLESCENT
PSYCHIATRIC CLINICS
OF NORTH AMERICA

Relational Learning in Pediatric Palliative Care: Transformative Education and the Culture of Medicine

David M. Browning, MSW, BCD, FT[a,*],
Mildred Z. Solomon, EdD[a,b]

[a]Center for Applied Ethics and Professional Practice, Education Development Center,
Inc., 55 Chapel Street, Newton, MA 02458, USA
[b]Division of Medical Ethics, Harvard Medical School, 641 Huntington Avenue,
Boston, MA 02115, USA

I encourage you to see patients as your tutors and to ground your relationships with them in advocacy, mutual vulnerability and trust . . for this is the heart of medicine.
—Faculty covenant with students, University of Virginia Medical School [1]

Noting the difference between what we *say* and what we *do*, students learn that medicine is a profession in which you say one thing and do another, a profession of cynics.
—Thomas Inui, medical educator [2]

In recent years, medical educators have given increased attention to what has been diagnosed as a growing problem in the education of health care professionals: the discrepancy between what is taught in formal educational settings and what is learned by practitioners in the informal flow of everyday practice. This hidden curriculum in the culture of medicine has been aptly described by one educator as "what we actually do in our day-to-day work with patients and one another—not what we say should be done when we stand behind podiums in lecture halls [2]." From the standpoint of the learner, this aspect of medical culture has been depicted as follows:

It all goes back to that old adage, 'monkey see, monkey do'... The way you treat me as a student will set the tone for how I treat patients. So if you want me to take a personal interest in my patients and to treat patients as

This work was supported by funding from The Nathan Cummings Foundation and The Argosy Foundation.
* Corresponding author.
E-mail address: dbrowning@edc.org (D.M. Browning).

childpsych.theclinics.com

partners, the most powerful thing you can do is to treat me the same way [3].

A growing body of literature identifies the components of this informal learning, and analyzes its apparent ability to operate "under the radar screen" of educators and administrators [2,4–7]. Commentators have argued that the underlying premises of the hidden curriculum are built upon value-based assumptions such as

- Doctors must be perfect
- Uncertainty and complexity are to be avoided
- Outcome is more important than process
- Medicine takes priority over everything else
- Hierarchy is necessary [7].

Along with efforts to expose and address the hidden curriculum, a growing number of commentators, alarmed by the atrophy of professionalism in medicine, have implored medical educators to refocus on traditional virtues such as "altruism, accountability, excellence, duty, service, honor, integrity, and respect for others [4]." They argue that today's culture of medicine, which is increasingly shaped by powerful economic forces of commercialism and profit, is hostile to the development of these and other traditional virtues that are rooted in relationships between patients and practitioners. The literature also suggests that relational capacities that are intact at the beginning of a medical career may be undervalued by young physicians (A.L. Romer, unpublished dissertation), and then gradually unlearned in the course of professional training. Studies show that the empathy of physicians demonstrably declines throughout medical education [2,8], which prompts educators to conclude that "medical students come into medicine because they are caring, compassionate people and they want to heal—it gets bred out of them by about their third year [9]."

Albert Schweitzer is said to have emphasized in his teaching the idea that ethical practice, in medicine and in life, begins with a sense of solidarity with other human beings. Sadly, there is growing evidence that, for too many physicians, professional development contains, embedded within it, the erosion of this moral experience of solidarity. Indeed, the growing fear that the culture of medicine has lost its moral compass has led one bioethicist to warn, "A profession without its own distinctive moral convictions has nothing to profess [10]."

In this article, the authors apply a well-documented range of concerns about the hidden curriculum and the erosion of professionalism to the arena of pediatric palliative care education. Parker Palmer is a sociologist and educator who is recognized by the Accreditation Council for Graduate Medical Education's Courage to Teach Awards, and the authors agree with his proposition that *how* teaching occurs in professional settings has distinct moral implications. In Palmer's words,

Every epistemology has a moral trajectory. Every way of knowing takes us someplace in terms of the living of our lives. An epistemology that sets the known world at great length from the knower also sets the living actor at a distance of moral irresponsibility for the world in which he or she is living [11].

Palmer's insight can help pediatric palliative care educators resist the temptation to keep the suffering of children and families at a distance from the cognitive and emotional worlds of the clinicians entrusted with their care. The authors propose that educational initiatives must always be grounded in the charged existential space of relationships among children, families, and practitioners, because the learning that matters most occurs within these relationships. The authors present an educational approach, which they call relational learning, based on these principles, and offer some preliminary strategies educators may wish to consider in their own institutions, aimed at fostering this kind of learning.

From content and curricula to pedagogy and process

Since the release of the Institute of Medicine's landmark report, *When Children Die: Improving Palliative and End-of-Life Care for Children and Their Families*, several substantive educational initiatives focused on pediatric palliative care have been developed for health care professionals who work in hospitals, hospices, and community settings across the country [12–15]. There is consensus across these projects, which is reflected in the curricular material that has been produced, about important skill and content areas that need to be mastered by health care professionals who focus on pediatric palliative care. These include managing pain and symptoms, facilitating ethical decision-making, communicating effectively, managing prognostic uncertainty, responding to grief and loss, and integrating spirituality. Educational initiatives in pediatric palliative care have also been posed with an additional challenge: to make a difference, skills and knowledge must be successfully married to "ancient values and attitudes, such as compassion and mercy" [16].

The subject matter of pediatric palliative care has been well delineated in the aforementioned educational projects. This article focuses, therefore, on the educational challenge outlined above—the process and pedagogy by which practitioners can learn critical relational capacities such as compassion and mercy. There are, of course, some who argue that these relational virtues cannot be taught. The authors are uncertain as well about whether they can be taught, at least in the conventional sense. They are convinced, however, that they can be learned, and that health care organizations bear responsibility for creating cultures that nurture opportunities for such learning.

The rationale for focusing on relational capacities and how they are learned in medical settings is shaped partly by a particular negative outcome that must be avoided. Imagine a potential scenario in which new classes and curricula in pediatric palliative care produce measurable improvement in practitioner skills and knowledge, without changing how care is experienced by children and families. To have a meaningful impact on the lives of children with life-threatening conditions and their families, educational initiatives will need to be guided by pedagogy tied to the everyday relationships in which practitioners, children, and families are engaged.

The centrality of relationships in pediatric palliative care

> The significance of the intimate personal relationship between physician and patient cannot be too strongly emphasized.
> —Francis Peabody, 1927 [17]
> We are in need of medicine with a heart.
> —Salvador Avila, bereaved parent, 2003 [18]

When parents who have lived through the life-threatening illness or death of a child are asked what was most important to them about the medical care they received, they routinely identify their relationships with practitioners as primary [19–22]. On the positive side, parents often experience their practitioners as part of a loving, extended family, whose ongoing presence enables them to navigate their way through inordinate tragedy. On the negative side, they explain that their encounters with tactless or uncaring practitioners have a lifetime impact and compromise the course of their bereavement.

> One of the most striking findings in these studies was how a single event could cause parents profound and lasting emotional distress. Parents recounted incidents that included insensitive delivery of bad news, feeling dismissed or patronized, perceived disregard for parents' judgment regarding the care of their child, and poor communication of important information. Such events haunted them and complicated their grief even years later [20].

Whether describing inadequate pain relief [23], fragmented or discontinuous patterns of care [22], unclear or inconsistent communication [20,21], or agonizing end-of-life decisions [24], the common thread in all of these activities is that they occur in relationships. Clearly, families need something different, and something more, from these relationships than what they are presently receiving.

If it is true that the health care system must more adequately address the needs of these children and families, it is equally important to examine a parallel population of human beings whose emotional and spiritual needs have also been marginalized, if not denied altogether. Attuned to the high stakes inherent in clinical practice with highly vulnerable children and families, the practitioners—social workers, chaplains, physicians, nurses, child-life specialists, and others—who do this difficult work face daunting challenges, including moral distress [25,26], cumulative grief [27,28], and problems of conscience [24]. They must also contend with substantive occupational hazards that range from compassion fatigue [29] to vicarious traumatization [30] and secondary traumatic stress [31]. Indeed, this interdisciplinary group of professionals, by virtue of their common choice to serve this particular cohort of patients and families, bears witness—day after day, month after month, and year after year—to a distinctive anguish that, at least in the developed world, most people manage to avoid: the death of a child. In so doing, practitioners are involved in a kind of parallel suffering [32,33] that exacts an ethical claim of its own, one that warrants careful attention on the part of educators.

By asking the right questions and listening carefully to the stories of practitioners as well as children and families, one can begin to see the entire spectrum of relationships in pediatric palliative care settings, and begin to understand this complex world of relationships from each of the key vantage points:

- A child, relating disappointment with his team of clinicians: "It hurts me inside to think they're not listening" [34]
- A parent, reminding practitioners: "We need them—somebody that cares about us" [35]
- A physician, describing the impact of caring for patients and families: "No one prepares you for this—this assault on your sense of being" [36]

This more complete picture makes it possible to focus attention on the ebb and flow of everyday learning that determines how, when, and whether practitioners develop the relational capacities that are at the core of competent clinical practice.

Relational learning and clinical competence

What if we assumed that learning is as much part of our human nature as eating or sleeping, that it is both life-sustaining and inevitable, and that given a chance, we are quite good at it? And what if, in addition, we assumed that learning is, in its essence, a fundamentally social phenomenon, reflecting our own deeply social nature as human beings capable of knowing [37]?

By the time they enter the workplace in their respective disciplines, nurses, physicians, social workers, chaplains, and child-life specialists already have a substantial amount of education under their belts. For the most part, however, their academic achievements have been won in an educational system that tends to envision learning primarily as a process in which persons with expertise (teachers) deposit knowledge into the brains of those lacking that expertise (students), an approach Paulo Freire has called a banking approach to education [38]. Within this context, knowledge tends to be seen as a kind of possession, and teaching is understood primarily as something that is done to learners.

The inadequacy of this perspective is evident when applied to the multifaceted experience of learning to become a health care practitioner, a process in which competency depends on the ability to apply knowledge to a diverse range of practice settings, within a complex nexus of relationships. The development of professional expertise is a highly contextual process, which involves the accumulation and integration of a wide repertoire of learning experiences, all of which are situated firmly in relationships with patients, families, and colleagues. The relational capacities that accompany expertise are learned painstakingly, one human encounter at a time [39]. The crucial importance of these relational habits, skills, and attitudes in the development of clinical competence has been increasingly recognized by professional bodies such as the Accreditation Council for Graduate Medical Education [40].

To flesh out a more comprehensive understanding of the relational learning that leads to competence for pediatric palliative care practitioners, there is a robust literature on social learning [41], situated learning [42], and adult education [43]. These relational perspectives enable us to think about the education of physicians, nurses, and social workers less in terms of what is being taught in classrooms and lecture halls and more in terms of what is being learned, both in these formal educational settings and in the informal learning of everyday practice. By focusing on this expanse of relational learning, professional education can be viewed less as an independent process of acquiring knowledge that belongs to the learner, and more as an interdependent process of social participation to which learners belong.

The centrality of relational learning in pediatric palliative care can be concretized with a clinical example:

> Sometimes I feel pressure about 'getting it right.' It's not about getting it right. It's not how 'professional' I am. It's how I respond to this family as a human being, if I'm not sincere, that is what families will remember the longest. It's not really what I *say,* but more how I *am*, how I can *be* with them at the time [44].

These words are excerpted from a conversation with a veteran child-life specialist, in which she reflects on a memorable meeting with two young parents in the hours surrounding the death of their little girl. She is describing an experience that happened several years in the past, but in its telling it seems like yesterday to her. As she remembers the encounter, the pain she felt in the past is re-visited in the present. She is not certain why this particular experience stands out in her memory, having faced death with innumerable children and families through the years. It simply appears as a story she wants to tell, a story that seems to matter.

Of course, this practitioner, as is true with her colleagues in nursing, medicine, social work, and chaplaincy who have worked for any length of time with these vulnerable children and families, carries an anthology of such stories in the interior recesses of her being, somewhere between head and heart. Some of these stories are written down, but most are not, and few have been shared with others, even with close peers. In this conversation, she approaches the invitation to share with a mixture of apprehension and resolve, yet as she talks, the story begins to claim a kind of inalienable integrity of its own. It becomes, in its telling, a story that must be told. Furthermore, as she talks, it is evident that the learning embedded in the story does not exactly belong to her; rather, it lives in the unique relationship she established with this particular child and family.

Returning to the text of this practitioner's account from the perspective of relational learning, we might profitably explore several questions. How often do clinicians feel pressure, in high-stakes encounters with children and families, to get it right, even when there is no right answer? Where do practitioners learn how to respond to families as human beings while they simultaneously occupy the roles of physician, chaplain, or child-life specialist? What are they taught in their professional training about what they should say to children and families who face agonizing end-of-life dilemmas? Moreover, beyond learning about what words to use in these instances, where in their learning do practitioners integrate the more profound insight that what they say will in the long run be less important than who they are and how they can be with children and families at these remarkable times.

A relational pedagogy can provide these opportunities, because the development of professional competence is understood in its connection to the moral realm of human relationships and experience. Relational capacities that involve compassion, mercy, authenticity, or integrity become meaningful only as they become actualized in living relationships with children, families, and colleagues. In this process of actualization, the ethical quality of these capacities becomes palpable:

> Ethics should mean a process of continual learning: who one is (what values make a person who she or he is), who one wants to become (what values are worth cultivating) and how best to facilitate others in their process of becoming. The most significant aspects of this learning are recognitions of expanding interdependence. We should speak less of ethics as some activity or substantive content that appears to stand alone and more of ethical relations: living with ourselves, perpetually responsive to others [45].

Returning to the child-life specialist's story, we can see both the uniquely personal aspect of her learning as well as the archetypal nature of the lesson she draws from her experience. When practitioners find within themselves such morally salient stories, and then share them with colleagues, amazing learning can ensue. However, before such stories can be shared, they must first be discovered. To facilitate the process of finding these stories, we must take a careful look at the conversational world of everyday practice.

Conversations and everyday ethics

> Learning does not belong to individual persons, but to the various conver-
> sations of which they are a part.
>   —Richard McDermott, educator [41]

> How do we get a wedge in here, loosen the conceptual and linguistic
> cramps in our heads—and our hearts—so that we can see what is in front
> of us?
>   —Larry Churchill and David Schenck, bioethicists [46]

The daily panoply of conversations in which practitioners engage includes what we might call professional conversations (patient interviews,
family meetings, rounds, nursing report, in-service training) as well as the
more casual conversations with patients, families, and colleagues inter-
spersed throughout the day. Any of these conversations may, in one context,
be experienced as mundane or inconsequential, or in another, as an exhila-
rating opportunity for learning:

> Good conversation is mutual, it is interactive. There is something happen-
> ing back and forth, and it is building up and up and up. When my point is
> affirmed, and someone picks it up, it reaffirms me to say, 'okay, I'm giving
> this a shot,' and I will throw a different angle on it [47].

The capacity for practitioners to see conversations as a rich and largely
untapped source of learning is constrained by utilitarian understandings
that view communication largely as the transfer of information from one
party to another (physician to physician, nurse to nurse, physician to nurse,
nurse to physician, physician to patient, nurse to family member, and so on)
Although the need for efficient transfer of information in medical settings is
indisputable, relational learning is compromised when this mindset is generalized to the world of complex interactions that constitute professional practice. An illustration of this problem is evident in many educational efforts to
teach practitioners the communication skills necessary for "delivering bad
news", a construct that tends to convey a one-way, information-transfer
kind of image. The language we use to describe the subject matter of learning will impact substantially on how practitioners engage with that learning.
When one thinks of things that are delivered, one might picture the delivery
of pizza, or dry cleaning, or the day's mail [48]. From an educational standpoint, is this how we want practitioners to think of themselves as they enter
into these life-altering conversations with children and families?

It makes little sense to teach "communication skills" for end-of-life conversations with children and families, if that learning is not connected in concrete
and meaningful ways to the actual experience of the children, families, and
practitioners who engage in these conversations. Rarely are training programs
in these areas structured to promote the deconstruction of, and reflection
upon, these conversations from the inside out, so that the learning itself can
be informed and shaped by how these conversations are actually experienced

by the persons who engage in them [48]. One reason why educational efforts around communication skills tend not to use this kind of contextual, experience-based approach may be because it can be more challenging to measure the outcomes of this kind of relational learning. One prominent medical educator argues that the obsession with measurement in health care settings is one of the primary reasons for the medical profession's increasingly diagnosed failure to teach young physicians the fundamental virtues that traditionally have been considered essential to ethical practice in medicine [4].

To cultivate the essential relational capacities in practitioners, we must attempt to capture, educationally, the emotional depth and moral complexity embedded in these encounters. Helping practitioners derive wisdom from these conversations necessitates an approach to learning communication skills that situates those skills in the real-life moral and emotional worlds in which they are practiced. Moreover, the relational capacities necessary to practice competently in these conversations extend beyond the mastery of such necessary but insufficient knowledge as remembering to turn off beepers, sustain eye contact, and validate feelings. Consider a practitioner's conversation with two new parents, for example, who are faced with making a life-or-death decision on behalf of their infant daughter. When every available option seems impossible to imagine, practitioners need a certain kind of moral sensibility as much as they need communication skills. This situation calls for a sharing of moral burdens, aimed at helping these parents "to feel that how they acted was as good as it could have been, given the inherent impossibility of the situation [45]."

> What families need help with in many end-of-life situations is not a buffing up of their decisional capacities, but compassionate attention to how the events unfolding before them can be made meaningful or bearable. This is ethics, not on the decisional edge of big choices, but in the full human sense of how people get around their world and orient themselves in life-changing situations [46].

Helping parents get around their worlds when dealing with their child's life-threatening condition, and doing our best to ensure they are not left alone with anguish that is more than what human beings should have to bear, is a particular kind of moral challenge for practitioners, one that is not always captured in discussions about bioethics. Becoming skillful at accompanying families through these extra-ordinary times is tied to common sense ethics like trying to be a good person, or treating people as you would want to be treated, or striving to do the right thing. A focus on everyday ethics shines a kind of moral light on the learning of relational capacities that are fundamental in pediatric palliative care, and encourages practioners to explore more deeply together how to be with children and families, and who one is becoming in the process.

A robust perspective on relational learning can be a part of a larger effort to countermand and eventually transform the existing hidden curriculum in health care organizations. The process of transformation can begin by explicitly asserting relational values and capacities we want practitioners to learn, over and against extant organizational forces—tied to premises of the hidden curriculum—that are effectively opposed to this learning. These contrasting realities can be juxtaposed as follows: the expectation of perfection can be contrasted with the acceptance of vulnerability; the need for certainty can be balanced with the value of not-knowing; the focus on outcome can be counter-posed with the complexities of process; the need for hierarchy can be balanced by the value of learning from individuals and groups who are disenfranchised. When our educational strategies include a commitment to challenge the hidden curriculum, we increase the potential that our efforts will contribute to the organizational change that will be necessary to support relational learning in the long run. Left unaddressed, however, these powerful premises can defeat even our most ambitious and innovative educational efforts.

Below, the authors propose some steps that educators and organizational leaders in pediatric palliative care can take to promote relational learning in their institutions. These suggestions are intended to generate reflection about the constant flux of informal learning occurring in nursing stations and at the bedside, the "formal" learning that happens in lunchtime chats and grand rounds presentations, and the system of organizational learning in which all of our actions are embedded.

Fostering relational learning in health care organizations

1. Create an interdisciplinary team of leaders committed to pediatric palliative care

When it comes to organizational change, one of the most frequent mistakes a committed health care professional makes is thinking they can do it alone. The solitary champion inevitably burns out. The potential for burnout is likely to be even greater in pediatric palliative care, where the challenges are so profound and practitioners suffer alongside patients and families. For these reasons, the first step toward building a strong educational infrastructure to maintain excellence in pediatric palliative care to identify a leadership team comprised of between 5 and 25 individuals who are passionate about the issue and want to play a major role in securing organizational change. It is important that the group represent multiple disciplines, including medicine, nursing, social work, psychology, chaplaincy, and child-life, as well as, allied health practitioners, such as pharmacy or respiratory therapist. Equally important is the inclusion of family members who have experienced the life-threatening condition or death of a child and who are interested and invested in this kind of change effort. The leadership team will need public endorsement from senior administrators such as the chief of medicine, the vice president of nursing, and the director of social work.

The way to build support for the group's work over time is to ensure that the whole organization knows about its mission, scope, and reach. Therefore, announcements in hospital newsletters, on its website, at key grand rounds presentations, and at key unit meetings should all be considered. Since the work of the leadership team involves a significant commitment of time, it will be helpful for members to be granted release time, and for their efforts to be authorized as important components in their professional development and career advancement.

The first task of the leadership team is to define its purpose and scope. Some may begin as study groups. They may assign themselves literature to read and discuss together, in order to eventually develop a common understanding of how they define pediatric palliative care and its educational requirements. Others may wish to undertake needs assessment activities to discover and document gaps in the quality of pediatric palliative care at their institution, and then envision both quality improvement and educational remedies to help close those gaps. Many of the interdisciplinary teams involved in the Initiative for Pediatric Palliative Care (IPPC) developed action plans for improving pediatric palliative care [49], which included quality improvements they hoped to put in place as well as educational initiatives they thought would be necessary for the quality improvements to take hold.

2. Identify the formal learning activities you will want to support or create

Part of setting the educational agenda is figuring out who the target audience(s) will be, how they can be reached, and what curricular materials to use. Will the leadership team begin by targeting one or two units only, piggyback on existing department-sponsored grand rounds, try to get time within regularly scheduled meetings, sponsor a lunchtime brown bag series, host their own grand rounds, or run an offsite retreat? Will sessions be organized and offered by unit, so that the range of disciplines who work together can learn together as well, drawing upon their common experiences and the paradigmatic cases they have encountered as a work team? Will there also be an opportunity for uni-disciplinary learning by, for example, integrating pediatric palliative care content into residency education? Each and every one of these options can be effective, and the most powerful impact comes from combining strategies, so as to reach as broad a swath of the community as possible.

Formal learning activities provide a context for introducing practitioners to relevant subject matter, but they are also important venues for relational learning. For example, formal sessions can offer a protected time and place for clinicians to bring concerns they may have about the disconnect between espoused ideals and practices they actually see around them. A survey conducted by one of the authors [24], documented that a significant percentage of clinicians believe they have acted against their conscience when providing end-of-life care to children. When these data were presented at grand rounds, they helped to generate institutional commitment to improving pediatric palliative care. When they were brought up in small group seminars, participants were able to tell ethically salient stories of times they personally felt challenged when determining the right thing to do. The simple act of sharing these stories opened up a range of creative strategies for better handling future situations.

The leadership team also needs to decide what curricular materials [12–15] are best matched to the audience it wants to reach. Again, using the IPPC experience [12,13] as an example, the authors developed formal case-based seminars that ask learners to consider ways to engage authentically with children, adolescents, parents, and siblings. The cases raise such challenges as how to help families anticipate the likely course of their child's illness and the choice points they are likely to face along the way, and how to protect the desires of older children and adolescents who want to be involved in decisions about their own care. Discussion of such cases can bring attention to issues that may otherwise remain off limits, and signal to practitioners that this is an institution invested in addressing tough issues.

In addition to case-based seminars, formal sessions can also include role-play activities, where practitioners not only reflect on difficult conversations, but are able to concretely explore new ways of communicating. At Children's Hospital Boston, for example, medical educators have developed realistic case scenarios, which are enacted by professional actors and clinicians who practice their skills in front of their peers [48]. The pedagogy is explicitly relational and focuses on the everyday ethics and human authenticity that emerge in these conversations. In a range of challenging scenarios, clinicians are encouraged to find their own voice as they grow in their capacity to communicate bad news, bear witness to anger and despair, and tolerate a potent range of feelings within themselves.

3. Develop a cadre of teachers capable of facilitating relational learning

While working on defining an educational agenda, the interdisciplinary leadership team also needs to identify and develop a cadre of individuals— relational teachers— who have the necessary knowledge, values, and skills to facilitate the formal and informal learning activities prioritized by the leadership team. An essential quality to look for first in these individuals is the extent to which they can integrate experiential sources of knowing— their students' and their own—with cognitive understanding. If we want clinicians to learn how to bear witness to the suffering of children and families, we need teachers and mentors who can bring all of themselves as human beings to the educational process.

Sadly, academic cultures can be inclined to distrust the kind of personal knowing and self-integration that is at the heart of relational teaching. Yet this integration is increasingly recognized as critically needed, not only in pediatric palliative care, but in the broader culture of medicine as well:

> Acknowledging that the educational process in medicine changes—in some substantive sense—who we are as well as how we relate to others, may be the key to understanding why we need to be mindful, articulate, and reflective about the process. It also highlights the risk of substituting technological expertise for knowledge of self in relationship to others. In a field that demands as much of us as medicine, anything less than this integration of person and professional may be unsupportable in the long run [2].

Relational teachers strive to create and maintain learning atmospheres built upon safety, trust, and respect. For practitioners to be willing to enter into formal and informal learning with openness, honesty, and curiosity, they need to be convinced that the learning context is safe, trustworthy, and hospitable to intellectual risk-taking as well as emotional and spiritual exploration.

Relational teachers invite multiple perspectives into the learning process. This could mean bringing different people into the conversation, such as practitioners from different disciplines or disparate work settings (for example, hospital and hospice or community-based health care settings). It could also mean bringing diverse ways of knowing into clinical learning. For example, in discussing a case involving parental bereavement, one might weave together one learner's understanding of grief theory, a second learner's description of his friend's despair after losing a child, and a third learner's questions about the potential use of anti-depressant medicine, in the same conversation.

Relational teachers cultivate a range of facilitation skills to manage the group dynamics involved in learning. They learn to balance the need to provide important content with the need for spontaneity in the group's process. They encourage learners who talk very little, and set boundaries on those who talk too much. They convey the same respect for inexperienced learners as they do for veteran clinicians. This is an especially important skill when exploring areas like end-of-life communication, where it would not be unusual for some medical students, for example, to have access to greater empathy and personal insight than some senior physicians whose people skills have eroded over time.

The leadership team should consider ways to provide potential teachers and facilitators with opportunities to practice their skills in a supportive setting. Sometimes it can be helpful to pair individuals with different strengths and clinical backgrounds, such as a social worker with a physician, or a nurse with a chaplain. It can be especially valuable—and educationally powerful—to invite and prepare interested parents who have lost a child to co-facilitate learning activities with practitioners—a strategy described in greater depth below.

Finally, it is important to acknowledge that the best teachers in pediatric palliative care are not always those who occupy official faculty roles. Good teachers can emerge from every discipline, with a wide range of personal and professional experience. Some of the best, if encouraged to try out teaching in a practice context, will be rank-and-file clinicians who have never before imagined themselves in a teaching role. Because many of their relational capacities are directly translatable into teaching and facilitation skills, however, these clinicians often discover passion and new realms of competence in the role of relational teacher.

4. Maximize the involvement of patients and families on multiple levels

> Because many of our [patients and families] are powerless and oppressed, their knowledge has been subjugated, and their insights have been excluded from the discourse by those who are empowered to define the "truth." We must bring forth their wisdom, their lived experience, and their visions of the world [50].

In the world of pediatric palliative care, it is not uncommon to hear talk of family-centered care, parental involvement in treatment, the importance of listening to children, and the value of partnerships with parents in the provision of care. However, in reality, these espoused principles are often only that. Real family-centered care, real partnerships with parents, and real listening to children require institutional commitment, including a sustained willingness to confront many unstated rules within the hidden curriculum. In our view, change efforts in pediatric palliative care will be unsuccessful in the long run if they fail to incorporate the knowledge and expertise of children and families into clinical practice in meaningful ways. Real family-centered care will depend on a genuine commitment to include parents (and their children, when appropriate) in daily rounds and discharge planning meetings, and to treat them in actuality as full members of the health care team [51]; the system cannot change without them.

From the standpoint of relational learning, the integration of family members into educational efforts is pivotal. Input from family members makes it clear that, too frequently, they feel misunderstood, mischaracterized, and/or mistakenly seen to be less competent than they are. There is a simple and straightforward strategy for improving how practitioners view, characterize, and talk about patients and families, yet it is curiously underused. Since much of the negative learning about families occurs when families are absent, educators should look for opportunities to increase their presence. The interdisciplinary leadership team should brainstorm creative ways to include family members and integrate patient and family voices in as many formal and informal learning activities as possible. When family members join in learning activities as co-teachers and co-learners with practitioners, they routinely keep things honest, because the learning is held accountable, as it were, to the real-life experience of children and families.

Within the Initiative for Pediatric Palliative Care, the authors have attempted to be family-centered in several ways:

- Recruiting a family advocate, herself a bereaved parent, to provide ongoing leadership
- Producing a series of videotapes which present the experience and perspective of a diverse range of children and families, to ensure that family voices are represented in curricular materials
- Including bereaved family members (nearly 20%) who have experienced the life-threatening condition or death of a child as equals with health care professionals in the faculty development process
- Providing guidance and consultation to hospitals and hospices about ways to include family members in education and organizational change efforts
- Ensuring that a substantive number of family members are involved as co-teachers and co-learners in regional educational retreats
- Securing funding earmarked specifically for developing family members as pediatric palliative care educators.

The following comments, offered by participants at IPPC educational retreats, illustrate the inherent potential for transformative learning when an interdisciplinary group of practitioners come together with family members to teach and to learn.

"What stood out for me was having the parents present and having them share their experiences with our group. Also, the constant reminders that aside from our professional roles, we are humans."

Psychologist.

"What extraordinary people...I learned about the incredible range of emotions that medical professionals deal with daily and realized how challenging that must be. I learned beautiful ways to affirm my child's life."

Family member.

"What stood out for me was having a safe place to express emotions and insecurities about my work. I've never had an opportunity to learn from family members in this way, and I'm very grateful for it."

Physician.

"I felt as though, by far, the most meaningful aspect of this experience was having the parents here to give their sides of the story and help the interdisciplinary teams understand better the feeling and attitudes of those we care for. I will forever carry this with me."

Nurse.

"The most meaningful part was the open sharing and the humanness of the medical staff, and the feelings they experience that are so like the parents. I will carry with me the thought that our son helped change the lives of some medical staff and the care they will provide in the future."

Family member.

The authors have found that, when an open and honest learning context is created for practitioners and family members, there develops the opportunity, often for the first time, for a real experience of partnership and even, at times, a healing sense of solidarity.

5. Build organizational support for addressing the hidden curriculum through informal learning opportunities and "teachable moments."

Many of the chronic problems in hospitals and other health care institutions are difficult to solve because of unwritten rules that determine what can and cannot be said out loud. These problems can be on the level of practice, such as, repeated complaints from parents that their assessment of their child's pain is ignored by staff, as well as, at the organizational level, such as, a hospital's failure to make headway in reducing the incidence of medical error. Uncovering these obstacles to change, these elephants in the room, pose a familiar dilemma for health care leaders charged with addressing intransigent problems. When sufficient safety is provided and organizational support given, the hidden curriculum, previously considered impossible to identify or address, can be productively exposed. Relational learning can be a central part of this process.

When learners are authorized to address discrepancies between what we say we do and what we actually do, in health care settings, especially across lines of hierarchy, authority, or professional discipline, heretofore lackluster professional settings can become electric in their potential for new and transformative learning. For example, the careless practices such as, characterizing particular parents as over-involved, negligent, or in denial, or describing young patients solely as disease entities instead of as children, are rarely scrutinized. When this ethic of representation [52]—the ways children and families are talked about when they are not present—becomes the subject matter of learning in a safe and respectful environment, the education experience for practitioners involved in that learning is likely to come alive.

To support vigorous and meaningful exploration of the hidden curriculum, practitioners need environments imbued with safety, trust, and respect, as well as institutional mechanisms that support and reward those courageous health care practitioners who risk speaking out about less than-ethical behavior they witness in their institutional settings. These individuals, when operating as solo activists, are particularly vulnerable to repercussions in a medical culture. For example, the fear of a ruined career or being seen as a pariah can easily prevent a medical resident from reporting a pattern of unprofessional behavior on the part of an attending physician, especially when a positive evaluation from that same individual may be required to advance professionally. However, senior leaders in medicine, nursing and social work can counter this dilemma by taking a public stand that ethically questionable behavior should be brought into the open and scrutinized, without fear of personal reprisal or negative consequences. Some institutions might also consider creating a more formal ombudsman role, so that anyone concerned about unprofessional behavior has a protected venue in which to share their concerns.

6. Link the educational initiative to broader efforts in organizational learning

Robust educational initiatives in pediatric palliative care will develop strategies to address both formal and informal learning. To achieve maximal success, however, initiatives must also be linked to organizational practices that will support the setting of new educational priorities. For example, to help hospitals and other pediatric institutions undertake self-reflection and identify areas ripe for educational intervention, the authors participated in the development of the Pediatric Palliative Care Institutional Self-Assessment Tool [53], which includes quality indicators across key domains of pediatric palliative care, and enables champions to quickly determine the areas of strengths and weaknesses in their institutions. Another example is the implementation of routine audits to ensure that key aspects of pediatric palliative care are being fulfilled. Audits might include, for instance, unannounced spot-checks of patients' pain as reported on a visual analog scale at the bedside; chart reviews to establish the extent to which pain assessments have occurred and been documented; or follow-up bereavement calls in which emotional support is offered, bereavement services are reviewed, and parents are invited to share any lingering concerns they may have about their child's care.

In addition, to be effective, educational initiatives should not be too narrowly focused, but rather should connect to broader efforts in organizational learning. One such project, aimed at addressing the discrepancy between informal learning and the formal curriculum, was implemented recently at the Indiana University School of Medicine (IUSM) [54]. Guided by principles of relationship-centered care and relational learning, collaborative teams of students and faculty set out to create a new practice in which they reflect on issues of professionalism and the hidden curriculum in a variety of structured conversations throughout the institution.

The IUSM project is driven by the assumption that improved professionalism will be directly connected to changed behavior on the part of community members, especially those in positions of power or authority. Preliminary data indicate a renewed spirit of collaboration and institutional mission, which is reflected in the following observations:

- A senior faculty member spots a husband and wife who appear lost, and changes course on his way to the parking lot to escort them to their destination
- Committee members structure time on their agenda so they can express appreciation for each other's contributions to the meeting

- A faculty member, swept up in the excitement of positive change in the medical school community, comments, "I can't stop thinking about this new way of seeing" [54]

The emphasis on everyday ethics is central to the organizational learning strategy being implemented in this innovative project. One physician, reflecting on the growing trust and respect he experiences in the IUSM learning community, conveys what we might similarly hope to hear from pediatric palliative care practitioners engaged in a vigorous educational initiative focused on relational learning:

> "Now that I see how good we really are, I have to ask myself why we tolerate it when people aren't as good as this. I can't just look on quietly anymore when people are disrespectful or hurtful. It's no longer okay to be silent; this is too important [54]".

Summary: Cultivating the Garden

> What have you done with the garden entrusted to you?
> —Antonio Machado [55]

Within health care organizations that serve critically ill children and their families, there is a certain kind of moral gift-giving going on that is continuous, unrelenting, and operating in parallel relational worlds. The care of each young patient has been given—in trust and for safekeeping—to his or her parents, extended family, and health care professionals. The care of the child's mother and father, siblings, and loved ones has been given—in trust and for safekeeping—to an interdisciplinary team of health care professionals. The care of these nurses, physicians, social workers, psychologists, chaplains, and child-life specialists, has been given—in trust and for safekeeping—to those individuals in health care organizations who are responsible for professional learning. Accompanying the gift, in each of these interdependent worlds, is a simple but ethically demanding question addressed to all: What have you done with the garden entrusted to you?

Fostering learning that matters in pediatric palliative care will hinge on our capacity to see that, minute by minute and day by day, health care professionals are engaged in a complex process of learning, at the core of which is a lifelong effort to discover how they can be with children and families and who they are becoming as human beings who have chosen this sacred work. For educators committed to the professional development of these practitioners—this is our garden.

May we bring wisdom, compassion, and perseverance to its cultivation.

Acknowledgements

We would like to acknowledge several colleagues with whom we have discussed these ideas over the years, and with whom we have collaborated on projects that have grown out of the views expressed in this chapter: Loring Conant, MD; Elaine Meyer, PhD, RN; Cynda Rushton, DNSc, RN, FAAN; Deborah Sellers, PhD, and Robert Truog, MD. We are especially grateful to Deborah Dokken, MPA, whose family-centered wisdom and insights have deeply influenced our approach to education in pediatric palliative care. Lastly, we would like to thank Alise Brann for her assistance in the preparation of the manuscript.

References

[1] University of Virginia School of Medicine. Convocation for the entering class – covenants. Available at: http://www.healthsystem.virginia.edu/internet/ome/advoc/covenants.cfm. Accessed February 14, 2006.

[2] Inui TS. A flag in the wind: educating for professionalism in medicine. Washington, DC: Association of American Medical Colleges; 2003. Available at: www.regenstrief.org/Members/tinui/bio/flaginthewind. Accessed February 14, 2006.

[3] Skiles J. Teaching professionalism: a medical student's opinion. The Clinical Teacher 2005; 2(2):66–71.

[4] Coulehan J. Viewpoint: today's professionalism: engaging the mind but not the heart. Acad Med 2005;80(10):892–8.

[5] Wear D. On white coats and professional development: the formal and hidden curricula. Ann Intern Med 1998;129:734–7.

[6] Hafferty FW, Franks R. The hidden curriculum, ethics teaching and the structure of medical education. Acad Med 1994;69:861–71.

[7] Haidet P, Stein HF. The role of the student-teacher relationship in the formation of physicians. The hidden curriculum as process. J Gen Intern Med 2006;21(Suppl 1):S16–20.

[8] Bellini LM, Shea JA. Mood change and empathy decline persist during three years of internal medicine training. Acad Med 2005;80(2):164–7.

[9] Okie S. An act of empathy: 'Wit' star seeks to teach doctors the lost art of conveying emotions. The Washington Post; Health Section: October 21, 2003. p. HEO1.

[10] Churchill LR. Reviving a distinctive medical ethic. Hastings Cent Rep 1989;19(3):28–34.

[11] Palmer PJ. The courage to teach: exploring the inner landscape of a teacher's life. San Francisco (CA): Jossey-Bass; 1997.

[12] Solomon MZ, Browning DM, Dokken D, et al. The Initiative for Pediatric Palliative Care (IPPC) curriculum: enhancing family-centered care for children with life-threatening conditions. (Modules 1–5). Newton (MA): Education Development Center, Inc. 2003. Available at: http://www.ippcweb.org/curriculum.asp.

[13] Browning DM, Solomon MZ. The initiative for pediatric palliative care: an interdisciplinary educational approach for healthcare professionals. J Pediatr Nurs 2005;20:326–34.

[14] American Association of Colleges of Nursing. ELNEC pediatric palliative care training program. Available at: http://www.aacn.nche.edu/ELNEC/Pediatric.htm. Accessed February 14, 2006.

[15] National Hospice and Palliative Care Organization. Education and training curriculum in pediatric palliative care. Available at: http://www.nhpco.org/i4a/pages/index.cfm?pageid=3409. Accessed February 14, 2006.

[16] Carter B, Levetown M, editors. Palliative care for infants, children and adolescents: a practical handbook. Baltimore (MD): Johns Hopkins University Press; 2004.

[17] Peabody FW. The care of the patient. JAMA 1927;88:877–82.

[18] Hinds PS, Schum MS, Baker JN, et al. Key factors affecting dying children and their families. J Palliat Med 2005;8(suppl 1):S70–8.

[19] Solomon MZ, Browning D. Relationships matter and so does pain control. J Clin Oncol 2005;23(36):9055–7.

[20] Contro N, Larson J, Scofield S, et al. Family perspectives on the quality of pediatric palliative care. Arch Pediatr Adolesc Med 2002;156(1):14–9.

[21] Meyer EC, Burns JP, Griffith JL, et al. Parental perspectives on end-of-life care in the pediatric intensive care unit. Crit Care Med 2002;30(1):226–31.

[22] Heller KS, Solomon MZ. Continuity of care and caring; what matters to parents of children with life-threatening conditions. J Pediatr Nurs 2005;20:335–46.

[23] Kreicbergs U, Valdimarsdottir U, Onelov E, et al. Care-related distress: a nationwide study of parents who lost their child to cancer. J Clin Oncol 2005;23(36):9162–71.

[24] Solomon MZ, Sellers DE, Heller KS, et al. New and lingering controversies in pediatric end-of-life care. Pediatrics 2005;116(4):872–83.

[25] Rushton CH. The Baby K case: ethical challenges of preserving professional intergrity. Pediatr Nurs 1995;21:367–72.

[26] Jameton A. Dilemmas of moral distress: moral responsibility and nursing practice. Clin Issues Perinat Womens Health Nurs 1993;4(4):542–51.

[27] Papadatou D, Bellali T, Papazoglou I, et al. Greek nurse and physician grief as a result of caring for children dying of cancer. Pediatr Nurs 2002;28(4):345–53.

[28] Serwint JR, Rutherford LE, Hutton N. Personal and professional experiences of palliative residents concerning death. J Palliat Med 2006;9(1):70–82.

[29] Figley CR. Introduction. In: Figley CR, editor. Treating compassion fatigue. New York: Brunner-Routledge; 2002. p. 1–14.

[30] Stamm BH, Varra EM, Pearlman LA, et al. The helper's power to heal and to be hurt - or helped trying. Register report. Washington (DC): National Register of Health Service Providers in Psychology; 2002.

[31] Stamm BH, editor. Secondary traumatic stress: self-care issues for clinicians, researchers, and educators. Lutherville (MD): Sidran Press; 1995.

[32] Charon R. Compassion in the care of patients. In: Shea S, Rabkin M, editors. General medicine ambulatory care syllabus. New York: Columbia University Medical Center; 1997. Available at: http://cpmcnet.columbia.edu/texts/ambulatory/35COMPAS.html. Accessed February 14, 2006.

[33] Browning DM. Fragments of love: explorations in the ethnography of suffering and professional caregiving. In: Berzoff J, Silverman P, editors. Living with dying: a handbook for end-of-life healthcare practitioners. New York: Columbia University Press; 2004.

[34] Initiative for Pediatric Palliative Care. Big choices, little choices [Video]. Newton (MA): Education Development Center; 2003.

[35] Initiative for Pediatric Palliative Care. Speaking the same language [Video]. Newton (MA): Education Development Center; 2003.

[36] Kleinman A. The illness narratives: suffering, healing and the human condition. New York: Basic Books; 1989.

[37] Wenger E. How we learn. Communities of practice. The social fabric of a learning organization. Healthc Forum J 1996;39(4):20–6.

[38] Freire P. Pedagogy of the oppressed. London: Continuum International Publishing Group; 2003.

[39] Hartrick G. Relationship capacity: the foundation for interpersonal nursing practice. J Adv Nurs 1997;26(3):523–8.

[40] Epstein RM, Hundert EM. Defining and assessing professional competence. JAMA 2002; 287:226–35.

[41] McDermott RP. The acquisition of a child by a learning disability. In: Chailklin S, Lave J, editors. Understanding practice: Perspectives on activity and context. New York: Cambridge; 1993.

[42] Lave J, Wenger E. Situated learning: legitimate peripheral participation. Cambridge (UK): University of Cambridge Press; 1991.

[43] Brookfield SD. Understanding and facilitating adult learning. San Francisco (CA): Jossey-Bass; 1986.

[44] Initiative for Pediatric Palliative Care. I need it to make sense [Video]. Newton (MA): Education Development Center; 2003.

[45] Frank AW. Ethics as process and practice. Intern Med J 2004;34(6):355-7.

[46] Churchill LR, Schenck D. One cheer for bioethics: engaging the moral experiences of patients and practitioners beyond the big decisions. Camb Q Healthc Ethics 2005;14(4): 389-403.

[47] Baker AC, Jensen PJ, Kolb DA. Conversational learning: an experiential approach to knowledge creation. Westport (CT): Quorum; 2002.

[48] Browning DM. To show our humanness: relational and communicative competence in pediatric palliative care. Bioethics Forum 2003;18(3-4):23-8.

[49] The Initiative for Pediatric Palliative Care. Collaborating hospitals. Available at: http://www.ippcweb.org/hospitals.asp#Boston. Accessed February 23, 2006.

[50] Hartman A. Many ways of knowing. In: Professional writing for the human services. Washington (DC): NASW Press; 1993.

[51] Dokken D, Ahmann E. The many roles of family members in "Family-Centered Care." Pediatr Nurs, In press.

[52] Frank AW. First person microethics: deriving principles from below. Hast Cent Rep 1998; 28:37-42.

[53] Levetown M, Dokken D, Heller KS, et al. A pediatric palliative care institutional self-assessment tool (ISAT). Newton (MA): Education Development Center, Inc.; 2002.

[54] Suchman AL, Williamson PR, Litzelman DK, et al. Toward an informal curriculum that teaches professionalism: transforming the social environment of a medical school. J Gen Intern Med 2004;19(5 Pt 2):501-4.

[55] Machado A. Times alone: selected poems of Antonio Machado. Translated by Robert Bly. Middletown (CT): Wesleyan University Press; 1983.

ELSEVIER
SAUNDERS

Child Adolesc Psychiatric Clin N Am
15 (2006) 817–825

CHILD AND
ADOLESCENT
PSYCHIATRIC CLINICS
OF NORTH AMERICA

Index

Note: Page numbers of article titles are in **boldface** type.